Physiotherapy Practice in Residential Aged Care

For Butterworth-Heinemann:

Senior Commissioning Editor: Heidi Harrison
Associate Editor: Robert Edwards
Project Managers: Samantha Ross; Gail Wright
Senior Designer: George Ajayi

Physiotherapy Practice in Residential Aged Care

Edited by

Jennifer C. Nitz BPhty MPhty PhD

Division of Physiotherapy, School of Health and Rehabilitation Sciences, The University of Queensland, St Lucia, Australia

Susan R. Hourigan BPhty(Hons) BScApp(HMS-Ex Man)

Division of Physiotherapy, School of Health and Rehabilitation Sciences, The University of Queensland, St Lucia, Australia

BUTTERWORTH HEINEMANN

Edinburgh London New York Oxford Philadelphia St Louis Sydney Toronto 2004

BUTTERWORTH-HEINEMANN
An imprint of Elsevier Limited

ISBN 0 7506 8772 X

British Library Cataloguing in Publication Data
A catalogue record for this book is available from the British Library

Library of Congress Cataloging in Publication Data
A catalog record for this book is available from the Library of Congress

Notice
Medical knowledge is constantly changing. Standard safety precautions must be followed, but as new research and clinical experience broaden our knowledge, changes in treatment and drug therapy may become necessary or appropriate. Readers are advised to check the most current product information provided by the manufacturer of each drug to be administered to verify the recommended dose, the method and duration of administration, and contraindications. It is the responsibility of the practitioner, relying on experience and knowledge of the patient, to determine dosages and the best treatment for each individual patient. Neither the Publisher nor the editors and contributors assumes any liability for any injury and/or damage to persons or property arising from this publication.

The Publisher

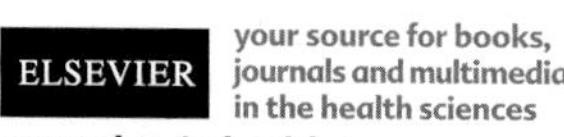

www.elsevierhealth.com

The Publisher's policy is to use **paper manufactured from sustainable forests**

Printed in China

Contents

Contributors

Susan R. Hourigan BPhty(Hons) BScApp(HMS-Ex Man)
Division of Physiotherapy, School of Health and Rehabilitation Sciences, The University of Queensland, St Lucia, Australia

Venerina Johnston BPhty(Hons)
Division of Physiotherapy, School of Health and Rehabilitation Sciences, The University of Queensland, St Lucia, Australia

Diane L. Josephson DipPhysio GradCertPhty(Geriatics)
Private Practitioner, Brisbane, Australia

Nancy Low Choy BPhty(Hons) MPhty
Division of Physiotherapy, School of Health and Rehabilitation Sciences, The University of Queensland, St Lucia, Australia

Jennifer C. Nitz BPhty MPhty PhD
Division of Physiotherapy, School of Health and Rehabilitation Sciences, The University of Queensland, St Lucia, Australia

Ann Rahmann BPhty GradCertPhty(Geriatrics)
Division of Physiotherapy, School of Health and Rehabilitation Sciences, The University of Queensland, St Lucia, Australia

Ruth Sapsford AUA DipPhty
Division of Physiotherapy, School of Health and Rehabilitation Sciences, The University of Queensland, St Lucia, Australia

Tina Souvlis BPhty(Hons) PhD
Division of Physiotherapy, School of Health and Rehabilitation Sciences, The University of Queensland, St Lucia, Australia

Introduction

Jennifer C. Nitz and Susan R. Hourigan

In 2002 there were 2.5 million older people (aged 65+) in Australia, representing 12.7% of the total Australian population. In 2031 older people will represent 22.3% of the total population (or 5.4 million people) and by 2051 they will represent over one-quarter of our population (Australian Bureau Statistics 2003). The increase in the older old (those 85 years+) is even more pronounced, rising from 9.1% of those aged 65 years and over in 1996 to 20.1% by 2051. The average age of people living in residential care homes in Australia is 83 years (AIHW 2002).

In Australia, at the latest census in June 2001, there were 136 608 people accommodated in 2977 residential aged care facilities (RACFs). Two per cent of these places were devoted to respite care but this accounted for 43 606 admissions during the financial year ending June 2001. In that time there were 46 545 admissions for permanent care. Most of the people admitted to RACFs were women (72%) and just over half of all people admitted were aged over 85 years. Only 6094 (4.5%) people admitted were less than 65 years of age. Twenty-three per cent of these younger people were admitted to high care compared to 63% of all older people admitted. The remaining admissions were to low care (AIHW 2002).

Prior to admission, 41% lived alone in a house or flat, 21% with a spouse and 12% with family members. Thus most people admitted to RACFs enter from the community. When in the community, many would have been the recipients of Community Aged Care Packages that were designed to enable older people to live independently in the community with assistance from community agencies such as meals on wheels, home help or community nursing (AIHW 2002).

Where does the physiotherapist fit into the residential aged care scene? This book was conceived to enable physiotherapists to define their role in this area of practice and to educate physiotherapy students (both undergraduate and postgraduate). It should assist our co-workers in aged care regarding the skills we bring to the workplace and how collectively we might offer best practice procedures that enable residents and carers to attain a quality living environment.

From here on in we will refer to residential *aged care* facilities even though young people are also cared for in these communities. In other countries the RACFs will be known as nursing homes, rest homes, hostels and retirement homes.

People entering RACFs often do so after losing the ability to manage independently in the community. It is often a culmination of events such as the loss of a partner or parental carer who made life at large in the community possible, or in other circumstances a catastrophic life event that has led to physical dependency. In many cases this ultimate loss follows a series of losses including driver's licence, home, friends through death and pets. To many individuals, entering a care facility means giving up self-determination, dignity and quality of life but this need not be the case with good management in a well-organized facility. Irrespective of whether the resident will spend their final days in the facility or have been admitted to provide respite for a carer or even for slow stream rehabilitation, it is the duty of the care providers to ensure best practice in all aspects of resident management. In many respects care providers are bound to take on an advocatory role to ensure residents are protected from injury and are able to access all necessities for the best quality of life possible to them. Physiotherapists possess numerous skills that enable them to assist residents and carers to achieve this goal.

Identification of the needs and risk factors a resident presents with on admission to a care facility allows development of the most appropriate care plan that will enable attainment of the best quality of life afforded by their circumstances. If all care staff adopt a clinical reasoning approach when drawing up a care plan that incorporates the stated desires of the resident, a harmonious and cooperative environment can be provided. By allowing the new resident and/or their family to participate in the planning process, trust is generated and communication of doubts and fears are encouraged, alleviating much anxiety.

New residents often come to residential care with preconceived ideas that are often of a negative nature. The very idea of something new is foreign to many as they have lived in the same house with the same people possibly all their life and to change brings fear of the unknown. A new environment without any of the familiar objects is very confusing to many older people. Often the change needs interpersonal skills that have not been developed due to previous isolation. If you consider the intimate interaction that occurs when assisting a totally dependent person with bathing and toileting some idea of the extent of adaptation necessary is gained. Not only is there a new physical environment for new residents, but also new carers, new routines, new faces, new procedures and new timetables. Add difficulty with communication to a physical dependency and we can begin to understand the mental turmoil of some new residents. Some lucky people come to a residential care facility after having mentally prepared themselves for the lifestyle change. However, there will be a level of stress that always accompanies anybody who moves from one place of residency to another. Limiting the number of new experiences can reduce stress. Therefore it is beneficial to have one carer undertake the admission process for the new resident. They should also continue to care for the needs of the resident at this time. To have a family member or friend who is accepted by the resident present during admission might help transition.

On admission, an interim care plan is drawn up for each new resident. This will enable a safe level of functioning to prevail until a full assessment of physical, communication and behavioural status is undertaken. In reality, this process takes a few weeks depending on the distress caused by the admission to the RACF. Therefore the initial care plan should not be seen as unchangeable nor should any care plan be considered finite. All residents will be liable to rapid change in their medical condition simply due to their age and frailty. Every person involved in the care of a resident should be aware of this and be able to adapt management strategies immediately. However, many carers lack the skill to be able to identify when the resident's condition changes let alone know how to adapt a care plan to suit the change. The physiotherapist is the appropriate practitioner to evaluate change in physical ability and to recommend appropriate care plan modification.

Clinical reasoning is the approach used to develop the care plan for a resident. It involves using theoretical knowledge related to ageing and pathological processes seen in the elderly, the assessment of these problems and intervention options to enhance function and quality of life for the residents. In this book we will look at physiological changes accompanying the ageing process as well as the physiotherapist's role in assessment, preventing residents' injuries and promoting life satisfaction. Major presenting problems relating to being immobile, barely mobile, or ambulatory will be examined physiotherapeutically. Information and strategies to assist with residents suffering from pain, osteoporosis, incontinence or palliation will be covered. A special chapter concerned with aquatic physiotherapy is also included as pools are becoming more prevalent in aged care facilities.

Appendices have been included to cover a number of issues which are important to physiotherapy practice. In a number of RACFs funding is linked to proof of efficacy; therefore choosing the appropriate outcome measurement that reflects the results of intervention (unique to an individual resident's care plan) is vital. The appendices include a table of useful outcome measures, assessment case studies, suggestions for successful case conferences, electrotherapy considerations in aged care practice and mobility aids.

We hope the ideas and topics contained in our book are informative as well as thought provoking for our readers. Working in residential aged care as a physiotherapist is extremely challenging as our skills in clinical practice, education, health promotion and research will be recruited and utilized frequently as we fulfil our role.

References

Australian Bureau Statistics 2003 Australian Social Trends, Cat 4102.0, p 2

Australian Institute of Health & Welfare (AIHW) 2002 Residential aged care services in Australia 2000–01: a statistical overview. AIHW Cat. No. AGE 22. Canberra: AIHW (Aged Care Statistic Series No. 11). http://www.aihw.gov.au

SECTION 1 AGEING AND ITS ATTENDANTS

1 Physiological changes with age

Jennifer C. Nitz and Susan R. Hourigan

This chapter aims to:

- overview the changes associated with ageing in all of the systems important to physical performance and functioning. This information will be referred to throughout this text as we examine clinical reasoning and physiotherapeutic treatment of elderly people living in residential aged care facilities.

Introduction

It is a common belief that both physical and cognitive function will decline with ageing and that people must accept these changes. In many respects this is true, but compensatory and preventive management can control the effects of system decline. An example of this is to use corrective lenses to accommodate for the presbyopia of middle age. Similar adjustments to lifestyle can slow or negate the effect of ageing in other systems. In this chapter the changes due to ageing will be investigated in the context of residents in aged care.

People generally reach their peak health and performance abilities between adolescence and 30 years of age. Functional capacity after this age then declines throughout the lifespan depending on genetics, lifestyle characteristics and health. All physiological measures that decline with age do not do so at the same rate. Heart rate at rest does not change dramatically with advancing years; however, heart rate at maximum physical exertion decreases significantly. Nerve conduction velocity slows 10–15% from 30 to 80 years of age and maximum breathing capacity declines by approximately 60% between 30 and 80 years. The rates of decline in the various functions differ and are significantly influenced by various factors including the level of physical activity and any associated pathology. There is no doubt that regular activity and physical training enables older persons to retain higher levels of functional capacity (McArdle et al 1996).

Decline in the special senses can be a most disabling aspect of ageing. As will be seen in later chapters, the resulting disability when vision, auditory and vestibular function and somatosensation diminish with age plays a major role in exposing the older person to an increased risk of injury from falling. In addition, interaction with the environment is decreased and opportunities for choosing modalities for entertainment are curtailed by loss of vision or hearing or the ability to safely mobilize in the community. Thus decline in the special senses can lead to a dramatic change in lifestyle and possibly a diminished quality of life. Therefore understanding the ageing effects on these organs is important when working with the elderly.

Special senses

Vision

As the eye ages the lens loses clarity owing to an increase in lens density (Jackson et al 2002). It becomes yellowed and crazed (Bron 1997). In addition, the ageing lens can form a cataract. Cataract formation is believed to be due to lens protein modification and reduction in antioxidants (Bron 1997). The retina at the back of the eye is also affected by ageing. Within the retina lie the rods that are responsible for vision in dim light and the cones that respond to bright light and colour. At the centre of the retina lies the macula. This is a specialized area comprising a central cone-rich fovea that is surrounded by a rod-dominated parafovea. The photoreceptor outer segment contains the proteins of the phototransduction cascade. The nutritional needs of this component are maintained by the retinal pigmented layer. This layer is responsible for maintaining photoreceptor health by helping to maintain ionic balance and hydration, transport and filtration of nutrients, by providing retinoid intermediates that replenish photopigment bleached by light exposure and also by absorbing stray photons (Jackson et al 2002). Blood flow to the retinal pigmented layer and the photoreceptors is via the choroidal system, which has the richest blood flow in the body. Between the choroid capillaries and the retinal pigmented layer lies Bruch's membrane. Age-related macular degeneration (ARMD) in the early stages is characterized by extracellular lesions and changes in the retinal pigmented layer morphology and damage to Bruch's membrane in the region of the macula (Bron 1997, Jackson 2002). Later extensive retinal pigment layer atrophy and vascular changes with in-growth of vessels in Bruch's membrane and under the retinal pigmented layer accounts for blindness in ARMD (Jackson 2002).

ARMD might be demonstrated in the early stages by an increased time for recovery of vision after exposure to bright lights. With ageing, dark adaptation after exposure to bright light increases by about 8 seconds per decade. Delays of an average 13 minutes have been seen in people with early ARMD (Owsley 2001). This can lead to a considerable increase in fall risk for older people when moving from light to dark environments or from dark to light as the time for clear vision to return increases with age. Thus older people should be made aware of this delay in order to include into their lifestyle safety practices that will reduce the risk of injury. Older people with early ARMD (Scilley et al 2002) also experience night driving problems.

Eventually with ARMD, there is central visual field loss that affects the ability to read and perform activities requiring fine manipulation such as sewing. Distortion of colour and shapes can occur. Together this can affect edge perception where contrast is minimal. From a functional viewpoint, the person is placed in danger of not seeing steps or thinking there is a step up or down because of colour change or shadow. A door that is ajar if it is the same colour as the surrounding walls may not be seen nor the edge of the chair seat or the edge of the bed if contrasting colours are not used. The older person is therefore at risk of a fall through errors of judgement induced by decline in visual acuity or depth perception (Carter et al 1997, Pinto et al 1997). Changes in visual acuity can affect depth perception, especially when stereopsis cannot be attained with corrective lenses. It can also contribute to visual illusions such as not perceiving moving repeated patterns such as on escalators (Harwood 2001).

With ageing, the ciliary muscles are less able to change lens curvature, thereby slowing the ability to rapidly change focus from close work to distance. This becomes a problem when ambulating when near and distant sections of the environment require scanning to navigate safely through environmental hazards.

The pupillary light reflex is slowed with age. This means that it takes longer for the elderly to be able to see clearly when there is a change in light conditions from dark to light or light to dark. ARMD also plays a role in this presentation. In the younger person light accommodation takes a few seconds. As a person ages, the time interval extends and might take as long as 15 minutes to occur. Not allowing for the slowed light accommodation by standing still and waiting for the vision to clear can increase the risk of a fall. The typical time when this becomes critical is at night when putting on the light to get up to go to the toilet or during the day when moving from indoors to outdoors, especially on a bright sunny day (Pinto et al 1997).

Visual acuity changes with ageing. Presbyopia can increase but more commonly ARMD and lens pathology interfere with the ability to read or perform close work (Pinto et al 1997). The use of coloured print or paper should be limited if using the print medium to communicate to residents via notice boards or newsletters. Many of the oldest old residents may find it difficult to discern coloured letters on coloured paper due to the cumulative effect of these eye changes and so might become isolated from the community activities. Larger font and bold black print on white paper can limit this possibility even if it is not as attractive to the eye.

Pathological conditions that can affect vision are more common in the elderly. These include complications arising after cataract surgery, retinal detachment and glaucoma. All can contribute to diminished sight or blindness. Conditions such as stroke and multiple sclerosis can also cause visual field loss and are relatively common in residents.

Visual conflict occurs when what the person interprets they are seeing is at odds with proprioception, touch and pressure and vestibular sensory input. Difficulty in discerning reality in visual conflict situations is often related to decline in the vestibular and proprioceptive systems as well as central integrative systems within the central nervous system (Harwood 2001). In these instances the older person is at more risk of a fall.

Hearing and vestibular function

Age-related hearing loss is known as presbyacusis (Seidman et al 2002). Cochlear degeneration occurs with ageing and signs of degeneration begin with decline in the ability to hear high frequency sound, followed by progressive loss of lower frequency hearing. There is also loss of the ability to discriminate between sounds, which leads to speech sounding muffled, and in some instances whole words become indiscernible. Hearing loss is not usually symmetrical and this causes difficulty in location of sound source. Functionally this difficulty in sound location can delay avoiding responses to danger such as moving aside to clear a skate boarder on the footpath or an approaching car. Delayed detection of the direction from which danger is approaching might require faster evasive movement than can be controlled by the elderly person and a fall can eventuate. Where possible, hearing should be tested and elderly people with hearing loss should be encouraged to wear hearing aids at all times.

Slowed nerve conduction from the ear and within the central nervous system can cause auditory response time to increase. This can lead to confusion in the elderly if multiple questions are fired at them without allowing for time to process the input and respond accordingly. Many professionals have been guilty of this and then misinterpreting the lack or inappropriateness of response by the older person as indicating dementia. Unfortunately such labelling can stick, with far-reaching consequences.

The vestibular apparatus comprises the utricle, saccule and three semicircular canals that enable orientation of the head with respect to gravity and enable response and perception of head movement (Guyton 1991). Thus normal vestibular function is needed for a person to maintain head stability during any movement task, to allow conjugate eye movement for reading and the integration of visual and proprioceptive information for environmental interaction (Di Fabio & Emasithi 1997). By the age of 70 years there has been a reduction of 40% in the number of vestibular hair and nerve cells (Rosenhall & Rubin 1975). Ageing of the components of the vestibular apparatus leads to a reduction in vestibular sensory input that causes the older person to rely more on vision and less on proprioceptive information to continue to move and interact in the environment. The impact of vestibular decline with age will be covered in more detail in the chapter dealing with balance (Chapter 9).

Taste and smell

With ageing there is a decline in ability to taste food. Because of this diet is often changed by the elderly to increase taste needs. Unfortunately this is often by increasing the sugar and salt content, thereby raising the likelihood of glucose intolerance and hypertension. The sense of smell also declines. Since the aroma of food and taste are intimately connected to enhance enjoyment of eating, the elderly often reduce nutritional intake due to the lack of interest in food that accompanies the decline in these senses. A potential danger associated with loss of smell is the inability to smell smoke. This functional decline might be a factor in the number of elderly people injured or killed in house fires each year. In a recent study undertaken in the USA, which examined olfactory decline in people aged 53 to 97 years, impaired olfaction was found in 24.5% of the participants. Impairment was more prevalent among men and was present in 62.5% of people over 80 years of age. Self-reported olfactory decline did not equate to test findings and this aspect became worse with age, thus confirming the importance of acknowledging the deficit and educating older people about safety precautions to compensate for the loss (Murphy et al 2002).

Table 1.1 summarizes the changes to special senses, the effect of these changes on function, and management strategies that might be employed to minimize the impact on daily life.

Table 1.1
Special sense changes with ageing

Special sense	Change due to ageing	Functional impact	Management strategy
Vision	Lens: yellowed and crazed cataract ARMD Glaucoma Acuity	Decreased ability to discern colour, perceive an edge and do close vision activities	Use strongly contrasting colours in decor so edges are defined Large black print and increased wattage for light bulbs Encourage use of spectacles for close or distance
	Slowed reflexes: pupillary light reflex lens accommodation	Increases risk of falls	Pause until vision is clear when focus or light conditions change Remove clutter on the floor
	Visual conflict	Inappropriate balance correction leading to increased fall risk	Identification of the problem and instigation of a strategy suitable for the individual resident
Hearing	Cochlear degeneration: loss of high frequency sound unilateral hearing loss	Social isolation Increased risk of falling	Encourage hearing aid use and help change batteries Face the deaf person at their height so they can see you clearly. Speak slowly and clearly. Do not shout. Be aware your approach might not be heard and sudden appearance in line of sight can disturb balance

table continues

Special sense	Change due to ageing	Functional impact	Management strategy
Vestibular	Otolith and endolymph function declines Hyposensitivity to head position and movement in all planes	Delayed balance response and increased risk of falls Greater reliance on vision and somatosensation for balance	Ensure good lighting and correction of acuity so vision can be used efficiently to maintain balance
Taste and smell	Decline in taste and smell	Lack of interest in eating and consequent nutritional lack Inability to detect a fire	Prepare visually appealing food to stimulate the appetite. Use spices to enhance taste Installation of smoke-detecting fire alarms

Gastrointestinal system

Age changes can occur in the gastrointestinal tract from the mouth to the anus. These changes can have a major bearing on the health of the elderly resident and thereby directly or indirectly affect the role of the physiotherapist.

Nutritional deficiency has been identified as one of the factors contributing to frailty (Campbell & Buchner 1997). The diet of elders contains decreased protein, fruit and vegetables; thus problems relating to vitamin and mineral deficiencies are common. Such deficiencies can adversely affect tissue health, with all organs being affected, but the main effects are evident in the skin and neural tissues. Anaemia is common in the elderly and affects the oxygen-carrying potential of the blood. This in turn can lead to reduced metabolic function in all tissues with particular consequences of declined cognitive function, muscle weakness and increased falls risk.

A number of factors can contribute to poor nutrition. Inability to shop for fresh food, lack of financial capacity to buy fresh food as well as lack of the cognitive and physical capability to prepare and cook the food can compound the physiological changes due to ageing that reduce the nutrition gained from food ingested. Residents of care facilities should not be disadvantaged nutritionally as all the factors identified to contribute to malnutrition should be countered.

The changes due to ageing of the gastrointestinal system affect the alimentary tract and also the related organs including the liver and pancreas. It is therefore important to understand the ageing effect on these organs as the resident can present with major health ramifications from these changes.

The mouth

Atrophy of the gums and bone that occurs with age and poor dental hygiene can lead to tooth loss. Many elders have no teeth and often do not wear false teeth. The most common reason for not using dental prostheses is poor fit because of gum atrophy. The consequence of not having teeth relates not only to cosmesis but to inability to enunciate words so that communication is impaired. Most importantly nutrition suffers, as the first part of digestion when salivary enzymes are mixed with the food bolus is inefficient. Nutrition is further reduced by reduction in saliva production with age. In response to these deficiencies, mastication of food is reduced in efficiency and most elders adapt their diet in response.

Swallow

During swallowing aspiration and nasal regurgitation can occur due to age-associated decline in the efficiency of the oropharyngeal control of the food bolus. The texture and consistency of the food might need to be changed to prevent these occurrences in order to prevent lethal outcome from aspiration pneumonia. If aspiration or nasal regurgitation is suspected, a swallow assessment by the speech pathologist should be requested urgently.

Digestion

Preliminary protein digestion by salivary amylase might be deficient in the elderly, thus reducing the efficiency of the digestive process in the stomach, duodenum and small intestine. Other factors that can affect digestion include the delayed gastric emptying that occurs with ageing. This can cause an uncomfortable bloated feeling and cause the elderly person to eat less. An advanced thoracic kyphosis can add to this discomfort by its effect of reduced abdominal volume capacity.

In general, as the gastrointestinal tract ages it becomes less efficient at absorbing nutrients and maintaining fluid balance. Apart from the nutritional aspect this will also impact on drug and mineral absorption. In addition to gut malabsorption, excretion is impaired, especially where there is impaired liver and renal function.

The liver

The liver is a discrete organ the basic functions of which are related to the metabolism of carbohydrates, fats and proteins. The liver stores vitamins A, D and B_{12} as well as iron. The liver has an excretory function that forms bile. Also the liver filters and stores blood (Guyton 1991). As a person ages, the liver loses weight. Between the age of 20 and 80 years this weight loss has been shown to be around 24% in men and 18% in women. However, liver weight loss does not appear related to morphological changes, as liver function tests remain normal with ageing (Zeeh & Platt 2002). Change in hepatic blood flow is most likely responsible for decline in liver function. There is a consequent reduction in bile salt formation, bile flow and alteration in hepatic enzyme activity. Thus metabolism and excretion of many drugs is impaired and this can lead to overdose, especially of drugs such as some antibiotics, tricyclic antidepressants and benzodiazepines. However, drug excretion can be influenced by factors other than reduced liver function and bile excretion such as tissue distribution, protein binding and renal excretion. Hormones are also excreted in the bile after chemical alteration in the liver. Therefore any reduction in efficiency of this system can lead to endocrine dysfunction (Guyton 1991).

In addition to excretion of waste products in the bile many are transported in the circulation to be excreted in the urine. It is therefore important to consider renal function alongside liver function.

The kidney

The kidney functions to maintain fluid balance in the body and to assist in the process of excretion of metabolic waste products. However, with normal ageing the efficiency of these functions decreases as there is a reduction in kidney plasma flow of around 45% by the age of 80 (Guyton 1991). Chronic and acute renal failure are relatively common in the elderly. There is also a decrease in renal weight due to decline in nephrons. Accompanying this is a decreased filtration rate and impaired excretion, specifically of urea and creatinine, as well as less efficient fluid balance control. Also of importance is the effect of reduced renal function on drug excretion. This will result in high plasma levels and potential side effects that might increase the risk of falls for the resident. An important function of the kidney is the second stage of conversion of vitamin D into 1,25-dihydroxycholecalciferol after initial conversion in the liver so that calcium can be absorbed from the intestine. Obviously this is important for maintenance of bone mineral density by allowing access to dietary calcium.

Although ageing changes in renal function alone will not need to be considered a problem, the prevalence of renal failure in residents in aged care is such that physiotherapists must understand the implications in the context of functional capacity. Mechanical problems relating to micturition and bladder function are covered in more detail in the chapter that addresses continence (Chapter 14).

The skin

The skin of elderly people undergoes changes that make it more susceptible to injury. These include a decrease in strength, and the thickness of the dermis declines with loss of subcutaneous fat, blood vessels, hair follicles, sebaceous glands and free nerve endings. There is a loss of collagen and elasticity, and the skin becomes fragile and tears rather than stretching and returning to shape as it does in younger people. The epidermis can, however, become thickened in areas of hyperkeratosis. Fingernails and toenails can also become hyperkeratotic, making it more difficult to keep the nails cut. Long toenails can cause problems with footwear, leading to foot pain and gait instability, and in turn to immobility. The elderly have difficulty in reaching their toenails and so need assistance in regular pedicure if this cause of mobility problems is to be controlled.

Ultraviolet light damage over a lifetime damages the skin and many elderly people will have skin cancers or scars where skin cancers have been removed. Ageing changes the distribution and amount of melanin in the skin. Exposure to the sun should be limited in the elderly and sun block, broad-brimmed hats and sunglasses applied when going outdoors to reduce skin damage potential and glare.

The reduction in blood vessels in the dermis also poses a problem for thermoregulation due to the reduced ability to sweat to reduce body temperature, and heat stroke can occur easily in hot weather. Thermoregulation in the elderly is considered related to a reduction in physical activity and fitness (Van Someren et al 2002). There is a normal circadian regulation of body temperature that leads to a core temperature that is maximal in the late afternoon and minimal in the early morning. Deviations from this circadian rhythm come from physical activity and environmental modification. Age-related changes may affect thermoreception, central integration and thermogenesis. Thus older people are more at risk of hypothermia or heat stress than younger people. This is attributed to the slower perception of environmental temperature change and a lesser ability to generate heat to warm core temperature through shivering or physical activity or to cool the body by sweating (Van Someren et al 2002). Reduced arterial compliance has been related to decreased ability of older people to change skin perfusion to conserve or lose heat. Dehydration also plays a major role in thermoregulation in the elderly. Adequate fluid intake and environmental temperature control are mandatory in hot weather to counteract this problem. However, hydration and environmental temperature control are also vital in cold climates for older people.

Musculoskeletal system

Skeletal muscle function

Muscle cross-sectional area is generally the largest at around 20–30 years of age for both men and women; this coincides with the highest strength levels within the lifespan. Thereafter, strength in most muscle groups declines, progressing slowly at first and then more rapidly after middle age. Most people notice the effect of skeletal muscle ageing in middle age when there is a perceived loss of strength and endurance (Tseng et al 1995). Strength loss among elderly individuals is directly associated with their limited mobility and physical performance as well as to the sequelae of the increased incidence of accidents suffered by those with muscle weakness and poor balance (Brookes & Faulkner 1994, Chakravarthy et al 2002).

Motor unit remodelling is a continual and natural process in the normal individual. It occurs by selective degeneration of muscle fibres, followed by terminal sprouting of axons from adjacent motor units. Researchers have hypothesized that with age this process gradually becomes a ‘denervation muscle atrophy’ and an irreversible degeneration of muscle fibres and endplate structures, especially in the type II muscle fibres. This leads to a progressive decrease in cross-sectional area of muscle (Brookes & Faulkner 1994). However, skeletal muscle size is not the only determinant of functional ability. Synchronized motor unit recruitment is vital for efficient function (Booth & Criswell 1997). Improvement in both these aspects of skeletal muscle decline that are found with ageing can be addressed by functional resistance activation of the muscles (Booth et al 1998).

A 40–50% reduction in muscle mass between 25 and 80 years of age, due to motor unit losses and muscle fibre atrophy, is the primary factor responsible for the age-related decline in muscle strength, even among healthy active men and women (McArdle et al 1996). The loss of muscle fibres becomes particularly apparent around the fifth decade. The loss of muscle volume is due to reduced fibre size, especially in the fast twitch fibres in the lower extremities. This results in a proportionate increase in the area occupied by slow twitch (type I) muscle fibres (Larsson et al 1979).

Decreased strength is the result of several factors that are believed to contribute to decreased muscle hypertrophy and diminished function in human muscle tissue with ageing. These include a loss of alpha motor neurons, atrophy of type I and II myofibres, diminished oxidative capacity of exercising muscle, and a subsequent reduction in ability to produce torque (Craik 1993). These progressive neuromotor responses coupled with a decrease in the daily level of muscle loading lead to a decline in strength (Lexell 1993). Lower extremity muscle strength can be reduced by as much as 40% between the ages of 30 and 80 years (Anniansson et al 1986). Weakness is even more severe in older nursing home residents with a history of falls. Whipple et al (1987) found a marked reduction in measures of mean ankle and knee strength in fallers compared to non-fallers. The importance of skeletal muscle strength to function is large. Buchner & deLateur (1991) concluded that over 20% of the variance in functional status is explained by relative strength. Interestingly, very little research is available which reports on eccentric muscle strength and age-related changes although this type of contraction is important in maintaining postural stability (Lord et al 1995).

Flexibility

The length of soft tissues including skeletal muscle, fascia, nerves, blood and lymph vessels in addition to joint capsule and ligamentous structures determines flexibility or suppleness of the body. Adaptive shortening of all soft tissues ensues if regular lengthening and shortening to the available limits with active movement does not occur. Tissue length and joint range of movement are lost with ageing.

With advancing age the normal curvature of the spine changes. In the thoracic spine, up to the age of 40 years women have a slightly straighter curve than men but after this age the increase in thoracic curvature is similar for both men and women. Similarly, there is loss of range of both flexion and extension in the lumbar spine with age (Loebl 1967). In the cervical spine, for example, the loss of range of active neck extension declines by 5 degrees each decade while flexion, lateral flexion and rotation to each side declines by 3 degrees each decade (Youdas et al 1992).

Peripheral joint range is also lost with age. In the ankle loss of range becomes of considerable importance when the contribution of ankle dorsiflexion and plantarflexion is considered. This ankle range is essential for strategies adopted in balance reactions, sit-to-stand activities and when walking on the flat or up and down hills or stairs. A significant decrease in ankle dorsiflexion range has been demonstrated to occur between the ages of 35 and 85 years in women (Nitz et al 2004, Spanevello & Nitz 1999). The biggest decline was shown between the 55–65 age cohort and the 75 years and over cohorts, with no significant difference in range between the women up to 55 years of age.

A major component in the soft tissues is collagen. With ageing collagen has been shown to undergo glycation that is due to non-enzymatic cross-linking and is responsible for the loss of elasticity and dysfunction of this tissue with age (Bailey et al 1998). Functionally, these changes lead to joint stiffness and a decrease in tensile strength of tendons (Johnson et al 1994) and thus increased susceptibility to injury (Dressler et al 2002).

An important consideration for physiotherapists working in aged care is adverse neuromechanical tension. Due to changes outlined herein there is a greater susceptibility of aged persons to develop neural tension and neuromechanosensitivity. This may well lead to a syndrome of pain, immobility, decreased movement and related postural change (Wright 1998).

Nervous system

Age-related decrements in neuromuscular performance are demonstrated by studies that examine both simple and complex reaction and movement times. The decline in performance of these activities with age results largely from a 37% decline in the number of spinal cord axons and a 10% decline in nerve conduction velocity (Clarkson 1978). 'When reaction time is split into central processing time and muscle action time it is the time required to detect a stimulus and process the information to produce a response that is affected most by the ageing process' (McCardle et al 1996, p 641, Spirduso 1975).

Because reflexes (such as the knee jerk response) are controlled at the spinal level these are less affected by ageing than voluntary responses such as reaction and movement times. Interestingly in all instances of one study at least, the active groups (both young and old) were far swifter than those people in the non-active group, irrespective of age (McCardle et al 1996).

Slowed reaction time is a usual deficit produced by ageing (Spirduso 1975). The time interval between application of a stimulus and initiation of movement is increased (Stelmach & Worringham 1985). This finding is also linked to degenerative changes in the motor unit. In addition, pre-motor time (time interval between application of a stimulus and initiation of electromyographic (EMG) activity) and motor time (time interval between onset of EMG activity and initiation of movement) are lengthened with normal ageing (Craik 1993, Welford 1984). Impairments of central sensory processing and organization may occur with ageing. Although accurate sensory inputs may be available, this may cause the central nervous system (CNS) not to recognize or incorporate accurate information into determinations of position and movement (Allison 1995). The decline in ability to divide attention and accurately perform multiple tasks, whether they are motor or a combination of motor and cognitive tasks, has been demonstrated in older people with no obvious pathology (Brauer et al 2001, 2002, Mulder et al 1993).

Cognition

Cognitive function is dependent on cerebral oxygenation and glucose levels which in turn are dependent on cerebral blood flow (Guyton 1991). Oestrogen levels are also considered to play a major role in both neurodegenerative events and non-degenerative events that lead to age-related cognitive and memory decline (Morrison & Hof 1997).

When considering cognitive state, however, we must acknowledge the importance of sleep and the disturbances to sleep that are encountered as well as memory loss, confusion and dementia, which are also prevalent in residents. These problems worry the resident and can lead to stress-related conditions. Care planning and strategies for managing residents with cognition-related disorders depend on understanding aspects of sleep, memory and confusion that can be improved. Therefore these topics will be considered in more detail.

Sleep

Disorders of sleep are common in the elderly. Although the reason why we sleep is still unclear, changes in sleep patterns and the effects of these changes are obvious and can be disturbing in the elderly. Most adults require between 7 and 8 hours of sleep each night. Although some adults routinely sleep as little as 3 hours with no detrimental effect on functional capacity, others need as much as 10 hours nightly. Sleep has two components, rapid eye movement (REM) and non-rapid eye movement (NREM). On falling asleep there is a period of NREM sleep that progresses to REM sleep. During NREM sleep, muscle relaxation occurs and the breathing and pulse rate drops. REM sleep has been described as having four stages during which there is characteristic eye movement and changes in muscle tone, respiratory and heart rate. REM sleep occupies about 25% of the sleep cycle. With ageing, the cycle of NREM and REM sleep decreases and may contribute to nocturnal waking and daytime drowsiness and snoozes. Some researchers have connected this pattern to cognitive decline especially in people over 75 years. Elderly men have been identified as demonstrating this pattern and thus have more cognitive decline. Another sleep disorder that commonly presents in later life is REM sleep behaviour disorder, which is distinguished by the sufferer enacting dreams. This disorder has been connected with nocturnal falls (Morfis et al 1997). Care should be taken not to discount this condition when investigating falls during the night. REM sleep behaviour disorder has been connected to vascular lesions in the pontine tegmentum. As vascular lesions become more prevalent in older people, it is important to be aware of the contribution of such lesions to nocturnal falls as medication management can effectively overcome the REM sleep disorder (Morfis et al 1997).

Disruption to the circadian sleep rhythm can be intrinsic or extrinsic. Extrinsic examples of disruption include the effect of jet lag or working night shift. In the elderly, an intrinsic circadian rhythm sleep disorder is the advanced sleep phase syndrome. This presents with excessive waking. This has been related to changes in the hypothalamic-suprachiasmatic nucleic function (Burney-Puckett 1996). Disorders of this area of the brain have also been linked to the 'sundown syndrome', where the elderly person shows increasing agitation in the evening.

Insomnia is another example of an intrinsic disorder of sleep. It is the chronic inability to obtain the amount of sleep needed to maintain functional capacity and wellbeing. Primary insomnia describes the disorder that has been present since childhood. Secondary insomnia is very common and is caused by pain, incontinence problems, stress, depression, alcohol and tobacco abuse, caffeine, dementia and normal ageing.

Sleep is considered within Chapter 4 ('Life satisfaction') in some detail as the authors acknowledge the important relationship between sleep and healthy function.

Memory

Many elderly people consider memory loss to be an inevitable part of the ageing process. This is not necessarily so as the ability to remember is determined by many factors. When an event is given undivided attention and during this process the event is related to some other experience that in turn gives the event meaning, a person is more likely to be able to recall the event (Rugg 1998). Memory is often thought of as short or long term. Durable or long-term memories are mostly related to the hippocampus and adjacent medial temporal lobe areas of the brain (Knowlton & Fanselow 1998, Rugg 1998). The early concept of short-term memory is now referred to as working memory. The working memory refers to the ability to manipulate and maintain information to enable reasoning, learning and understanding (Baddeley 1998). These short-term memory functions, exemplified by remembering a list of words and then recalling the list, involve the left prefrontal cortex (Baddeley 1998, Rugg 1998), left parahippocampal and fusiform gyri (Wagner et al 1998) for encoding including analysis of the meaning of the word and the right prefrontal cortex for recall (Baddeley 1998, Rugg 1998). When the items needing to be remembered are novel, the parahippocampal cortex is involved. This activity is known to be bilateral where verbal and pictorial memory encoding takes place (Rugg 1998). Other areas of the brain implicated in pictorial memory are the fusiform regions, caudate and anterior cingulate (Brewer et al 1998).

Decline in memory ability can be related to pathological changes in the specific areas of the brain that are responsible for the function. A factor that might contribute to poor memory is lack of use. Stimulation of neural pathways through practice of memory tasks might enhance function. Also the ability to remember is often contextual or requiring relevancy to be considered worthy of remembering. Residents in aged care often dismiss the importance of keeping abreast of the news if they believe there is no relevancy to the current life situation and so no effort is made to remember news items. The same can be said for other information such as daily routine. If care staff are there to remind the resident when and where to go to lunch, then there is no reason to remember at what time lunch is served or how to find the dining room. Encouraging residents to be self-sufficient in simple memory tasks such as this should help maintain functional memory.

Cardiovascular system

Identification of the changes in the heart and arterial system that are only attributable to ageing and not to pathology is difficult as very few older people are free from pathologies such as hypertension, diabetes, hyperlipidaemia or a smoking history. With ageing, morphological changes to the heart include increasing thickness of the ventricular walls, dilation and stretching of the valves, with calcification of the valves and coronary arteries a common occurrence, as well as increased deposition of epicardial fat (Roffe 1998). There is a decrease in myocardial maximal oxygen consumption. Systolic function is preserved but diastolic function declines. The decline in diastolic function is due to a reduction in rate of calcium reuptake after depolarization in the sarcoplasmic reticulum. This reuptake is required for relaxation of the myocardium. Structural changes such as increased fibrosis of the pericardium and myocardium lead to increased stiffness that also affects diastolic function (Bounhoure 1997). There is reduced sympathoadrenergic responsiveness in the aged to the need for increased cardiac output. Collectively these lead to a rise in diastolic pressure (Roffe 1998). Those older people who undertake regular physical activity retain a pattern of left ventricular diastolic filling (though attenuated) that is similar to younger people but better than sedentary older people (Petrella et al 1996). The rise in cardiac output induced by exercise in the elderly is not achieved by raising the heart rate as occurs in young people. Rather it is due to increased left ventricular filling and reliance on the Frank–Starling mechanism (Roffe 1998).

The effects of ageing of the arterial system contribute to the changes seen in the heart with ageing. Although there is a reduction in number of small arteries and arterioles with ageing, there is a progressive increase in arterial volume due to the large arteries becoming dilated and tortuous (Roffe 1998). The arterial walls comprise elastin and collagen fibres in addition to smooth muscle. They become thickened in the media and intima due to deposition of lipid thus decreasing the lumen of the vessels. With ageing the elastin fibres transfer their distensibility to the collagen, which is less elastic, and so the arterial wall becomes stiffer (London & Guérin 1999). Parallel to this change is an increase in systolic blood pressure. Hypertension presents commonly with ageing. Blood pressure is usually expressed as the systolic and diastolic pressure. The product of the total peripheral resistance and the cardiac output defines the mean blood pressure. With ageing the diastolic blood pressure increases up to about 70 years of age then decreases due to the increased volume in the large central arteries. On the other hand, the systolic blood pressure and pulse pressure amplitude continually increase with age in response to increasing arterial stiffness. The change in stiffness of the aorta causes an increased pulse wave velocity and increase in amplitude of the component pressure wave from ventricular ejection and these waves are reflected back towards the heart faster. The reflected wave tends to reach the heart during left ventricular ejection rather than after aortic valve closure (as occurs in younger people with normal arteries), thereby raising central systolic pressure. This in turn lowers mean diastolic pressure and coronary perfusion instead of the opposite effect seen in young people. The result of this in the elderly is an increase in cardiac muscle oxygen consumption, ventricular afterload and left ventricular hypertrophy (London & Guérin 1999).

Another consequence of the dilatation of large arteries is a decline in the baroreceptor responses to change in blood pressure. This contributes to the symptoms of postural hypotension experienced by a number of older people when dizziness, lightheadedness and syncope are experienced on changing position from lying to sitting or sitting to standing (McLaughlan 2001). Prolonged standing can also precipitate syncope from orthostatic hypotension (Carey & Potter 2001). Also at rest and during exercise the heart rate slows in older people. This can cause dizziness, increase the potential for a fall and generally decrease exercise tolerance. Carotid sinus syndrome is considered to result from altered central processing of baroreflex responses. It can result in syncope when mechanical stimulation of the carotid sinus occurs in situations such as turning the head or straining (Carey & Potter 2001).

Hypertension will increase the risk of cardiovascular disorders such as myocardial infarction, disorders of rhythm and arterial disease, stroke and renal dysfunction. Normal ageing in the cardiovascular system is exacerbated by additional pathologies including arteriosclerosis and chronic heart failure (McLaughlan 2001).

Respiratory system

Static and dynamic lung measures both deteriorate with age. There is a significant slowing of ventilation and gas exchange kinetics during the transition from rest to exercise, for example. The three most important changes that occur within this system with age are a gradual increase in the size of the alveoli, the disintegration of the support structure of the lungs, and a weakening of the respiratory muscle. The normal lung enjoys a large reserve capacity that can meet ventilation requirements even during maximal exercise. This reserve capacity begins to diminish after the age of 30 and then accelerates after 60 years of age (Brooks et al 2000).

Ageing induces intrinsic and extrinsic mechanisms that affect the respiratory system. The extrinsic mechanisms relate to the chest wall and ventilation mechanics while the intrinsic mechanisms include the lung tissue and pulmonary circulation.

Chest wall changes with ageing

The ability of the chest to increase in volume, enabling the development of negative intrathoracic pressure during inspiration, reduces with age. The contraction of the inspiratory muscles elevates the ribs and sternum, extends the thoracic spine and lowers the diaphragm, thereby increasing the thoracic volume (Webster & Kadah 1991). Muscle strength and joint range of movement determine the size of movement. In the older person, the muscles become less efficient due to morphological change and the joints become stiffer. The thoracic kyphosis is often increased due to poor postural muscle activity or vertebral crush fractures from osteoporosis so the potential for thoracic extension to increase the vertical volume of the chest in conjunction with rib elevation is diminished. Also the increased thoracic kyphosis and loss of the lumbar lordosis that occurs with age contributes to the abdominal contents being pushed up under the diaphragm. This inhibits the amount of diaphragmatic descent available and further reduces respiratory mechanical efficiency. Thus attention to postural correction in lying, sitting and standing is vitally important for the older person.

Age effect on the lung

The contribution of inhaled environmental pollutants to the ageing effects on the lung makes it difficult to identify the true effects of age on the lung. Ageing of the lung should be viewed in conjunction with an individual's occupation, diet and where they lived during different periods of their life. Normal values of lung function tests might overestimate the normal values for the elderly simply from the 'survivor effect' or because these values might have been extrapolated from normal data from younger age cohorts. Acquired lung pathology also interferes with ventilation in any age group but with ageing the likelihood of some pathological lung changes being present increases.

The physiological changes that have been identified in lungs from older people include a reduction in elasticity that is postulated to reduce lung compliance and recoil, with an increase in collapse of small airways during expiration. Thus although total lung volume is considered not to change, inspired volumes are reduced due to decreased lung elasticity, chest wall stiffness and muscle weakness, and there is an increase in residual volume (Dyer & Stockley 1999).

Within the lung the large airways maintain their diameter but there is loss of small airways and alveolar dilatation. Thus surface area over which gaseous exchange can take place is reduced.

Oxygen transport from the inspired air to the tissues is also affected by age. Ventilation–perfusion mismatch increases with age. Pulmonary arterial wall thickening due to fibrosis and collagen deposition within the media causes loss of arterial compliance. There does not appear to be a loss of alveolar capillary density but there is a decrease in alveolar area. This might explain the decrease in ventilation–perfusion mismatch that causes reduced arterial oxygen pressure and saturation with ageing.

With ageing there is a reduction in the ventilation response to hypoxia and hypercapnia. This presentation might cause the older person to not feel breathless until considerably incapacitated by hypoxia or hypercapnia. However, there is an increased response to hypercapnia during exercise in the elderly. This should be considered when undertaking an exercise programme.

Other changes that occur with ageing within the lung include a decline in mucociliary clearance ability that can increase susceptibility of the older person to infection (Dyer & Stockley 1999). Thus an increase in retention of lung secretions combined with reduced immunity can account for this state. Parkinson's disease has been associated with an increased production of lung secretions that can exacerbate the decline in mucociliary clearance ability and further increase the potential for lung infection.

Endocrine system

Decline in endocrine function with ageing becomes clinically important when involving the pancreas and the thyroid and indirectly via the effect of hypothalamic-pituitary decline leading to the menopause and andropause (Lamberts et al 1997). Pancreatic, insulin receptor and post-insulin receptor changes that occur with ageing lead to impaired glucose tolerance or diabetes mellitus (DM). DM is present in 40 to 50% of people over 65 years of age and is responsible for considerable morbidity and mortality. It is often associated with poor diet, decreased activity levels, increased abdominal fat and decreased lean muscle mass. Exercise plays a major role in control of DM, in addition to diet and oral hypoglycaemic drugs and insulin.

Thyroid dysfunction due to ageing is revealed by a slight decline in pituitary thyroid-stimulating hormone (TSH) release and a decreased peripheral degradation of thyroxine (T_4) which results in a decline in triiodothyronine (T_3) concentration (Lamberts et al 1997).

Thyroid disorders are relatively common in older people (Finucane & Anderson 1996). Reduced thyroid function (hypothyroidism) is manifest by a number of symptoms including inertia with consequent reduction in activity levels, cognitive impairment, depression, reduced cold tolerance, constipation, bradycardia, leg cramps, skin changes to name a few that are most problematic for the older person. Hyperthyroidism is also found in the elderly. The most significant problems associated with this state include heat intolerance, leg oedema, tremor, tachycardia, anxiety or apathy, cognitive impairment, and psychosis (Finucane & Anderson 1996). Finucane & Anderson (1996) point out that thyroid dysfunction can be overlooked in the older person as many of these symptoms can be confused with normal ageing presentations.

There is a decline with ageing in the level of growth hormone release by the pituitary. This leads to a decrease in insulin-like growth factor

(IGF-1) by the liver and other organs. It is implicated in the somatopause, which is associated with decrease in muscle mass and strength, bone mass and ultimately quality of life from the resultant decline in physical ability and possible morbidity related to falls.

Hypothalamic-pituitary decline also leads to menopause in women and andropause in men as well as a decline in adrenal production of dehydroepiandrosterone (DHEA) and dehydroepiandrosterone sulphate (DHEAS). Adrenal cortisol levels remain unchanged with age. The decline in oestrogen has been shown to increase the incidence of atherosclerosis, bone mineral loss and decline in cognitive state (Compton et al 2002, Lamberts et al 1997). The decline with ageing of DHEA, which is a precursor for oestrogen or testosterone in both men and women, can be related to decline in muscle mass and muscle strength. High physical activity levels have been associated with maintenance of DHEAS levels in women (Nitz et al 2002) and support the importance of maintaining physical activity capacity in the elderly.

Hormonal levels under the control of the hypothalamic-pituitary axis and associated with the ageing process are responsible for change in body composition. This is expressed by increased adiposity, especially in the abdominal area, and reduction in lean muscle mass in addition to reduction in bone mass due to loss of bone mineral density. The consequences of these changes are a decline in physical ability and bone fragility. Both of these are responsive to intervention, the simplest of which is exercise. Physiotherapists should be able to design an exercise programme that addresses these aspects as well as the problem of balance decline that accompanies muscle function decline.

Immune system

The immune system is responsible for defending the body from infection. It is closely associated with the endocrine and nervous systems (Mariani et al 1998) with which it communicates via hormones, cytokines and neurotransmitters. There are two components, the innate and the adaptive, that comprise the immune system. The innate systems aim at lysis and phagocytosis of the pathogen by the leucocytes and neutrophils, thereby trying to resolve the infection. The natural killer (NK) cells attack intracellular infections, such as viruses, by inducing apoptosis of the cell. If the infection is not resolved within 4–5 days the second immune response, the adaptive immune response, has developed. This involves the activation of the T cells into Th1 and Th2 effector cells. The Th1 cells help the macrophages clear intracellular bacterial infections and the Th2 cells help the B cells to produce high affinity antibody (Lord et al 2001). With ageing both the innate and adaptive immune responses can decline but owing to the cooperative interaction between the two systems at a number of levels, decline in either system compromises the immune response. The increased susceptibility of the elderly to bacterial infection is considered to relate to this decline.

Poor nutrition has been identified as a contributing factor for decreased immunity in the elderly. One result of poor nutrition is low zinc bioavailability. Zinc is required as a catalyst in the immune response and reduced immunoresistance in the elderly may be due to low zinc bioavailability (Mocchegiani et al 2001). Studies of zinc supplementation for a short period of 1 to 2 months in the elderly have shown improved general health and cognition up to a year post intervention (Mocchegiani et al 2001). Also important in the maintenance of homeostasis of the immune system is the calcium ion regulating hormone 1,25-dihydroxy-vitamin D_3 (Mariani et al 1998). Reduced vitamin D availability is common in the elderly residing in aged care facilities due to dietary deficiency and decreased sun exposure that facilitates vitamin D production by the skin (Ravaglia et al 1994). Vitamin D levels have been shown to be significantly associated with NK cell activity. NK cells increase in number with age. This helps to compensate for the decline in the number of T cells in the immune response (Mariani et al 1998).

Stress is a factor that is known to change immunoregulation. Stress can be physical or psychological and affects the cortisol levels in the hypophyseal-adrenal axis. Acute or chronic stress can have different immunological effects.

Humour or laughing has been shown to reduce the effect of stress on immunosuppression (Kamei et al 1997). Therefore incorporation of 'humour therapy' might be of use in reducing the disease susceptibility.

Absence of depression has been associated with increased physical ability and cognitive function in the oldest-old and depression was not correlated with NK cell numbers or function (Mariani et al 1998). This finding supports the importance of participation by residents in physical and cognitive activity programmes in RACFs. Physiotherapists in collaboration with occupational therapists and speech pathologists play an important role in the implementation and design of such programmes.

Conclusion

Exacerbation of the ageing effect on many of the body systems can come about intrinsically from poor nutrition, hydration and oxygenation ability and lack of physical activity. Extrinsically environmental pollutants, excess sun exposure, thermal stress and potential for trauma from other environmental influences such as people and machines can hasten the ageing effect on the body tissues. Collectively there is a cascade effect from intrinsic and extrinsic influences that results in loss of quality of life from acquired morbidity. The ageing responses are also determined to some extent by the individual's genetic make-up, thus accounting for the variability and heterogeneity of older people. These factors also identify possible avenues for controlling the ageing effect. Physiotherapists can provide interventions that affect most intrinsic ageing contributors and can assist in limiting the effect of environmental influences that might lead to trauma, for example from a fall that is injurious.

During the ageing process, the maintenance of a positive equilibrium in the intrinsic contributors for good health is crucial. In order to achieve optimal function for enhanced quality of life and the prevention of physical and cognitive decline this balance must be preserved. The interaction between different intrinsic components of good health may be visualized as a wheel of good aged health as pictured in Figure 1.1. It is important to note that no component is more important than any other. Therefore, failure in any component may lead to total collapse of the system, resulting in bad health or an inability to function well.

The functional consequences of the changes in various physiological systems have been summarized in Table 1.2. These changes need to be considered when evaluating the status of residents in aged care facilities. Therefore the next chapter, which looks at the physiotherapist's contribution to assessment of the resident, acknowledges these changes and incorporates them into the assessment and shows how the age changes influence performance and interpretation of findings. Normal ageing is also incorporated into Chapter 3, which deals with resident injuries, as many injuries occur due to increased susceptibility to injury that is related to circulatory, neural and tissue structural decline. In this chapter, for example, circulatory changes are discussed in more detail in the context of injury and healing in the presence of additional pathological changes, thereby increasing the relevancy of the information.

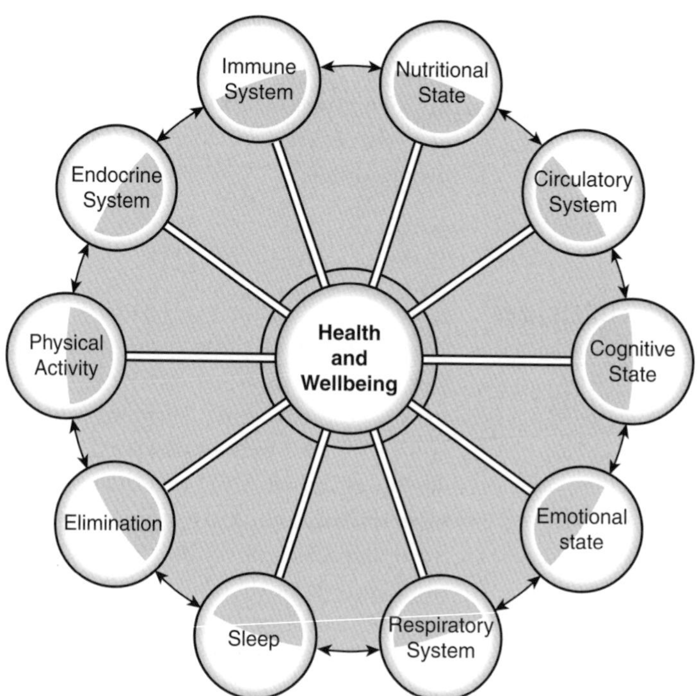

Figure 1.1 *The wheel of good aged health: intrinsic components of healthy ageing.*

Table 1.2
Summary of the physiological effects of ageing

System	Functional consequence
Gastrointestinal system	
Atrophy of the gums and bones, tooth loss and poorly fitted dentures	Impaired mastication, enunciation and communication
Reduction in saliva production	Reduced preliminary digestion
Swallow inefficiency	Nasal regurgitation or aspiration
Delayed gastric emptying	Bloated feeling and decreased appetite
Decline in intestinal absorption	↓ vitamin, mineral, fat, carbohydrate and protein for normal tissue maintenance and metabolism
Slowed gut motility and fluid balance ability	Constipation and poor excretion of waste products
Liver	
Reduced hepatic blood flow	Reduced bile formation and flow, altered enzyme activity
Decreased metabolic and storage capacity with decreased size	Poor drug absorption, mineral, vitamin and glycogen storage
Kidney	
Decreased plasma flow, decreased renal weight, decreased number of nephrons, decreased filtration rate and impaired excretion	Chronic and acute renal failure
Less efficient fluid balance control and drug excretion	Drug toxicity and increased risk of falls
Skin	
Decreased thickness and strength of the dermis, ↓ collagen elasticity, areas of hyperkeratosis	Skin fragility and tears and increased ulcer risk Nail changes
Decreased subcutaneous fat, hair follicles, blood vessels, sebaceous glands and nerve endings	Sensory loss, dryness and poor thermoregulation and increased risk of bruising Decreased touch and temperature perception and risk of burns and shear injury
Decreased melanin	Increased risk of sunburn
Muscles and joints	
Muscle mass ↓ due to ↓ number and size of type IIa and IIb fibres and ↓ type I fibre size	Decreased strength and postural stability
Insulin sensitivity ↓	Decreased muscle glycogen utilization, weakness
Oxidative enzymes ↓, size and number of mitochondria ↓	Decreased muscle metabolic function, weakness and ↓ endurance
Size of motor units ↓	Decreased strength
Stiffness of connective tissues in joints ↑	Decreased joint stability and mobility
Water content in intervertebral cartilage ↓	Atrophy and increased chance of disc protrusion and compression fractures in spine
Increased cross-linkages in collagen	Increased susceptibility of tendon rupture
Loss of soft tissue compliance	Decreased flexibility Increased potential for adverse neural tension presentation

table continues

System	Functional consequence
Body composition and stature	
Abdominal fat deposition ↑	Coronary heart disease, hyperlipidaemia
Body fat ↑	Impaired mobility and increased risk of disease
Lean body mass ↓	Decreased metabolic rate and ↓ strength and exercise tolerance and thermoregulation
Kyphosis ↑	Loss of height, decreased postural stability, impaired respiratory mechanics and decreased abdominal volume
Endocrine/Bone	
Bone minerals ↓	Osteoporosis – increased risk of fracture
Impaired glucose tolerance and insulin sensitivity	Increased incidence of diabetes mellitus
Changes in thyroid function	Confusion, inertia, constipation and leg cramps or cognitive impairment, heat tolerance, apathy and psychoses
Growth hormone decline	Decreased muscle strength and bone mass
Gonadal hormone decline	Oestrogen level decline → loss of bone minerals, decline in cognitive ability and increased atherosclerosis
Immune system	
Innate and adaptive system decline	Increased susceptibility to bacterial infection
Poor nutrition	Low vitamin, zinc and iron bioavailability
Respiration	
Increased stiffness of the thoracic cage	Decreased static and dynamic lung volumes
Maximum breathing capacity ↓	Decreased lung volumes, less respiratory reserve and lower exercise capacity
Elasticity of lung support tissues ↓	Increased work of breathing, decreased lung elastic recoil
Size of alveoli ↑	Decreased diffusion capacity and increased dead space
Number of pulmonary capillaries ↓	Decreased ventilation/perfusion ratio and mismatch
Decreased mucociliary clearance	Increased retention of secretions and increased susceptibility to infection

Summary

- Changes do occur in all systems with ageing.
- It is difficult to quantify the effects of ageing on physiological function and physical performance.
- Disease may complicate our understanding of the ageing process itself.
- Changes associated with ageing are difficult to extrapolate on for a number of reasons. Ageing itself is a variable process and individuals vary considerably in their capacity for longevity and wellness, which makes the elderly quite a non-homogeneous group.
- Many aspects of ageing are exacerbated by poor nutrition, hydration and oxygen delivery to tissues.
- Knowledge of changes due to ageing leads to logical assessment of disabilities related to older people and well-integrated care plans.

References

Allison L 1995 Balance disorders. In: Umphred D A (ed) Neurological rehabilitation. Mosby-Year Book, St Louis

Anniansson A, Hedberg M, Henning G 1986 Muscle morphology, enzymatic activity and muscle strength in elderly men: a follow up study. Muscle Nerve 9:585–591

Baddeley A 1998 Recent developments in working memory. Current Opinion in Neurobiology 8:234–238

Bailey A J, Paul R G, Knott L 1998 Mechanisms of maturation and ageing of collagen. Mechanisms of Ageing and Development 106(1–2):1–56

Booth F W, Criswell D S 1997 Molecular events underlying skeletal muscle atrophy and the development of effective countermeasures. International Journal of Sports Medicine 18(Suppl 4): S265–S269

Booth F W, Tseng B S, Fluck M, Carson J A 1998 Molecular and cellular adaptation of muscle in response to physical training. Acta Physiologica Scandinavica 162(3):343–350

Bounhoure J P 1997 Heart failure in the elderly. Annales de Cardiologie et D'Angiologie 46:473–478

Brauer S G, Woollacott M, Shumway-Cook A 2001 The interacting effects of cognitive demand and recovery of postural stability in balance-impaired elderly persons. Journal of Gerontology Medical Sciences 56(8):M489–496

Brauer S G, Woollacott M, Shumway-Cook A 2002 The influence of a concurrent cognitive task on the compensatory stepping response to a perturbation in balance-impaired and healthy elders. Gait and Posture 15(1):83–93.

Brewer J B, Zhao Z, Desmond J E, Glover G H, Gabriele J D E 1998 Making memories: brain activity that predicts how well visual experience will be remembered. Science 281:1185–1187

Bron A J 1997 Loss of vision in the ageing eye. Age and Ageing 26:159–163

Brookes S V, Faulkner J A 1994 Skeletal muscle weakness in old age: underlying mechanisms. Medicine and Science in Sports and Exercise 26:432

Brooks G A, Fahey T D, White T P, Baldwin K M 2000 Exercise physiology: human bioenergetics and its applications. Mayfield Publishing, Mountain View, CA

Buchner D M, deLateur B J 1991 The importance of skeletal muscle strength to physical function in older adults. Annals of Behavioural Medicine 13:12–21

Burney-Puckett M 1996 Sundown syndrome: etiology and management. Journal of Psychological Nursing 34:40–43

Campbell A J, Buchner D M 1997 Unstable disability and the fluctuations of frailty. Age and Ageing 26:315–319

Carey B J, Potter J F 2001 Cardiovascular causes of falls. Age and Ageing 30(S4):19–24

Carter S E, Campbell E M, Sanson-Fisher R W, Redman S, Gillespie W J 1997 Environmental hazards in the homes of older people. Age and Ageing 26:195–203

Chakravarthy M V, Joyner M J, Booth F W 2002 An obligation for primary care physicians to prescribe physical activity to sedentary patients to reduce the risk of chronic health conditions. Mayo Clinic Proceedings 77(2):165–173

Clarkson P M 1978 The relationship of age and level of physical activity with the fractionated components of patellar reflex time. Journal of Gerontology 3:650

Compton J, van Amelsvoort T, Murphy D 2002 Mood, cognition and Alzheimer's disease. Best Practice and Research in Clinical Obstetrics and Gynaecology 16(3):357–370

Craik R L 1993 Sensorimotor changes and adaptation in the older adult. In: Guccione A A (ed) Geriatric physical therapy. Mosby Year Book, St Louis

Di Fabio R P, Emasithi A 1997 Ageing and the mechanisms underlying head and postural control during voluntary motion. Physical Therapy 77(5):458–475

Dressler M R, Butler D L, Wenstrup R et al 2002 A potential mechanism for age-related declines in patellar tendon biomechanics. Journal of Orthopaedic Research 20(6):1315–1322

Dyer C A E, Stockley R A 1999 The ageing lung. Reviews in Clinical Gerontology 9:103–115

Finucane P, Anderson C 1996 Thyroid disease in older patients: diagnosis and treatment. Current Therapeutics 4:72–79

Guyton A C 1991 Textbook of medical physiology, 8th edn. W B Saunders, Philadelphia, p 679–684

Harwood R H 2001 Visual problems and falls. Age and Ageing 30(S4):13–18

Jackson G R, Owsley C, Curcio C A 2002 Photoreceptor degeneration and dysfunction in ageing and age-related maculopathy. Ageing Research Reviews 1(3):381–396

Johnson G A, Tramaglini D M, Levine R E et al 1994 Tensile and viscoelastic properties of human patellar tendon. Journal of Orthopaedic Research 12(6):796–803

Kamei T, Kumano H, Masumura S 1997 Changes in immunoregulatory cells associated with psychological stress and humor. Perceptual and Motor Skills 84:1296–1298

Knowlton B J, Fanselow M S 1998 The hippocampus, consolidation and on-line memory. Current Opinion in Neurobiology 8:293–296

Lamberts S, van den Beld A W, van der Lely A-J 1997 The endocrinology of aging. Science 278:419–424

Larsson L, Grimby G, Karlsson J 1979 Muscle strength and speed of movement in relation to age and muscle morphology. Journal of Applied Physiology, Respiratory, Environment, Exercise Physiology 46:451–456

Lexell J 1993 Ageing and human skeletal muscle: observations from Sweden. Canadian Journal of Applied Physiology 18:2–9

Loebl W Y 1967 Measurement of spinal posture and range of spinal movement. Annals of Physical Medicine 9(3):103–110.

London G M, Guérin A 1999 Influence of arterial pulse and reflective waves on systolic blood pressure and cardiac function. Journal of Hypertension 17(Suppl 2):S3–S6

Lord S R, Anstey K J, Williams P, Ward J A 1995 Psychoactive medication use, sensori-motor function and falls in older women. British Journal of Clinical Pharmacology 39:227–234

Lord J M, Butcher S, Killampali V, Lascelles D, Salmon M 2001 Neutrophil ageing and immunosenescence. Mechanisms of Ageing and Development 122(14):1521–1535

McArdle W D, Katch F I, Katch V L 1996 Exercise physiology: energy, nutrition and human performance. Williams & Wilkins, Baltimore

McLaughlan M A 2001 The ageing heart: state-of-the-art prevention and management of cardiac disease. Geriatrics 56:45–49

Mariani E, Ravaglia G, Meneghetti A et al 1998 Natural immunity and bone and muscle remodelling hormones in the elderly. Mechanisms of Ageing and Development 102(2–3):279–292

Mocchegiani E, Giacconi R, Muzzioli M, Cipriano C 2001 Zinc, infections and immunosenescence. Mechanisms of Ageing and Development 121 (1–3):21–35

Morfis L, Schwartz R S, Cistulli P A 1997 REM sleep behaviour disorder: a treatable cause of falls in elderly people. Age and Ageing 26:43–44

Morrison J H, Hof P R 1997 Life and death of neurons in the aging brain. Science 278(17 October): 412–419

Mulder T, Berndt H, Pauwels J, Nienhuis B 1993 Sensorimotor adaptability in the elderly and disabled. In: Stelmach G, Homberg V (eds) Sensorimotor impairment in the elderly. Kluwer, Dordrecht, p 413–436

Murphy C, Schubert C, Cruickshanks K J et al 2002 Prevalence of olfactory impairment in older adults. JAMA 288:2307–2312

Nitz J C, Low Choy N L et al 2002 How physical activity level affects balance, bone activity markers and some sex hormone levels in women over 40. Abstract, Australasian Menopause Society Conference, Sydney, Australia

Nitz J C, Low Choy N L et al 2004 Ankle dorsiflexion range in women aged 20 to 85 years. New Zealand Journal of Physiotherapy (In review)

Owsley C, Jackson G R, White M, Feist R, Edwards D J 2001 Delays in rod-mediated dark adaptation in early age-related maculopathy. Ophthalmology 108:1196–1202

Petrella R J, Cunningham D A, Nichol P M, Paterson D H 1996 Effects of regular physical activity on left ventricular filling in the elderly. Cardiology in the Elderly 4:201–206

Pinto M R, De Medici S, Zlotnicki A et al 1997 Reduced visual acuity in elderly people: the role of ergonomics and gerontechnology. Age and Ageing 26:339–345

Ravaglia G, Forti P, Pratelli L et al 1994 The association of ageing with calcium active hormone status in men. Age and Ageing 23:127–131

Roffe C 1998 Ageing of the heart. British Journal of Biomedical Sciences 55:136–149

Rosenhall U, Rubin W 1975 Degenerative changes in human vestibular sensory epithelia. Acta Otolaryngology 79:67–81.

Rugg MD 1998 Memories are made of this. Science 281:1151–1152

Scilley K, Jackson G R, Cideciyan A V et al 2002 Early age-related maculopathy and self-reported visual difficulty in daily life. Ophthalmology 109(7): 1235–1242

Seidman M D, Ahmad N, Bai U 2002 Molecular mechanisms of age-related hearing loss. Ageing Research Reviews 1(3):331-343

Spanevello M, Nitz J C 1999 Ankle dorsiflexion range of motion in different aged women. Honours Thesis, Department of Physiotherapy, The University of Queensland

Spirduso W W 1975 Reaction and movement time as a function of age and physical activity level. Journal of Gerontology 30:435

Stelmach G E, Worringham C J 1985 Sensorimotor deficits related to postural stability. Clinics in Geriatric Medicine 1(3):679-694

Tseng B S, Marsh D R, Hamilton M T, Booth F W 1995 Strength and aerobic training attenuate muscle wasting and improve resistance to the development of disability with ageing. Journal of Gerontology Medical Sciences 50:113-119

Van Someren E J W, Raymann R J E M, Scherder E J A, Daanan H A M, Swaab D F 2002 Circadian and age-related modulation of the thermoreception and temperature regulation; mechanisms and functional implications. Ageing Research Reviews 1:721-778

Wagner A D, Schacter D L, Rotte M et al 1998 Building memories: remembering and forgetting verbal experiences as predicted by brain activity. Science 281:1188-1191

Webster J R, Kadah H 1991 Unique aspects of respiratory disease in the aged. Geriatrics 46:31-43

Welford A T 1984 Between bodily changes and performance: some possible reasons for slowing with age. Experimental Aging Research 10:73

Whipple R H, Wolfson L I, Amerman P M 1987 The relationship of knee and ankle weakness to falls in nursing home residents: an isokinetic study. Journal of the American Geriatrics Society 35:13-20

Wright A 1998 A reappraisal of the 'adverse neural tension' phenomenon. In: Adverse neural tension reconsidered. Australian Journal of Physiotherapy Monograph No 3

Youdas J W, Garrett T R, Suman V S et al 1992 Normal range of motion of the cervical spine: an initial goniometric study. Physical Therapy 2(11):770-780

Zeeh J, Platt D 2002 The ageing liver: structural and functional changes and their consequences for drug treatment. Gerontology 48:121-127

2 The physiotherapist's contribution to resident assessment

Jennifer C. Nitz and
Susan R. Hourigan

This chapter aims to:

- prepare the physiotherapist for the role of assessing the level of dependency of the resident by identifying how much and what type of assistance is needed by the resident on admission to the RACF
- encourage the physiotherapist to assess all aspects of resident function and through the process of clinical reasoning develop a treatment programme for the individual
- prepare the physiotherapist for working in a multidisciplinary team whose primary aim is to enhance the quality of life of the residents
- prepare the physiotherapist to take a leadership role within the team and to always ensure adequate and appropriate assessment takes place.

Introduction

Ideally all residents should be thoroughly assessed on admission to the RACF. The physiotherapist's assessment should be undertaken as soon as possible so that a realistic care plan can be developed. Of most importance is the evaluation of functional ability and potential for falls and injury from other sources. This information will enable a safe transition from the community to the RACF. A more thorough team assessment can then be made over the ensuing days and the care plan finalized. All team members must realize that this care plan has to be flexible to accommodate the changes occurring in the resident from day to day. The rate at which these changes occur can be swift but at other times the condition of the resident can remain stable for many years.

The team should consider assessment findings in the context of the social, cultural, spiritual and emotional background the resident brings with them to the RACF.

The diversity of residents in care facilities will be reflected in the problems the physiotherapist will encounter and be required to manage. As a general rule, most residents will be elderly. There will generally be a small percentage of residents who are younger and because of physical or mental disability are unable to cope independently in the community. Disabilities throughout the facility range from acquired brain injury, spinal cord injury or degenerative disease of the nervous system to arthritis, other musculoskeletal disorders and intellectual disability. Pathologies may be newly acquired such as a recent stroke, and the resident might not have received rehabilitation owing to various circumstances but might benefit from an intense rehabilitation programme. Conversely, the pathologies might be long-standing and the effect of ageing with the disability has led to the inability to cope in the community. Physical disability or intellectual impairment puts a person of any age at greater risk of injury in any environment. Physiological age changes augment the level of injury risk in the presence of physical disability. For these reasons residents of care facilities have a high risk for accidental injury. Those that are most traumatic primarily occur from a fall. Physiotherapists are often required to identify potential risk of injury to the resident by initially assessing dependency and development of the personal care plan and in so doing also address the important aspect of injury prevention for personal carers. The other aspect of assessment by the physiotherapist that is extremely important is the evaluation of disability that is potentially reversible and for which a rehabilitation programme should be developed.

Probably the most common physical problems encountered in residents are pain, incontinence, balance and mobility difficulties. Dementia and intellectual disability are also commonly encountered. Pain, incontinence and balance are such specialist areas that they warrant separate chapters devoted only to those topics and only passing reference will be made to their assessment in this chapter because it forms part of the holistic resident evaluation.

Principles of assessment

It is desirable to have information that relates to the most recent medical history so that all staff members are aware of any precautions for handling management. An example would be a recent total hip replacement where a flexed and adducted position of the hip such as might occur when rising out of a low chair is likely to facilitate dislocation of the joint and so needs to be avoided. The past medical and surgical history provides important information as it helps determine falls risk as well as other injury risk in addition to identifying a possible reason for pain. For example, past femoral-popliteal bypass surgery will indicate the presence of significant arterial disease and this will increase the potential for skin laceration and poor healing if minor bumps should occur in the lower limbs during transfers. It also indicates there will be less efficient perfusion of muscles and this will affect the type of exercise chosen to improve fitness, balance and function. A history of cardiorespiratory disease will also be a factor used in the clinical reasoning process that determines exercise prescription. Most residents will be elderly but residents who are younger generally have physical or mental disability that has prevented ambulation, so all residents will be likely to have some degree of osteoporosis. Where there is a history of cancer or surgery for cancer there is always the possibility that bony metastases and pain will become a problem. For the physiotherapist this knowledge enables appropriate choice of pain-relieving treatment after considering the contraindications to some electrotherapy modalities, for example. We also know that the greater the number (three or more) of significant medical and surgical co-morbidities presenting in the resident the greater the risk of a fall. Some specific conditions alone have been identified as significant risk factors for falls. These include dementia, with Parkinson's disease dementia (Waite et al 2000) being the most likely to lead to falls, neurological and musculoskeletal disorders and hypotension (Tinetti et al 1988). All the medications taken by the resident including those prescribed by the doctor and those bought over the counter should be identified as 4 or more medications increase the likelihood of recurrent falls (Leipzig et al 1999, Yip & Cumming 1994). Sedatives, psychotropic drugs and opioid analgesics are specific medications that have been shown to increase the risk of a fall (Neutel et al 1996, Weiner et al 1998). Other drugs that might contribute to a fall are antihypertensives, antiarrhythmics, anti-Parkinson's disease drugs and hypoglycaemic agents (Yip & Cumming 1994).

If the new resident is taking a course of antibiotics this will usually indicate the presence of an acute infection that in older people can cause confusion, weakness and reduced functional ability. Therefore the level of dependency shown during the illness might be expected to change once the resident becomes well. This exemplifies the need for review of function within the first few weeks of residency so that the true picture of the resident can be found and the care plan adjusted to reflect the presentation. If the new resident is accompanied by a family member or community carer at admission to the RACF, this person should be asked about usual functional status, what the resident likes and dislikes and any needs peculiar to them so as to ease the transition to care. Even if the new residents are able to speak for themselves, it is good to get this information from the relative to corroborate the story as the presence of confusion or dementia often clouds the picture.

The past history will also provide information on newly acquired medical conditions that might be reversible with more intensive physiotherapy intervention. Such a situation is the new resident who has suffered a recent stroke and has been slow to demonstrate recovery. These people often respond to slow stream rehabilitation that was not possible in the primary health care facility and the resident should not be denied the opportunity to achieve recovery. In many cases these residents will have the potential to return home to the community or at least achieve a better level of independence but remain in the RACF.

Table 2.1 *Key factors in an assessment*

Key factors	Rationale
1. Immediate medical and surgical history	Indicates need for special precautions
2. Past medical and surgical history: $\geqslant 3$ increase risk of a fall	Potential for improvement in condition
3. Complete medication list: $\geqslant 4$ increase risk of recurrent falls	Needed to complete the clinical reasoning process for all physiotherapeutic interventions and recommendations for manual handling issues
4. Communication ability	Trust and determination of needs
5. Vision and hearing	Safety
6. Swallowing ability	Prevention of aspiration
7. Cognitive state	Affects communication, memory and level of anxiety and stress
8. Functional level	Determines safety and amount of assistance needed for activities of daily living
9. Posture and any structural deformities need to be identified and measured	Thoracic kyphosis, scoliosis, joint arthrodesis or significant joint range loss should be noted and prevention of further deformity instigated
10. Skin integrity and circulation status	Presence of pressure areas or potential for pressure area formation must be evaluated, peripheral pulses or skin atrophy noted
11. Pain presentation	Type and cause of pain needs to identify cancer, osteoporosis, arthritis, vascular and neural causes of pain
12. Continence	Some continence problems can be improved by physiotherapy intervention

It is clear there are many factors a thorough assessment will include. Table 2.1 highlights the major factors necessary in an assessment.

Communication

Before embarking on a physical assessment of the resident, the physiotherapist needs to determine the most appropriate method of communication. This enables the development of a trusting relationship that can grow to mutually benefit the resident and care staff. There are times when the resident will arrive with comprehensive referral notes and this happy circumstance allows you to proceed with the assessment having a fairly accurate idea of communication ability. This is rarely the case and generally time must be spent in establishing communication. The cognitive state of the resident will determine whether they can understand instructions and how complex those instructions can be before understanding interferes with the ability to comply.

Depending on your impression regarding communication, evaluating the impact of cognitive decline or dementia might need to be undertaken prior to the physical assessment.

Be aware that the change from home to the RACF can cause confusion and alteration in the behaviour of the new resident. This might present as shortened attention span and the person being easily distracted. Memory might also appear poor. Re-evaluation needs to be undertaken after a short adaptation period so that this aspect is accounted for in the definitive care plan.

There are times when a comprehensive speech pathology and audiology assessment is indicated to determine the factors affecting communication difficulties. In these cases the physiotherapist might instigate the referral. Simple methods of communication other than with speech include writing and picture boards.

Functional ability and level of dependence

The starting point for this assessment will often be directed by where you find the resident. They could be in bed, sitting in a chair or wheelchair or walking in the corridor. Begin the assessment by evaluating the functional requirements of the situation where you encounter the resident. For ease of covering the items that need to be evaluated, the functional activities will be addressed in sequence.

Bed mobility

Independence in bed mobility enables the resident to remain comfortable by changing position during the night to relieve pressure, reduce joint stiffness, change the amount of bed clothes in response to air temperature and ultimately to achieve a good night's sleep.

Rolling

Evaluate rolling ability to each side. This should be done with the bed clothes up and down to see what effect this restriction has on the resident. If unable to roll independently identify what assistance is needed to achieve independence. This could be by supplying a bed pole (Fig. 2.1), bed rope or overhead ring or by elevating the bed rails so the resident can pull on them to roll. A sturdy bedside table might be a suitable substitute aid. Physical assistance might be needed for more disabled residents. This assistance might only require help to position the lower limbs once the roll has been achieved to prevent pressure from bone-on-bone contact or to place pillows under the upper knee to support a total hip replacement. In some cases full assistance is needed to roll. A slide sheet and one or two carers might be required depending on the individual resident's needs. Before indicating this level of dependency the physiotherapist

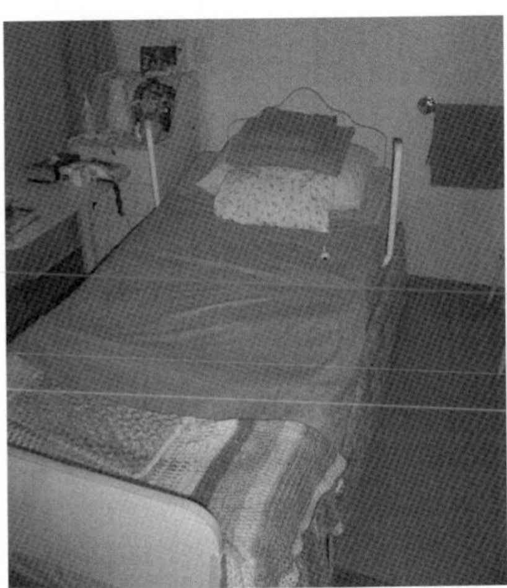

Figure 2.1 *Bed pole positioned for a frail elderly resident.*

should allow the resident to try out a range of devices that might assist independent activity to see if they can enable the resident to participate in the roll. This reduces the staffing numbers for this activity and will ensure the resident is helped to turn as frequently as is needed. It also allows retention of self-efficacy that is so important for life satisfaction.

Moving from lying to sitting on the side of the bed

The transition from lying to sitting on the side of the bed is undertaken by individuals in many ways. There are no rules regarding the best or appropriate method of achieving the movement except that safety must be maintained. Ask the resident to perform the movement and observe the way it is done. If the resident successfully performs the movement, decide if it could be made easier or safer by supplying an aid such as a bed pole. Your aim should be to enable residents to maintain independence with least effort expended so they have more energy to impart to other activities. Another aspect that you need to consider when evaluating the movement is how the execution of the movement might be aggravating pain or co-morbidities. An example of this would be if the resident had osteoporosis and sat up through a sit-up manoeuvre. This action applies a strong flexing moment to the thoracic and lumbar spine that could potentiate a crush fracture and increased pain. In such a situation the physiotherapist might encourage rolling to the side and then moving to sitting from the side lying position. Provision of an aid might help the adoption of a safer practice. If the resident had a diagnosis of dementia the carer might need to remind the resident to move in the new sequence, so standby supervision and instruction might be added to the care plan. However, do not forget to identify the specific instructions you want given so all participants (resident and care staff) are informed appropriately.

Residents who need physical assistance to achieve this movement need to be identified and the physiotherapist must nominate how the assistance should be given. Examples might include hands-on stability support once the sitting position has been achieved to ensure safety when postural hypotension is a problem and the resident is likely to faint and fall to the floor. The movement can cause considerable vestibular stimulation and this too can cause sitting balance to be precarious until the effect has subsided, so the resident might need hands-on assistance to maintain stability once they have moved to sitting independently. In each of these situations residents should not be left alone until they report they have balance control or a fall will result. More assistance might be needed when a resident has difficulty controlling the lower limbs during the transfer. In this case the carer might need to shift the legs for the resident. Care must be taken to prevent skin trauma by not bumping or scraping the heels or legs on the bed or other furniture when moving. A hoist transfer is the chosen option if the resident is completely unable to perform the movement with help and sitting balance is poor or very unreliable, therefore requiring full assistance.

Sitting balance

There are many levels of sitting balance required for daily function. The physical problems that can interfere with balance include ataxia, paralysis, spasticity or rigidity, weakness, pain or a combination of these. Often the safety of balance in sitting is determined by the ability of the resident to divide their attention between balancing and balancing whilst doing a task. It is important to find out whether the resident can sit on the edge of the bed holding on in safety for at least 10 seconds. This time allows the carer to ensure a shower chair or wheelchair is positioned appropriately for the transfer. This might be the situation with an ataxic resident who is reasonably strong, stable and able to perform tasks and transfers as long as they can hold on. Other residents might demonstrate various levels of sitting balance and ability to perform quite complex tasks safely while sitting unsupported. Sitting balance should be assessed in other situations such as on the toilet, when dressing or being dressed. Perhaps for safety the resident should be dressed while lying on the bed if the large perturbations that occur during dressing are likely to cause the resident to fall over. Finishing dressing the top half and putting on shoes could be done in the wheelchair.

What effect does having the feet firmly supported on the floor have on maintenance of balance? Should there be a specific mention in the care plan about bed and chair height to allow foot support and safer independent or assisted activity. Many residents use the sitting position when conversing, eating, drinking and participating in recreation or entertainment activities. Therefore appropriate support needs to be provided to enable a safe, balanced upright position. This support comes from the backrest, armrests, the seat and the feet.

In other words you need to identify seating requirements from this sitting assessment so you can recommend which chair is suitable for the resident to use. Which type of chair a resident should use needs to be identified in the care plan. Further discussion of seating requirements is found in the chapters dealing with the immobile or barely mobile resident (Chapters 5, 6 and 7).

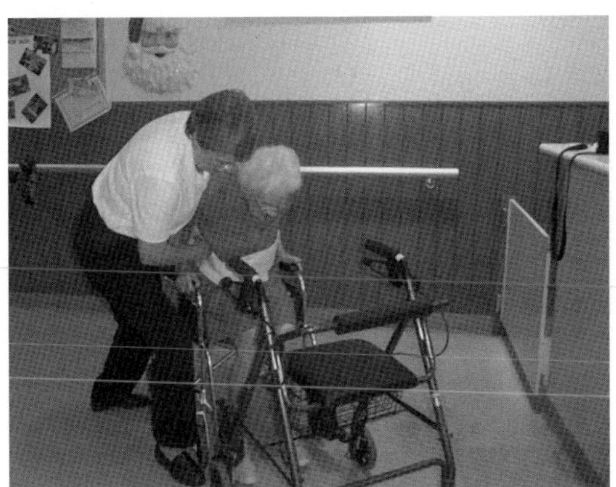

Figure 2.2 *Sit-to-stand transfer assistance using one person and a walk belt for stability.*

Seated transfer

If the resident is unable to take their weight through the legs and perform a standing transfer, their ability to perform a sliding transfer to a wheelchair independently or with assistance should be evaluated. Slide boards are commonly used to assist people to transfer to and from a wheelchair. If a resident has good upper limb function and some sitting balance this might be an option worth trying before settling for a hoisted transfer. If the resident can achieve this degree of ability the potential for outings and social integration are expanded.

Transferring from sitting to standing and standing to sitting

Can the resident do this independently with or without an aid? Do they need stand-by instruction to lean forwards and 'put nose over toes' to get up without physical help? Does the resident need some physical help from a carer using a walking belt? Is this help to ensure stability and safety due to the effect on blood pressure or vestibular stimulation from position change? Are one or two carers needed due to the resident's size or instability? Is the resident consistently reliable and not likely to collapse at the knees during the transfer? Can the resident control the sitting motion? Can they judge where the chair/bed is and safely sit? Does there appear to be a visual spatial disability, or is a difficulty with depth perception interfering with safe judgement? Would the resident benefit from some intervention to improve transfer ability? Figure 2.2 illustrates the use of a walking belt to assist a sit-to-stand transfer with a frail resident.

When maximal assistance is required to enable a standing transfer, a standing hoist might be employed as a safer option for staff and residents. The prerequisites for using a standing hoist are that the resident can take some weight-bearing through their lower limbs and the upper limb function is not restricted by shoulder pain and loss of range since the resident has to hold on to the standing hoist during the transfer.

Standing ability

Standing up is a tremendously valuable ability to maintain. In some instances the only way a resident can achieve this position is by pulling up on a wall bar (Fig. 2.3) or pushing up on some very secure piece of

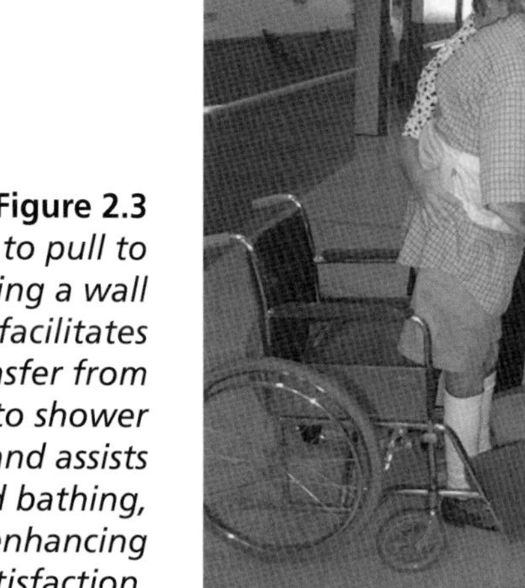

Figure 2.3 *Ability to pull to standing using a wall bar facilitates transfer from wheelchair to shower chair, and assists dressing and bathing, thereby enhancing life satisfaction.*

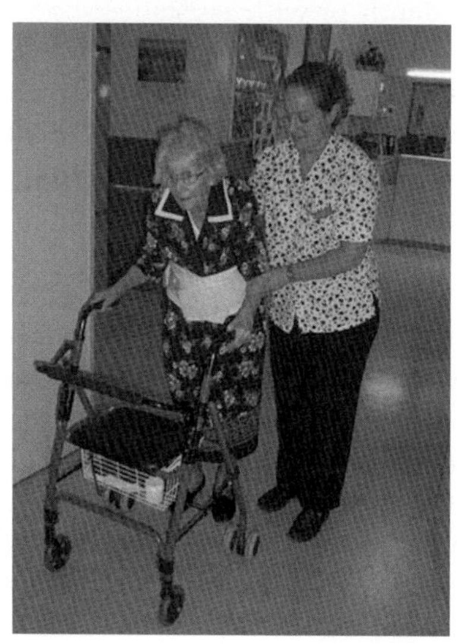

Figure 2.4 *Walking using a wheeled walker for support. Note the use of a walk belt for additional security.*

furniture. The assessment should investigate if the resident can do this and for how long. Carers need at least 10 seconds to dry the bottom or pull up the pants. These care tasks can be done on repeated stands. The participation by the resident during such activity provides major benefits that support the continuation of this activity for as long as possible.

It is important to determine the ability to stand unsupported and perform a simple task. An example of when this would be required is when walking using a pick-up walking frame (otherwise known as a hopper or Zimmer frame).

Gait assessment

The most important aspect of gait to evaluate is safety. If the resident uses a walking aid (Fig. 2.4), observe whether it is being used appropriately.

Are the rubber stoppers worn or safe, are the wheels jamming or running smoothly and are the brakes working and able to be applied easily? Ensure urgent maintenance is applied if the equipment is faulty as a fall could occur if you delay intervention.

Environmental distraction that divides the attention of the resident from the task of walking can cause a fall. Distractions can be people talking to the resident while they are trying to walk (Lundin-Olsson et al 1997, Nitz & Thompson 2003), people moving quickly through the visual field, environmental decor such as paintings, vases of flowers or notices. Brown et al (1999) have shown that decline in cognitive function prevents older people from maintaining safe balance when having to divide their attention between tasks. Many residents have some level of cognitive decline and so are at risk of falls when mobilizing. A simple method of testing falls potential is to see if the resident has to stop walking to talk. The conversation should involve some recall component as this appears to be more discriminatory for falls risk (Nitz & Thompson 2003).

The resident should be encouraged to wear supportive and protective shoes when walking. This practice will help prevent falls due to slipping and injury to the feet, and might help sensory input to enable better balance. Wearing shoes might rely on ability to put the shoes on easily. A long-handled shoe-horn is very useful for assisting the foot into the shoe and preventing the counter from becoming bent under the heel. Provision of a shoe-horn might prevent a fall or foot injury.

Wheelchair mobility

Residents using wheelchairs should be encouraged to maintain or gain independent mobility. The ability to propel a manual wheelchair in a straight line, turn corners and reverse should be assessed. The same manoeuvres should be evaluated for motorized wheelchair users. This is important for determining user safety as well as protecting other pedestrians. Efficient wheelchair users should be told to be careful when moving along corridors as walking residents could be at risk of falling if they move past them too quickly. On the other hand, residents who use wheelchairs for long distances might be encouraged to propel themselves so that they benefit from the fitness training this provides.

As with walking aids, the physiotherapist should check the resident's wheelchair for safety. Brakes, tyres, tip-up and removable footrests and removable armrests should be checked for function and any repairs or maintenance requirements attended to urgently. This maxim also applies for wheelchairs owned by the RACF that are used for resident transfers over long distances.

The cushion used on the wheelchair should be looked at to make sure it is positioned correctly and that extra covers such as plastic sheets are not being used as 'protection' from damage due to incontinence as this will negate the pressure-relieving function of the cushion. Care staff must be educated about the inadvisability of this habit.

Upper limb function

The physiotherapist should assess the functional ability of the upper limbs by noting whether the resident can hold a cup of water and drink without spillage, can do up and undo buttons or zips, hold a pen and write, turn the pages of a book as well as a magazine. Grip strength and endurance might be useful to test if the resident needs to pull up to standing and hold on firmly to maintain the standing position.

Shoulder range of movement needs to be evaluated for dressing and hygiene, especially in highly dependent residents. Any pain associated with arm movements must be noted and treatment implemented by the physiotherapist as well as due care being taken by carers during activities of daily living. Functional loss should also warrant treatment by the physiotherapist, as the potential to participate in care activities is highly reliant on retaining upper limb functional capacity.

Swallow safety

A number of conditions found in residents can contribute to swallowing problems that if not identified could cause aspiration pneumonia. Stroke, traumatic brain injury, Parkinson's disease, motor neuron disease, multiple sclerosis, muscular dystrophy, Huntington's chorea and Friedreich's ataxia are just a few such medical conditions. Admission notes might identify a swallowing problem but sometimes this is overlooked. In some medical conditions deterioration in motor function can lead to the development of swallowing problems. Care staff should be advised to report signs of dysphagia. When observing swallowing, the ease of swallow should be noted; also if a cough spontaneously follows the swallow of a drink, inefficiency in airway protection should be suspected. Similarly, if the voice sounds 'wet' after the swallow, there might be pharyngeal pooling of fluid that is then silently aspirated. If any of these presentations are apparent, it is wise to obtain a formal assessment from the speech pathologist and in the meantime recommend thickened fluids if swallow of more solid food boluses is effective.

Factors contributing to functional difficulties

Poor vision and hearing problems should be identified and how the carer should accommodate for them noted in the care plan.

Akinesia or 'freezing' can interfere with movement in the resident with Parkinson's disease. If medication is used well, this might not be a problem but the occasional occurrence should be pre-empted by providing strategies for the carer to follow close at hand, so that regular referral to the care plan reinforces how to intervene to protect the resident from a fall or injury.

Reduced attention-sharing ability must be noted and care staff warned not to talk to the residents while assisting walks between destinations in the building so as to reduce the risk of a fall.

Pain

Pain can interfere with all aspects of life by affecting mobility, sleep, rest and the enjoyment of entertainment or hobbies. It may be the only symptom that precipitates a fall by causing an arthritic knee to catch and give way during gait. Therefore pain in this instance becomes the primary problem that needs to be treated but in order to do so you need to assess the resident to determine the factors causing the pain. Avascular necrosis in the arthritic knee joint might have produced a small bone fragment that becomes a loose body in the joint. Loose bodies can jam between joint surfaces and cause acute pain, muscle inhibition and the fall potential. Similarly, if the patella is not tracking correctly due to arthritis affecting the joint, this too can cause painful catches that could lead to a fall. All pain from arthritic joints should be assessed and the appropriate treatment of the joint instigated. This treatment might include peripheral joint mobilizations, exercise and thermal or electrotherapeutic modalities. Interestingly, exercise and movement are the most beneficial interventions (Minor & Lane 1996).

Continence

Incontinence is a major physical disability that contributes considerably to the decision to place a person in an RACF. Consequently a very large proportion of new residents will have incontinence of urine and faeces. Management programmes for incontinence should be determined by examination of the medical and surgical history of the resident in conjunction with a thorough examination of the person. In some cases specific strategies can be put into place that will reduce the embarrassment and care needs of the individual and make them less reliant on a carer to remain dry. The physiotherapist should work with the nursing staff and the dietitian to develop the continence care plan. The reader is referred to Chapter 14 for more detailed discussion of continence.

Dementia

There are a number of types of dementia: Alzheimer's disease (AD), vascular dementia (VaD), dementia associated with Lewy bodies, Parkinson's disease dementia, AD plus vascular dementia and a miscellaneous group that might, for example, include adults ageing with the sequelae of traumatic brain injury or Down's syndrome (Fromage & Anglade 2002). To be classified as dementia, cognitive impairment needs to be such that it interferes with the person's ability to function independently in daily life. People with dementia present with impairment to memory, orientation, problem-solving ability, judgement, abstract thinking and the ability to perform complex physical activities such as personal hygiene independently. In addition the personality can change in ways that are evident in social behaviour (Jorm 1994). A person suffering mild dementia is still capable of functioning independently in the community although social interaction might be slightly impaired. People with moderate or severe dementia require care. Those with moderate dementia are unsafe to live independently as they can forget to turn off appliances and fire becomes a significant risk. In a hot climate forgetting to put food in the refrigerator can lead to food poisoning becoming a major health concern. There might also be a risk of poisoning from inappropriate medication use. People with severe dementia require constant supervision in order to maintain personal hygiene and function safely in the environment (Jorm 1994). Thus it is usually people with moderate to severe dementia that are admitted to RACFs because they are no longer safe to live in the community. However, examples of mild dementia are encountered where the person also has some degree of physical disability that interferes with independent living and has necessitated admission to the RACF.

When assessing the disability imposed by the dementia, three areas require attention: personal care ability, instrumental activities of daily living such as using money or the telephone, and behaviour. A large amount of information regarding these functional areas can be obtained from family and previous carers. However, there are times when this information is not available and the assessment will rely solely on current observations. The physiotherapist or occupational therapist undertakes the component of assessment relating to spatial perception, attention-dividing ability and mobility. The doctor or neuropsychologist best evaluates the cognitive components.

Recording assessment findings

Other things to note are the environmental requirements for the individual resident that enable them to function optimally. For example, the room of a person who is blind should be set up in the best configuration dictated by the physical and behavioural needs of that resident. Care and cleaning staff should understand that furniture items should not be shifted and obstacles not left in walkways so that the resident maintains safe independence. In other words, if you move something in the course of your duty you should immediately replace it in the position you found it. A photograph of the room layout might facilitate compliance with this very important need for the mobile blind resident.

Interpretation of assessment findings and the clinical reasoning process

Knowledge of the effects of ageing on all body systems in addition to an understanding of the pathological processes of medical conditions and the consequences of surgical procedures enables the physiotherapist to use the processes of clinical reasoning to guide assessment, problem identification, problem-solving, goal-setting and intervention. It enables the physiotherapist to adapt the process to the individual rather than requiring the individual resident to fit the process. Adaptability and flexibility during the assessment process, due to the skill in movement analysis and interpretation of the meaning of movement observations, enables the physiotherapist to bypass tests of basic functional skills when the ability to perform at a particular level has been indicated by observation during the initial interview phase. We are able to analyse how much assistance is required to achieve a particular functional level whether it be physical or from adaptation of the environment to allow independence. This thinking, reflective, deductive and decision-making process is the clinical reasoning process. It puts this skill into the context of the individual person by incorporating into the process the emotional, spiritual, behavioural and social components of life that particularly relate to that person. It also incorporates the individual person in the problem identification and decision-making processes, thereby encouraging self-efficacy and empowerment in the individual. In the case of people entering residential care, the process should include the family or previous carers as this enables them to retain worth in a process that might otherwise carry a feeling of failure. Such feelings of failure to continue to care for a family member can have a considerable effect on the health of these people. It can also affect the new resident who might have feelings of letting the carer down by not being able to help as much as was needed to enable them to stay at home. Therefore to incorporate family and carers in the admission process to the RACF and to value and use the input relating to their loved ones is vitally important.

Additional knowledge required to use the clinical reasoning process successfully includes a broad arsenal of intervention modalities, knowing when and how to use these interventions, how to evaluate the effect of the intervention and when it is appropriate to discontinue or change an intervention. Continual surveillance of the resident's status is needed in order to maximize the resident's function but also to enable early identification of change in ability before the person is put at risk of injury. It is often the untrained carer of the resident who is first to notice a decline in functional motor ability. They might say the resident is getting slower to walk from bed to shower or is more distracted during a task. These observations should trigger reassessment by the team as they could indicate physical or cognitive decline that might be amenable to a burst of physiotherapy or psychological intervention.

An important component of the process of assessment is the development of communication channels with the resident, their family and other staff members. This enables the interactive discussion of problems and care plan decisions. By discussing the assessment findings, the implications of these findings and the possible interventions that might address them with all participants, this education, negotiation and collaborative decision-making process helps all participants to maintain their worth and not feel excluded (Higgs & Jones 2000). Exclusion from decision-making is likely to cause feelings of dissatisfaction, dismissal and uselessness. In the case of the resident this can decrease motivation and increase depression.

Examples of cases are provided in Appendix 1 to enable the reader to appreciate more fully the clinical reasoning process through its application to real life situations.

Documentation and accountability

It is of paramount importance to keep accurate and timely reports of all assessment and treatment (Table 2.2). These notes will be the foundation of best practice and enable clinical reasoning such that the resident

Table 2.2 *Essentials of assessment and documentation*

Assessment should include:
Primary current diagnosis
Current medical conditions
Medical history
Surgical history
Medications
Social history/personal factors
Reason for admission
Resident's main goal/wish
Cognition
Hearing/vision
Communication
Pain
Swallowing
Global assessment
Physical:
- Compliance/cooperation
- Skin condition – pressure area risk
- Continence
- Respiratory/chest
- Tone
- Strength
- Range of motion
- Balance – sitting and standing
- Endurance

Chair prescribed
Mobility aid prescribed
All other aids used (wheelchair (manual or electric), mobility aids, hoists, slide sheets, bed poles, splints, compression stockings, orthopaedic devices, catheters, feeding devices/tubes, continuous oxygen, CPAP)
Mobility and dexterity assessment (functionally based)
Gait assessment
Falls risk assessment

Documentation should include:
Results of a thorough assessment as listed above plus:
Physiotherapy progress notes
Mobility/transfer plan (to instruct nursing staff on the method of choice)
Individualized exercise programme (usually conducted by the nursing staff daily)

receives the optimum care available. Ongoing progress notes will allow the therapist to review any changes and adjust the care plan accordingly. For example, on admission the priority for treatment with a given resident may be to provide assistance with active exercises targeting strength gain in the lower limbs and sit-to-stand practice. As the resident improves given the appropriate environment and treatment, the plan may change to target mobility and standing balance exercise. Ongoing assessment and adjustments enable a system which is sensitive to change and which ensures maximum gain with respect to a resident's mobility and dexterity, thereby contributing to independence and life satisfaction. It is just as important to note that changes may reflect the worsening status of a resident. A usual scenario would be the person who has had a sudden change of status leading to immobility such as a stroke or other neurological insult. The changes in this case may well lead to a new exercise care plan that incorporates passive exercise, massage and positioning where previously the aim was to maintain mobility or transfer ability.

In today's society of health care there is a great deal of interest in legal obligations with respect to documentation. Most practitioners are highly aware and concerned about ensuring they have covered themselves in respect of litigation. The accuracy and completeness of the resident assessment by the physiotherapist and the manner in which it is recorded in the individual's file is the professional responsibility of the physiotherapist. All resident files become a legal document that cannot be changed or added to retrospectively. Perhaps the most important details which need to be included in notes are as follows: time, date, resident's name, date of birth, assessment findings, treatment provided, reassessment, and plans. The notes should be signed, with surname printed and designation indicated, for example *JDBloggs* (BLOGGS) PT. Inclusions should be objective, indicate the source of the information, show goals of intervention, the intervention prescribed, any warnings or results of specific tests undertaken such as skin sensory testing prior to application of a hot pack or electrotherapeutic modality and the response to the treatment. Any adverse occurrence should also be recorded along with any action taken in response to such an occurrence.

Where possible, outcome measurements should be utilized to indicate the change in status of the resident. It is important, therefore, to have considered which clinical tests are available to monitor your plan. These tests should be valid, reliable and reproducible and therefore provide good objective measurement of how a resident is travelling with respect to the identified aims and goals of treatment. Some countries have specific recording tools that are required by law. In other places it is up to the individual facility and physiotherapist to choose an outcome measure that is most appropriate for the individual resident. Appendix 2 identifies some simple and complex assessment measurement tools, most have been scientifically validated; references to sources have been included where possible.

Perhaps the most important reason for good documentation in the mind of facility managers, accreditation bodies and government agencies will be to provide accurate levels of funding required to fulfil the directions prescribed. In Australia at least, the exercise programmes written and prescribed by the physiotherapist will often have to be implemented by nursing staff in the absence of physiotherapy supervision. In these situations exercise programmes need to be very clear and as simple to follow as possible. The key points which need to be included are as follows: resident name, date of birth, identified aims and goals, frequency of programme, staff assistance required, intensity, type of exercise, clear instructions as to given exercises (perhaps pictures), time or number of repetitions required, and signature. Often another major role of the physiotherapist working in RACFs will be to train staff in the supervision and implementation of exercises, both passive and active.

Summary

- The physiotherapist working in RACFs needs a broad range of assessment skills as residents' conditions and problems in this area are diverse.
- Functional assessments are very important as they relate to activities of daily life, useful goals and generate information relating to how much assistance a resident may require with daily tasks.
- The key factors requiring assessment were highlighted throughout this chapter along with the rationale for their inclusion within practice.
- We discussed the importance of good clinical reasoning and the interpretation of assessment findings within the context of the aged care setting.

References

Brown L A, Shumway-Cook A, Woollacott M H 1999 Attentional demands and postural recovery: the effects of aging. Journal of Gerontological Medical Sciences 54A(4):M165–171

Fromage B, Anglade P 2002 The ageing of Down's syndrome subjects. Encephale-Revue de Psychiatrie Clinique Biologique et Therapeutique 28(3):212–216

Higgs J, Jones M 2000 Clinical reasoning: an introduction. In: Higgs J, Jones M (eds) Clinical reasoning in the health professions, 2nd edn. Butterworth Heinemann, Oxford, p 3–14

Jorm A F 1994 Disability in dementia: assessment, prevention, and rehabilitation. Disability and Rehabilitation 16:98–109

Leipzig M, Cummings R, Tinetti M 1999 Drugs and falls in older people: a systematic review and meta-analysis: 1. Psychotropic drugs. Journal of the American Geriatrics Society 47:30–39

Lundin-Olsson L, Nyberg L, Gustafson Y 1997 'Stops walking when talking' as a predictor of falls in the elderly. Lancet 349:617

Minor M A, Lane N E 1996 Recreational exercise in arthritis. Musculoskeletal Medicine 22(3):563–577

Neutel C I, Hirdes J P, Maxwell C J, Patten S B 1996 New evidence on benzodiazepine use and falls: the time factor. Age and Ageing 25:273–278

Nitz J C, Thompson K 2003 'Stops walking to talk': A simple measure of predicting falls in the frail elderly. Australasian Journal on Ageing 22(2): 97–99

Tinetti M E, Speechley M, Ginter S F 1988 Risk factors for falls among elderly persons living in the community. New England Journal of Medicine 319:1701–1707

Waite L M, Broe G A, Grayson D A, Creasey H 2000 Motor function and disability in the dementias. International Journal of Geriatric Psychiatry 15:897–903

Weiner D K, Hanlon J T, Studenski S A 1998 Effects of central nervous system polypharmacy on falls liability in community-dwelling elderly. Gerontology 44:217–221

Yip Y B, Cumming R G 1994 The association between medications and falls in Australian nursing-home residents. Medical Journal of Australia 160:14–18

3 Resident injuries

Jennifer C. Nitz

This chapter aims to:

- identify mechanisms and consequences of injury
- identify precipitating factors for injury
- identify factors that interfere with recovery from injury
- describe interventions that might prevent injury
- discuss treatment suitable for injury management.

Introduction

One of the major problems in RACFs is the potential for the resident to sustain injury. Whilst in most instances injury is preventable, familiarity with factors that predispose a resident to injury or increase the likelihood of accidents is paramount for carers. This knowledge will enable preventive action that will enhance quality of life to be implemented. Physiotherapists have a major responsibility to ensure residents are protected from injury but are still able to function at their maximum level of ability. There also is a responsibility to care staff to protect them from injury and to enable confident participation in care procedures that facilitate maximum participation by the resident. In this way residents and carers maintain enthusiasm and quality of life.

Mechanisms of injury to residents

Every resident is at risk of injury at some stage during his or her stay in the RACF. For those residents who have retained some mobility a fall is highly likely to occur. The mobile resident is at additional risk from injuries such as bumps, shear stress, pressure, maceration and thermal mechanisms which are the common causes of injury seen with immobile residents. Increased morbidity and mortality is the consequence of any of these injuries. Table 3.1 lists mechanisms and consequences of injury.

Falls

The definition of a fall is when a person unintentionally comes to rest on the floor or at a lower level than before (i.e. not when this occurs due to a major intrinsic event such as a stroke or a faint or an overwhelming

Table 3.1
Injury mechanism and consequence

Mechanism	Consequence or source of injury
Falls	Major cause of fractured neck of femur Head injury Pelvic fractures Lacerations Loss of confidence and transition to immobility Increased morbidity and mortality
Bumps	Shins by wheelchair foot plates during standing transfers Elbows and forearms during transportation in wheelchairs Any body part during hoisted transfers Can cause lacerations that potentially might become infected and become life-threatening
Shear forces	Chair seats and backrests that offer little support and encourage sliding to gain comfort Toilet seats Poorly applied slings for hoist transfers Potentially allowing infection and life-threatening septicaemia
Unrelieved pressure	Wrinkles in socks inside tight shoes Wrinkles in bed clothes the resident is lying on Unprotected feet on wheelchair footrests Elbows on inside of chair armrests Occiput and ears are at risk, especially where the leg of spectacles are pressed against the head or ear due to the inability of the resident to lift their head All can produce pressure areas (decubitus ulcers) that can become life-threatening
Thermal injury	Shower and bath water burns Spills of tea or coffee Hot pack or ice pack treatment Electrotherapy modalities, e.g. ultraviolet light, infrared, ultrasound, electrical burns from short wave diathermy Potentially life-threatening if infected

environmental hazard) (Tinetti et al 1988). In the community, around 30% of people over the age of 65 will fall in any one year (Lord et al 1993).

Forty per cent of RACF residents enter because they have become unsafe to remain living in the community due to having sustained a fall (Tinetti et al 1988) or have developed a medical condition that predisposes them to falling. Such an admission often presumes that the person has entered a safe environment where supervision is available and therefore the possibility of falling is reduced. Unfortunately this is not the case as many extra factors that predispose a person to a fall immediately enter the equation and increase the potential for a fall. More than 50% of nursing home residents will fall each year (Runge et al 2000).

Falls can be due to factors intrinsic to the person such as postural instability, weakness, a neurological condition, cardiovascular instability, cognitive status, number of medications ingested, sensory decline or more commonly multifactorial in presentation (Ashburn et al 2000, Tinetti et al 1988). Extrinsic factors contributing to falls can be caused by environmental hazards such as poor lighting, uneven, wet or icy surfaces, traffic or moving walkways or escalators. The environmental hazards can be in the home or in the community and generally affect the person in a manner that relates to their level of activities of daily living (Nevitt et al 1989). Therefore if a person is able to go to the shopping centre independently then they are at greater risk of a community fall than those people who are unable to venture out. All people who have any of the intrinsic factors that can precipitate a fall and are homebound are more at risk of falling when moving around the house, especially if there is clutter, scatter rugs, stairs and poor lighting (Tinetti et al 1988). Many residents in low care facilities still retain community mobility and look after personal requirements for activities of daily living, and therefore are subject to the same risks as those people still living at home. Table 3.2 provides a list of intrinsic factors associated with increased risk of a fall. Differentiation between syncopal and non-syncopal causes of falls is necessary (Nevitt et al 1989, Runge et al 2000) because of the need for a different approach to prevention for these residents.

The relationship between musculoskeletal problems and falls

Arthritic conditions affecting lower limb joints and the associated pain, muscle weakness and lack of joint range of movement reduce the efficiency of balance and gait to such an extent that they have been implicated as a major predictor of falls (Nevitt et al 1989). Often lower limb arthritis is the main contributing factor to the inability to rise from a chair without using the armrests with or without physical assistance. Difficulty associated with chair rising has been shown to predict fallers in the community (Nevitt et al 1989, Tinetti et al 1988), so extrapolation to the RACF situation is not unreasonable since most residents will be more frail than community dwellers. In fact, falls are very commonly associated with residents who are no longer independently mobile and who try to get up and walk by themselves. This is often a dilemma for carers when deciding how to prevent falls from occurring whilst endeavouring to maintain mobility and resident autonomy.

Pain from musculoskeletal origins such as arthritis, polymyalgia rheumatica, fibrositis or osteoporosis has a potent muscle inhibition action that has the potential to precipitate a fall. Physiotherapeutic interventions can alleviate some if not all of the problems that contribute to the pain found in the arthritic and soft tissue conditions nominated and should be instigated, with due regard to concomitant pathologies, in all

Table 3.2 *Intrinsic factors associated with increased risk of a fall*

Category	Factors
Musculoskeletal	Arthritis Postural abnormalities (kyphosis, scoliosis) Polymyalgia rheumatica Cervical spondylosis Foot disorders Lower limb amputation Weakness
Special sense decline	Cataract Macular degeneration Depth perception difficulties Blindness Hearing loss
Neurological disease	Stroke Parkinson's disease Multiple sclerosis Peripheral neuropathy Autonomic dysfunction Menière's disease Vestibular disorders Dizziness Seizures
Nutritional and endocrine disorders	Dehydration Malnutrition Anaemia Vitamin B_1 and B_{12} deficiency Alcohol abuse Diabetes mellitus Hypothyroid or hyperthyroid disorder
Cognition	Multi-infarct dementia Alzheimer's disease Depression Delirium
Cardiovascular disease	Arrhythmias Ischaemic heart disease Peripheral arterial disease Postural hypotension Vertebrobasilar insufficiency
Medication	Antihypertensives Diuretics Cardiac medication Antipsychotics Tranquillizers Sedatives Anti-Parkinsonian Baclofen Narcotic analgesics

	NSAIDs Diabetic medication Anticonvulsants
Acute illness and other	Urinary tract infection Respiratory infection Incontinence Obesity Activity level Walking aid use Pain History of at least one fall

residents so that falls from these causes can be reduced. Chapter 15 provides information regarding management options for pain control and the reader is encouraged to access this information.

Postural deviations are common in the elderly, especially where osteoporosis has contributed to vertebral crush fractures. A kyphosis from this cause can drastically change the orientation of the centre of mass of the body in relation to the feet, thus leading to postural instability and difficulty in correcting postural perturbations. With the inevitable pull of gravity these kyphotic deformities progress further and put the resident at greater risk of losing balance. Ideally intervention would realign posture. However, in these cases this solution is not appropriate and adaptive methods need to be chosen. Back-strengthening exercises might help but an appropriate walking aid that provides effective support without encouraging further forward flexion is indicated.

Muscle weakness has been identified as a major contributor to a fall (Runge et al 2000, Tinetti et al 1988). It rarely occurs independently of neurological, arthritic or nutritional causes but can be present due to disuse. Examples of acquired weakness in the absence of pathology that would directly affect muscle are seen commonly in the person who through fear of falling has restricted movement to the extreme (Vellas et al 1997) or in the frail elderly person after an acute illness. Lower limb muscle weakness is implicated in the decline in function that leads to a fall. Research findings generally identify the quadriceps, dorsiflexors, plantarflexors and hip extensor muscles (Hauer et al 2002, Nevitt et al 1989). These findings coincide with anteroposterior instability and falls in these directions. More recently it has been shown that owing to mediolateral stability requirements for efficient gait and balance, weakness in the hip abductors and adductors also plays an important role in fall potential (Low Choy 2002). Trunk and upper limb weakness plays a major role in stability and gait performance when a walking aid is utilized, so a frail, generally weak resident is likely to be at risk of sustaining a fall. However, it can be argued that limitations in research protocols have only identified those muscles assessed in the elderly fallers for weakness and it is most likely that all muscles are weak and could benefit from general strengthening programmes that aim to improve functional mobility.

Foot problems that include rigidity of joints, deformities such as hallux valgus, hammer toes and dropped arches, calluses and corns as well as muscle weakness and sensory loss are prevalent in the elderly (Menz & Lord 2001a, 2001b). Tinetti et al (1988) identified foot problems as an independent risk factor for falls. Rarely are these foot problems considered in balance evaluations but they are often the reason for elders wearing inappropriate shoes or walking in socks. The safety issues accompanying these habits are many and all can contribute to a fall. Physiotherapists can contribute to the management of foot problems by improving foot joint mobility and increasing muscle strength, thereby allowing better accommodation to uneven surfaces and balance reactions that accompany foot–ground contact. Close liaison with a podiatrist is also warranted.

Decline in the special senses and falls

This topic has been covered in the chapter dealing with ageing (Chapter 1). Rarely will the problems associated with the decline in vision and hearing be present without some other risk factors due to pathology. The important implication for controlling risk associated with vision and hearing deficits is to ensure where possible that the resident is using spectacles and hearing aids effectively. The physiotherapist should also assess whether depth perception and other visual perceptual problems exist and ensure that care staff are aware of methods of overcoming these problems. When supervision or assistance is required for safety in transfers or walking, the carer can help the resident with judging how far away a chair is before sitting down or that the shadow on the floor or a change in floor colour is not a step up or down. These are common occurrences that are misinterpreted by the elderly resident and potential contributors to a fall. Environmental fall risk factors due to visual perceptual dysfunction are rarely identified in the literature but play a frequent role in falls in the elderly.

Neurological disease and falls

Neurological disorders (Tinetti et al 1988), specifically Parkinson's disease (Ashburn et al 2000, Nevitt et al 1989), have been identified as increasing the risk of a fall in the elderly. Seizures, dizziness and vertigo in addition to syncope and drop attacks have been identified as responsible for around 5% of falls (Runge et al 2000). Physiotherapists can assess whether there are aspects of balance dysfunction that present in residents with any of these neurological conditions. Intervention programmes that have been shown to be effective in improving balance and function (Low Choy et al 2003, Nitz & Low Choy 2004) should be instigated so that these residents can improve their quality of life through fall reduction and enhanced self-efficacy. Information concerning exercise prescription and ideas for appropriate exercises which may be helpful in designing a programme to suit individual residents can be found in Chapters 10 and 11.

Autonomic dysfunction plays an important role in increasing the risk of a fall due to orthostatic hypotension. Orthostatic or postural hypotension is a major cause of syncopal falls and is found in residents with diabetes, peripheral vascular disease, heart failure, Parkinson's disease, stroke and dementia to name a few. We generally think of postural hypotension causing syncope when moving quickly from sitting to standing, a situation that can be aggravated on a hot day or when slightly dehydrated. The drop in blood pressure can occur in elderly residents when standing up or even when hoisted from a lying position and sat upright in a chair. To prevent this occurrence position changes of the resident should be done slowly whilst continually monitoring for effect. A postural drop in systolic blood pressure of 20 mmHg or more is pathological. Consultation with the doctor managing the resident will assist with determining whether the drop in blood pressure is due to over-medication with antihypertensives or to reduced cardiac output. Either finding will respond to medication change and possibly reduce the likelihood of a fall.

Cognitive impairment and falls

Dementia has been singled out as a high risk factor for a fall (Nevitt et al 1989, Pomeroy 1993, Shaw & Kenny 1998, Tinetti et al 1988). Often residents with dementia will present with multiple pathologies such as cerebral infarcts and cardiac arrhythmias that will contribute to falls risk. Psychotropic drugs and drugs from other classes known to increase falls risk are commonly prescribed for residents with dementia (Thapa et al 1995), thereby increasing the potential to fall. Therefore in order to reduce the risk of a fall in residents with dementia a multidimensional approach to a falls risk assessment is needed. This should investigate medication administration for drug interactions and whether medications with greater likelihood of precipitating a fall can be replaced by ones less likely to do so. Nutrition and hydration need to be controlled so as to ensure they play no role in causing a fall. The physiotherapist and possibly a neuropsychologist will also assess the balance and attention ability of the resident. Inability to divide the attention between tasks has been shown to reduce balance ability and precipitate a fall (Brown et al 1999). Lundin-Olsson et al (1997) identified a simple assessment of this for residents with dementia: if they are unable to continue walking when talking, they are at risk of a fall.

Delirium is an acute confusional state common among elderly people residing in RACFs. The delirious resident must be differentiated from the resident with dementia as delirium is often the result of a treatable condition. Residents with delirium will present with reduced ability to concentrate, sustain focus or be diverted from an activity (perseverance). Often they have a poor awareness of the surrounding environment and their level of consciousness may be changed (Samuels & Evers 2002). The resident might become hypoactive or hyperactive in his or her delirium and depending on behaviour might be labelled quite erroneously as having a good or bad day. Delirium is often found in the frail elderly with numerous co-morbidities but can also present in the relatively healthy elderly. The most common causes for this acute confusion are polypharmacy especially when new drugs have been added within the previous few weeks, electrolyte abnormalities, dehydration, hypoxia, acute infection, acquired brain injury, myocardial complications, urinary retention and faecal impaction (Samuels & Evers 2002). Physical restraints have also been identified as contributing to delirium. Delirium can be present in a demented resident due to any of the causes already identified. Any sudden change in behaviour should be regarded as suspicious. The astute carer will recognize delirious behaviour and seek the cause. However, the physiotherapist is often the person to notice the relationship between the signs of heart failure, hypoxia or pneumonia and decline in cognitive behaviour in a resident and to instigate closer investigation by the doctor. Most of the causes of delirium can be reversed through appropriate medical intervention. It is the recognition of the cause and effect that enables this action and the ultimate prevention of a fatal outcome (Samuels & Evers 2002).

Depression can occasionally be confused with the hypoactive presentation of delirium. However, depressive signs in residents who have not been clinically diagnosed with depression should have an identifiable cause. Fluctuations in concentration and attention levels, symptoms of delirium, are not found in the depressed resident (Samuels & Evers 2002).

Cardiovascular disorders and falls

Syncopal episodes culminating in a fall are commonly related to cardiac arrhythmias, myocardial infarction, vasovagal attacks, aortic stenosis and vertebrobasilar insufficiency (VBI). Any or all of these pathological problems can be encountered in residents, so should be identified as possible risk factors and appropriate measures taken to reduce the contribution they can make to the resident sustaining a fall. This management might take the form of altering medication while closely monitoring responses.

It is important to educate residents and carers regarding the risks associated with sustained extended neck postures to eliminate contribution to injury from circulatory factors such as vertebrobasilar insufficiency. Also of note is the risk associated with the performance of a Valsalva manoeuvre during tasks requiring concentration or effort. Older persons with hypertension who use this breath-holding technique risk a dangerous elevation in blood pressure. It is relatively common for people with chronic lung disease to be in the habit of holding their breath during functional tasks such as stair climbing or dressing. The physiotherapist should monitor how residents perform difficult tasks and be vigilant with regard to this phenomenon in addition to analysing the movement during task performance. Older men with an enlarged prostate tend to hold their breath during micturition to assist bladder emptying. This might lead to a syncopal episode and a fall, so individuals should be made aware of this possibility and appropriate action taken to reduce the fall risk.

Hypotension is also common in residents who have a long history of hypertension and heart disease (Busby et al 1994). These residents are generally frail and in poor health. They are at greater risk of syncope with positional change. Also they will be more at risk of falls in hot weather and if they become dehydrated.

Medications and falls

Non-compliance or inability to comply with dosage requirements as might occur with a community-dwelling elder should not be a problem for residents as care staff usually take responsibility for timely provision of the prescribed dose to each resident. This allows better control of medication and should reduce the possibility of drug interactions from prescribed and off-the-shelf medications. On admission to an RACF, each resident should have a review of current medication by the doctor to limit the potential for drug interactions and overdose.

Drug interactions and the slowed metabolism and clearance that leads to high serum drug levels are major contributors to falls related to medication. Confusion and hypotension are two most likely consequences arising from medication ingestion that will result in a fall. Drug groups that need to be carefully monitored because of these effects are identified in Table 3.3.

Table 3.3 *Drugs commonly responsible for confusion or hypotension*

Confusion	Tricyclic antidepressants: imipramine (Tofranil) doxepin (Sinequan) amitriptyline (Tryptanol) nortiptyline (Allegron) Phenothiazines: chlorpromazine (Largactil) thioridazine (Melleril) prochlorperazine (Stemetil) Barbiturates: phenobarbital Narcotic analgesics Anticonvulsants
Hypotension	Anti-Parkinsonian: L-dopa Diuretics and other antihypertensives Phenothiazines Tricyclic antidepressants Benzodiazepines Antispasmodics: baclofen Narcotic analgesics: codeine MS contin

Nutritional and endocrine disorders and falls

Dehydration is a major problem for residents who live in warm climates. The confusion and hypotension associated with dehydration are the main reasons these people fall. Many aspects of the physiotherapist's practice in RACFs such as management of continence problems, fitness education and raising carer and resident awareness of the dangers of dehydration will work to reduce the prevalence of the problem.

Malnutrition with the consequent anaemia, protein, mineral and vitamin deficiencies will result in musculoskeletal and neurological dysfunction. Muscle weakness and slowed reaction time are the most obvious functional deficits from malnutrition. The contribution these deficits make to falls is obvious. However, what is not as obvious is the need to address nutritional deficiencies as well as introducing an exercise programme that is designed to improve balance, muscle strength and reaction time and prevent a fall.

Diabetes mellitus can contribute to a fall in various ways. Hypoglycaemic attacks (low blood sugar) can lead to drowsiness, incoordination and a fall. Long-term diabetes can lead to neurological damage of somatosensory and autonomic nerves, thereby affecting balance reactions and controlling postural hypotension, both of which can contribute to a fall. Vision is also commonly affected in the end stages of diabetes and this deficiency can also increase the risk of a fall.

Only about 5% of falls cause a bone fracture. More commonly the skin is lacerated or bruised. In young people who are healthy, injuries that break the skin undergo a healing process that is determined by the depth and size of the break. Normal wound healing depends on adequate arterial, venous and lymphatic circulation to provide nutrients to rebuild tissue and to clear metabolites from the area. Most elderly residents have deficits in the circulation that inhibit fast wound healing and in some cases precipitate chronic wounds that will never heal. In fact it has been suggested that close to 90% of nursing home residents will have some element of undiagnosed arterial obstructive disease (Paris et al 1988).

Ulcers and chronic wounds

Bumps, lacerations, shear forces, unrelieved pressure and thermal injuries can precipitate chronic wounds. Thus trauma is the initiating factor in these cases and is potentially preventable. Spontaneous skin breakdown can occur where the circulation is compromised by arterial or venous disease. *The differentiation between ulcers originating from arterial, venous or pressure causes is vital as this aspect determines the management* (Thomas 2001a). The causative pathology cannot be assumed by site of occurrence, as more than one pathology can contribute to the ulcer and not all treatment modalities are compatible with all pathological diagnoses (Thomas 2001a). This section will identify the differences in cause and the implications for management.

Ulcers of vascular origin

Ulcers are often encountered in people residing in aged care facilities. There are three main types of ulcer, pressure, arterial and venous, named for the different origins. Tissue and vascular changes associated with ageing put elderly and chronically ill people more at risk of developing all three types of ulcer. Other factors that increase the risk of ulcer development include nutritional deficiencies, paralysis, suppressed immunity, immobility, dementia, joint contractures and multiple co-morbidities causing functional dependency.

In order to understand how to prevent and treat each type of ulcer, it is necessary to explore how the age changes in skin and the blood vessels can precipitate ulceration.

There are two main causes of ulcer formation. Firstly, failure of the cardiac or venous pump is responsible for arterial or venous ulcers. Occlusion of an end artery is also a factor in arterial ulceration. Pressure, which inhibits circulation locally to the tissues under the area of pressure, ultimately leads to necrosis and ulceration.

Arterial ulceration

Peripheral vascular disease (PVD) or occlusive arterial disease (OAD) is the most common pathology that has the potential to cause arterial ulceration. Depending on the primary pathology large or smaller arteries are affected. Arteriosclerosis commonly resulting from hypercholesterolaemia (Khan et al 1999) mainly affects arteries of large lumen although it can also cause atheromatous plaques to stenose and/or occlude smaller diameter vessels. Diabetes mellitus generally is responsible for stenosis or occlusion of smaller diameter arteries. Renal disease is often a precursor of OAD. OAD leads to a chronic ischaemic state in the tissues supplied by a diseased artery. This puts these tissues at greater risk in the event of injury, where healing is compromised due to impaired arterial circulation, and chronic ulceration eventuates.

Pathologies that can present with arterial inflammatory states that have the potential to cause occlusion and necrosis of the tissues normally supplied by the artery include rheumatoid arthritis and systemic lupus erythematosus (SLE). The endarteritis seen in these conditions often only affects the nail beds but might on occasion affect any medium to small peripheral artery in any part of the body such as in the upper or lower limbs or gut. Deprived of its blood supply the tissue necroses and is seen as small black patches on the skin that generally progresses to an ulcer. Healing of ulcers of arterial origin is almost impossible without arterial reconstructive surgery. Often infection, presenting as cellulitis, complicates the condition and this includes local soft tissue; in some cases osteomyelitis is present. Pain is a major accompaniment to arterial ulcers and can be extreme since it is due to varying causes including ischaemia, inflammation and pressure from oedema. The management of pain from arterial ulcers is vital for the comfort of the resident. Very strong pain relief is generally required and needs to be constant not 'as required'. Referral to the chapter in this text that considers pain (Chapter 15) will assist in choosing appropriate physiotherapeutic modalities to treat pain from vascular origin.

Most elderly people who need to be admitted to an RACF have some degree of arterial insufficiency and residents who have had lower limb amputations as a result of OAD are often present. A study by Paris et al (1988) supports this statement; they found that 88% of residents had OAD but only 5% had been previously diagnosed with OAD. They concluded that elderly residents were at high risk of morbidity related to OAD. The presenting signs and symptoms of OAD should be easily identified by care staff and appropriate risk management measures adopted. In OAD the peripheral pulses are absent or weak, and the skin is shiny, hairless and tissue-paper thin. Evidence of the extent of OAD will be demonstrated on elevation as the limb will blanch quickly and on hanging dependent it will become engorged and purplish-red. In addition to the skin changes, there is muscle weakness, sensory loss and loss of thermoregulation in the region supplied by a diseased artery. The peripheral neuropathy is not always clinically obvious in the early stages of ischaemia but nerve conduction studies have indicated it is an early manifestation in conditions such as diabetes mellitus (de Wytt et al 1999). Thus the usual protective responses for noxious stimuli such as heat or pressure are absent or diminished (Table 3.4). Therefore substantial tissue trauma will occur before the person becomes aware of a problem. Resting pain or claudication is a warning sign of severe OAD. Acute arterial occlusion is also possible due to thrombosis or embolism. The signs are excruciating pain, pallor, muscle paralysis, paraesthesia and extremely cold skin distal to the site of occlusion. This is a situation that should be identified and managed immediately, otherwise irreparable damage will have occurred and limb amputation is the only option to remove the pain and life-threatening toxicity. Occasionally the decision is made to 'just keep the resident comfortable' in this situation. Usually a decision such as this is made because of the imminence of death from other causes. Large doses of analgesia are then required to control pain to keep the resident comfortable. Unnecessary moving of the resident out of a comfortable position is not recommended as at this stage prevention of complications from immobility is not the primary goal. Comfort is paramount in the last hours or days for this resident.

Injury prevention and risk identification

Prevention of injury should be the primary goal in the management of residents with OAD or connective tissue diseases. Attention should be paid to protecting the feet and shins from injury and this should involve the removal of potential risk factors from the resident's environment. Figure 3.1 shows the clinical signs of skin fragility in an older adult and the use of a sheepskin to protect the skin from injury.

It must be remembered that usual first aid treatments for simple injuries can be contraindicated and if applied to people with OAD can cause irreversible tissue damage.

A swollen foot or hand should never be elevated above the heart level in a person with OAD to try and reduce swelling. This only leads to less arterial perfusion of the tissues that will complicate the cause of the swelling. Clinical reasoning principles must be applied to understand why elevation is contraindicated even though it is the usual treatment choice for the presenting condition. Peripheral oedema in the elderly can be due to many aetiologies. Simple assessment principles can indicate the

Table 3.4
Key points relating to occlusive arterial disease (OAD)

Signs and symptoms of arterial insufficiency	Clinical presentation	Implications for management
Absent or diminished peripheral pulses	Dorsalis pedis and posterior tibial arteries in the foot and popliteal and femoral arteries proximally in the leg	Decreased healing potential of accidental injury, need to control environmental risk factors
Skin changes	Tissue paper thin, shiny, hairless, necrotic patches, e.g. nail bed necrosis	Easily traumatized by minimal pressure or shear contact. Spontaneous ulceration of necrotic patches
Autonomic dysfunction	Thermoregulation loss, loss of sweating Baroreceptor insensitivity leads to poor arterial adaptation to postural change causing blood pressure to drop	Susceptible to burn injury in bathing. Ice and heat treatments contraindicated Hypothermia or hyperthermia is common in cold or hot weather Postural hypotension leading to falls
Sensory neuropathy	Diminished light touch; pressure, pain, hot and cold sensation loss; decreased vibration sense and proprioceptive loss	Increased risk of injury from loss of protective reactions Balance loss and incoordination of movement, gait problems
Motor neuropathy	Absent or diminished tendon reflexes, muscle weakness, slowed reaction time	Balance loss and inefficient balance reactions, increased risk of falls, difficulty with gait and activities of daily living

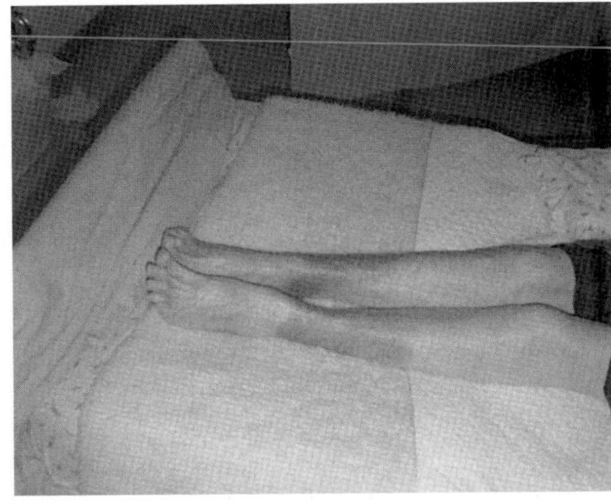

Figure 3.1
Skin fragility and the use of sheepskins for protection against injury.

most likely cause and so point to the most appropriate management choice. It should be determined if the oedema is present in one or both limbs. If oedema is present only in one limb (arm or leg) the most common precipitants include deep vein thrombosis, lymphoedema, cellulitis, muscle paralysis leading to loss of the muscle pump and circulatory stasis, complex regional pain syndrome or injury such as ankle sprain. Knowledge of the resident's medical and past surgical history will allow elimination of some options as well as identification of the likely cause. For example, a history of mastectomy might account for a swollen arm and further examination will often confirm the presence of lymphoedema. In this case elevation is one management option. On the other hand, palpation and observation of the limb might reveal heat and erythema, which are signs of cellulitis where antibiotic therapy is indicated.

If oedema is present bilaterally, the cause is more likely to be failure of the cardiac or peripheral pump. It can also be a complication of some medications such as non-steroidal anti-inflammatory drugs. In any case consultation with the resident's doctor should be made to confirm diagnosis and to allow appropriate treatment to commence.

Never treat a swollen joint or soft tissue injury such as a bruise or sprain with ice or heat when OAD is present. The circulatory response needed to cope with the temperature changes is inefficient and tissue damage will occur. Be particularly careful with residents who have rheumatoid arthritis or SLE as arteritis can be present and will contraindicate the use of many thermal modalities when treating painful swollen joints. Another precaution should be considered when prescribing exercise for residents with OAD. Muscle contraction during exercise or any movement compresses the arteries adjacent or contained within the muscle compartment. Complete closure of the arterial bed and interruption of blood flow ensues (Coffman 1988). This compromises the supply of nutrients to the muscles during contraction. In a situation of isometric contraction that is maintained for any length of time, this ischaemic state can aggravate tissue ischaemia already present owing to the reduced circulation due to the OAD. Claudication pain indicates there is significant arterial insufficiency, with retention of metabolites and tissue irritation and damage occurring. Therefore the duration of muscle contraction and the closer to maximum voluntary contraction demand will be factors that can increase tissue damage in OAD and must be considered when decisions on exercise programmes are made. Low or no resistance is recommended, and practice of functional tasks such as walking or moving from sitting to standing in the barely mobile resident are appropriate exercise choices. Exercise training of this nature has been shown to facilitate collateral circulation and inhibit progression of atherosclerotic disease, changes in blood rheology and metabolic adaptations to ischaemia (Remijnse-Tamerius et al 1999). If weights are utilized in an exercise programme great care should be taken when attaching them to the limbs, especially round the shin area where skin damage is likely. You should always weigh up the consequences of skin trauma in the presence of OAD against the possible strength gains with weight training, particularly as in reality the gains might be greater if functional tasks were practised instead.

Stretches to maintain soft tissue length are commonly included in resident treatment programmes. Certainly, contracture prevention is desirable to assist hygiene needs but static stretches are not an appropriate method to maintain length in residents with OAD. Consider the situation of tight calf muscles. This muscle group commonly becomes shortened in barely mobile residents due to the relaxed plantarflexed positions adopted for most of the day when the resident is either lying on the bed or sitting in an easy chair with feet raised on a support. If sustained dorsiflexion is prescribed to lengthen the calf, the circulation to calf muscles can be severely compromised due to the compression of the arteries in the posterior compartment by the less inextensible fascia being stretched during the manoeuvre, which in turn compresses the muscles and vessels. Soft tissue length can be maintained or gained by passive, assisted active or active, reciprocal movements to the limits of range. This can be attained by positioning the feet on the floor when the resident sits out in a chair for meals or for periods during the day. Active movement is achieved when the resident is assisted from sitting to standing and during a walk. Utilizing these methods enhances the likelihood of increased tissue length due to stimulation of the muscle pump to improve circulation, thereby enhancing muscle mutability and resulting in greater length. The added benefits of using this approach to prevent contractures are that the resident maintains the ability to stand even if unable to mobilize. This makes life easier for carers and less stressful for the resident.

The most appropriate treatment to improve arterial circulation is gentle exercise. Gentle exercise that is reciprocal in motion stimulates collateral circulation and enhances tissue nutrition. Walking is a very easy way of achieving this goal. However, many residents are unsafe to walk alone or are unable to walk. In these situations assisted mobility is desirable for the unsafe resident and time should be set aside by the staff to provide this treatment. Similarly, treatment time should be provided for immobile residents when they are assisted with reciprocal movements that are prescribed by the physiotherapist to assist circulation.

Venous ulcers

Two of the main causes of venous hypertension are failure of the cardiac and/or muscle pump that in turn might precede a venous ulcer. In the normal upright position the venous pressure in the lower limbs is about 2 mmHg (Cavorsi 2000). This is insufficient to move the blood against gravity and back to the heart. Successful venous return to the heart is assisted by the strong leg muscle pump and the valves in the large lower limb veins that prevent back flow. In people who have lower limb muscle paralysis this muscle pump is lost and peripheral oedema with venous and lymphatic engorgement ensues. A similar situation occurs in unaffected people who sit with their legs dependent for extended periods of time without any movement.

Neuropathic ulcers

Diabetes mellitus is a common cause of peripheral neuropathy (de Wytt et al 1999). Therefore residents with insulin- or non-insulin-dependent diabetes are at risk of ulcer formation due to neuropathy and arterial insufficiency so should be specially singled out for preventive management whether ambulant or immobile. There are many other conditions that lead to peripheral sensory loss encountered in residents. These conditions include stroke, multiple sclerosis, rheumatoid arthritis, systemic lupus erythematosus, alcoholic neuropathy, metabolic neuropathies, traumatic brain injury and spinal cord injury. Many residents will present with multiple co-morbidities that make them more likely to suffer injury from any source.

Sensory, motor and autonomic dysfunction is present in neuropathic conditions and all elements must be considered during risk assessment and preventive and intervention treatments. Muscle weakness or paralysis will contribute to the potential to develop ulcers due to the loss of the muscle pump in the lower limbs. This leads to venous pooling and changed arterial response to thermal and postural change. Neuropathic ulcers are most common on the soles of the feet or other aspects of the foot subjected to pressure from the ground or shoes during gait. Pressure and shear forces cause the tissue damage that goes undetected owing to lack of sensation. Thus the precipitating cause of injury is not removed and a chronic wound develops. Prevention and management approaches for neuropathic ulcers are similar to those for decubitus ulcers and are covered in the following section.

Pressure or decubitus ulcers and pressure areas

The incidence of pressure ulcers occurring in people living in residential care facilities is recognized as being around 25% of residents (Bergstrom et al 1995). Pressure ulcers are associated with pain, suffering and decreased quality of life and because pressure areas are more common in the frail elderly, their contribution to premature death in these residents is often underrated (Tsokos et al 2000). The physiotherapist should be aware of all factors that might predispose a resident to pressure ulcer formation as we are involved in the education of carers in RACFs and this role should include pressure area prevention.

Pressure areas develop due to the inability of the body to overcome the effect of pressure load on tissue and thereby maintain circulation to the area (Bergstrom et al 1995, Brienza et al 2001). Shear stresses on cutaneous tissue also play a part in tissue breakdown (Bergstrom et al 1995, Sprigle 2000). Repetition of shear stress and time of loading increase the possibility of tissue damage (Sprigle 2000). The body parts most susceptible to pressure are the bony prominences and other poorly vascularized tissues such as the heels of the feet and ears (Edsberg et al 2001).

Table 3.5 *Pressure ulcer severity scale*

Stage	Descriptive criteria
1	Non-blanchable erythema
2	Break in skin integrity such as blistering or abrasion
3	Break in skin exposing subcutaneous tissue
4	Break in skin exposing and or extending into muscle or bone

Aggravating factors include cognitive status, medications, malnutrition, obesity or emaciation, chronic disease or neurological disorder, incontinence, moisture, heat and pressure duration (Edsberg et al 2001).

Pressure ulcers are graded on a scale from 1 to 4. Table 3.5 describes the ulcer presentation and scale. Stage 4 and some stage 3 ulcers are life-threatening owing to the likelihood of deep-seated infection, haematogenous spread of infection and septicaemia.

Prevention of ulcer development is ideal since the financial and personal cost of pressure ulcers is enormous. Therefore identification of residents who are at most risk of developing a pressure ulcer is vital.

Risk assessment for pressure ulcer formation

On admission to a residential aged care facility every person should be assessed for risk of acquiring a pressure ulcer. Previous studies have shown that it is within the first week of admission to a nursing home that the resident is most likely to develop a pressure ulcer (Bergstrom et al 1995). This underlines the importance of assessing pressure area risk at admission so that prevention measures can be instituted immediately and not after skin breakdown has already occurred. A person who is independently mobile is least at risk. It is the dependent resident who is most at risk from superficial trauma. This usually results from friction or shear forces applied to the skin which is often exacerbated by maceration from wetness due to incontinence (Taler 2002).

Two validated and reliable scales have been developed to identify pressure area risk. These are the Norton and Braden Scales. Both scales indicate highest risk by a low score. The Norton Scale has five domains evaluated. These include: the physical condition and the presence of acute or chronic medical or surgical conditions that would affect tissue integrity; mental condition where capacity to respond to discomfort is defined; activity with respect to ambulation; mobility relating to the ability to change position independently to relieve pressure; and incontinence. The Braden Scale evaluates six domains. These include: sensory perception where appropriate response to discomfort from pressure is evaluated; frequency of moisture exposure of the skin (including sweat, urine and faeces); level of independent activity; mobility relating to the ability to change position independently; nutritional intake including fluids; friction and shear exposure during movement with or without assistance. Each scale uses a severity score of 1 to 4 in each domain assessed where 1 means complete dependency or major impairment and 4 indicates complete control and independence.

A score of 14 or less on the Norton scale (Norton et al 1975) or 16 or less on the Braden Scale (Bergstrom et al 1995) indicates vulnerability to pressure ulcer development.

Preventive measures for pressure ulcers

Prevention requires an understanding of the causative mechanisms. In the frail elderly who reside in aged care facilities, tissue changes associated with the ageing process play a major role in predisposing the person to a pressure ulcer. Decreased nutritional status, poor circulation, decreased dermal thickness, decrease in collagen content and loss of elasticity, changes in fat distribution in subcutaneous tissue (Thomas 2001a), decline in sensation and neural conduction velocity, muscle weakness and loss of bulk, stiff joints and cognitive decline contribute to the effect of ageing on increasing pressure ulcer risk. Many residents have additional physical disabilities such as stroke, motor neuron disease, multiple sclerosis, Parkinson's disease, amputation or arthritis that have necessitated their admission to the care facility and contribute to predisposing them to pressure ulcers owing to the effect on mobility. Incontinence accompanies ageing and many of these disabilities, thus increasing predisposition.

A logical approach to prevention that is easy to understand from the cause and effect viewpoint is most likely to be adopted and followed by carers. Table 3.6 identifies situations that will cause pressure ulcers if not acted on and methods of alleviating risk. It should be noted that the regular position change is advocated for residents unable to move independently. In acute care facilities position change every 2 hours is advocated to prevent pressure ulcer formation. In the frail elderly, 2 hours in one position is too long. The tissue changes due to age and concomitant conditions increase the susceptibility to pressure area development and position changes should be as regularly as every hour or more frequently depending on evaluation of skin condition at every turn. It is important to keep the skin and bedclothes dry to reduce the heat retention and maceration that contribute to skin breakdown (Edsberg et al 2001).

Management of pressure ulcers

The cost of managing pressure ulcers is vast both in staff time and materials, not to mention cost in suffering by the resident. The first and logical step should be to remove the causes where possible and provide the most advantageous healing environment. Thus pressure and shear forces must be removed. Continence must be controlled. Nutrition must include protein, vitamin C and zinc (Thomas 2001b).

The physiotherapist can assist the care staff in pressure ulcer treatment by utilizing electrotherapeutic modalities that facilitate healing such as high voltage galvanic, direct current electrical stimulation and low level laser or ultraviolet light therapy. We can also help by encouraging carers to adhere to the prevention and treatment protocols and by rewarding carers when they are compliant.

Stimulation of circulation is vital in order to promote healing. If the resident is able to mobilize, every opportunity should be taken to encourage

Table 3.6
Causes or indicators of incipient pressure ulcer development and recommended preventive interventions

Cause	Recommended intervention
Pressure – bed	Pressure-relieving mattress (ripple, egg shell) A water-bed can relieve the problem Regular position change (at times more frequently than second hourly turns are needed)
Pressure – chair	Pressure-relieving cushions and regular position change
Shear stress – bed/chair	Inclined backrest often causes the resident to slide down in the bed or chair. Sheepskins under the sacrum, heels and spine can reduce the friction and shear forces. Tilt-in-space chairs also will reduce the forward slide of the buttocks on the seat of a chair
Moisture – sweat	Many elderly people have altered sweating and if the sheets are wet should have regular linen changes
Moisture – incontinence (urine and/or faeces)	Residents should be checked every hour if incontinent and unable to communicate. Sheets and/or clothing should be changed regularly to prevent the resident sitting or lying in wet clothes. The acidity of urine and faeces irritates the skin more than sweat and will precipitate skin breakdown. Since wetness from incontinence affects the areas most at risk from pressure and shear tissue injury, extra vigilance is necessary if pressure areas are to be avoided
Mental confusion or the unresponsive resident	These residents are unable to communicate their discomfort and rely on the carer to check for wetness and change position regularly
Immobility	These residents may not be able to communicate and so need regular checks for wetness and position changes. Residents able to communicate should be assisted to move and not considered demanding if they are asking for help to change position frequently. Two-hourly turns are not frequent enough to prevent pressure injury in the elderly
Behavioural changes	Noisy demented residents are often uncomfortable. Check for wetness and change to dry clothing as well as assisting to move. Take residents for a walk if they are able

movement and walking. All carers should be recruited to the cause to maximize movement. Passive movements of limbs by the care staff can assist circulation when there is paralysis or loss of self-initiated movement. Care must be taken when applying passive movement that the limbs are fully supported and the heels are not dragged up and down the sheets, thus endangering the skin integrity in this area. Handling of the limbs should be done carefully where the skin is fragile as skin tears are often caused by the hand grip. The hand should cradle the limb during assisted movements. Figures 3.2 and 3.3 show some handling techniques.

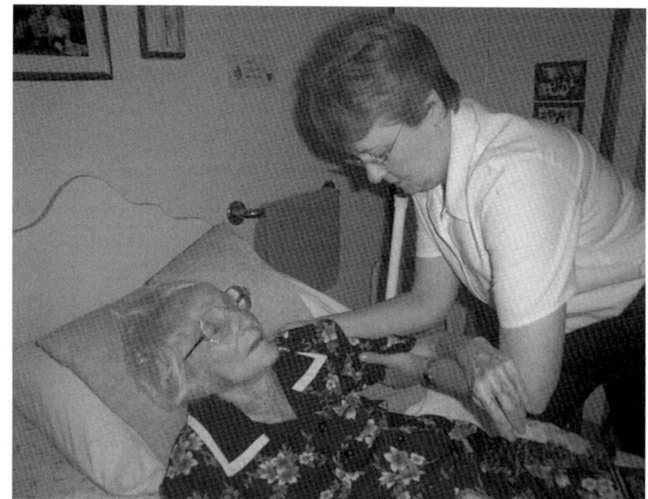

Figure 3.2
Careful handling of the upper limbs of a frail resident.

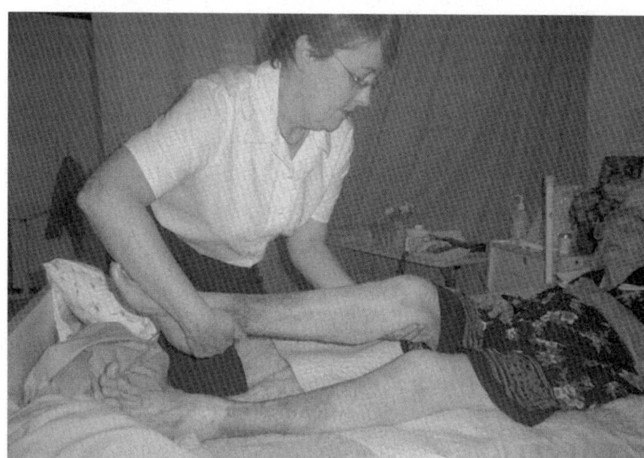

Figure 3.3
Careful handling of the lower limbs of a frail resident. Note the discoloration of the skin in the lower half of the legs due to circulatory changes.

Summary

- All residents are at risk of injury and need to be assessed and treated to reduce the likelihood of this occurrence.
- Injury leads to decreased mobility and movement that may accelerate morbidity and mortality.
- Falls are one of the greatest mechanisms of severe injury to older persons within RACFs. Prevention and risk management is vital.
- Ulcers and chronic wounds can be brought about by preventable injuries. Residents often have poor healing abilities and therefore increased risk of chronic wounds.
- Differentiation between arterial, venous or pressure ulcers is imperative in order to deliver appropriate treatment.

- Elevation is not always a treatment of choice with swollen limbs. You must consider occlusive arterial disease as in this case elevation may lead directly to poor perfusion and a worsening of the condition.
- Similarly, cold treatment or ice application to a body area in a resident who has occlusive arterial disease is an unwise application. Tissue damage might occur due to the circulatory insufficiency and inability to deal with thermoregulatory demands.
- Any exercise, stretch or position in which compression of arterial structures is likely or possible should be avoided with residents who have OAD, e.g. prolonged stretching and isometric muscle contractions.
- Physiotherapists should be involved in education relating to pressure area risk, prevention and treatment. There are several main causes of pressure ulcers, and interventions were suggested concerning how to deal with all of these within this chapter.
- Above and beyond all else – **think before you act and teach others to do the same. Most accidents are preventable.**

References

Ashburn A, Stack E, Pickering R M, Ward C D 2000 Predicting fallers in a community-based sample of people with Parkinson's disease. Gerontology 47:277–281

Bergstrom N, Braden B, Boynton P, Bruch S 1995 Using a research based assessment scale in clinical practice. Nursing Clinics of North America 30:539–551

Bergstrom N, Braden B, Kemp M, Champagne M, Ruby E 1998 Predicting pressure ulcer risk. Nursing Research 47:261–269

Brienza D M, Karg P E, Geyer M J, Kelsey S, Trefler E 2001 The relationship between pressure ulcer incidence and buttock–seat cushion interface pressure in at-risk elderly wheelchair users. Archives of Physical Medicine and Rehabilitation 82:529–533

Brown L A, Shumway-Cook A, Woollacott M H 1999 Attentional demands and postural recovery: The effects of ageing. Journal of Gerontology: Medical Sciences 54A(4):M165–M171

Busby W J, Campbell J, Robertson M C 1994 Is low blood pressure in elderly people just a consequence of heart disease and frailty? Age and Ageing 23:69–74

Cavorsi J P 2000 Venous ulcers of the lower extremities: Current and newer management techniques. Topics in Geriatric Medicine 16:24

Coffman J D 1988 Pathophysiology of arterial obstructive disease. Herz 13:343–350

De Wytt C N, Jackson R V, Hockings G I, Joyner J M, Strakosch C R 1999 Polyneuropathy in Australian outpatients with type II diabetes mellitus. Journal of Diabetes and its Complications 13:74–78

Edsberg L A, Natiella J R, Baier R E, Earle J 2001 Micro-structural characteristics of human skin subjected to static versus cyclic pressures. Journal of Rehabilitation Research and Development 38:477–486

Hauer K, Specht N, Schuler M, Bärtsch P, Oster P 2002 Intensive physical training in geriatric patients after severe falls and hip surgery. Age and Ageing 31:49–57

Khan F, Litchfield S J, Stonebridge P A, Belch J J 1999 Lipid lowering and skin vascular responses in patients with hypercholesterolaemia and peripheral arterial obstructive disease. Vascular Medicine 4:233–238

Lord S R, Ward J A, Williams P et al 1993 An epidemiologic-study of falls in older community-dwelling women – the Randwick falls and fractures study. Australian Journal of Public Health 17(3): 240–245

Low Choy N L, Isles R C, Barker R, Nitz J C 2003 The efficacy of a work-station intervention program to improve functional ability, flexibility and fitness in ageing clients with cerebral palsy. Disability and Rehabilitation 25:1201–1207

Lundin-Olsson L, Nyberg L, Gustafson Y 1997 'Stops walking when talking' as a predictor of falls in the elderly. Lancet 349:617

Menz H B, Lord S R 2001a The contribution of foot problems to mobility and falls in community-dwelling older people. Journal of the American Geriatrics Society 49:1651–1656

Menz H B, Lord S R 2001b Foot pain impairs balance and functional ability in community-dwelling older people. Journal of the American Podiatric Medicine Association 91:222–229

Nevitt M C, Cummings S R, Kidd S, Black D 1989 Risk factors for recurrent nonsyncopal falls. JAMA 261:2663–2668

Nitz J C, Low Choy N L 2004 The efficacy of a specific balance strategy training program for preventing falls among the frail elderly. A pilot RCT. Age and Ageing 33:52–58

Norton D, McLaren R, Exton-Smith A N 1975 An investigation of geriatric nursing problems in hospitals. Churchill-Livingstone, Edinburgh

Paris B E, Libow L S, Halperin J L, Mulvihill M N 1988 The prevalence and one-year outcome of limb arterial obstructive disease in a nursing home population. Journal of the American Geriatrics Society 36:607–612

Pomeroy V M 1993 The effect of physiotherapy input on mobility skills of elderly people with severe dementing illness. Clinical Rehabilitation 7:163–170

Remijnse-Tamerius H C, Duprez D, DeBuyzere M, Oeseburg B, Clement D L 1999 Why is training effective in the treatment of patients with intermittent claudication? International Angiology 18:103–112

Runge M, Rehfeld G, Resnicek E 2000 Balance training and exercise in geriatric patients. Journal of Musculoskeletal Interaction 1:54–58

Samuels S C, Evers M M 2002 Delirium: pragmatic guidance for managing a common confounding, and sometimes lethal condition. Geriatrics 57:33–38

Shaw F E, Kenny R A 1998 Can falls in patients with dementia be prevented? Age and Ageing 27:7–10

Sprigle S 2000 Effects of forces and the selection of support surfaces. Topics in Geriatric Medicine 16:47

Taler G 2002 What do prevalence studies of pressure ulcers in nursing homes really tell us? Journal of the American Geriatrics Society 50:773–774

Thapa P B, Gideon P, Fought R L, Ray W A 1995 Psychotropic drugs and risk of recurrent falls in ambulatory nursing home residents. American Journal of Epidemiology 142:202–211

Thomas D 2001a Age related changes in wound healing. Drugs and Aging 18:607–620

Thomas D 2001b Prevention and management of pressure ulcers. Reviews in Clinical Gerontology 11:115–130

Tinetti M E, Speechley M, Ginter S E 1988 Risk factors for falls among elderly persons living in the community. New England Journal of Medicine 319:1701–1707

Tsokos M, Heinemann A, Puschel K 2000 Pressure sores: epidemiology, medico-legal implications and forensic argumentation concerning causality. International Journal of Legal Medicine 113:283–287

Vellas B J, Wayne S J, Romero L J, Baumgartner R, Garry P J 1997 Fear of falling and reduction of mobility in elderly fallers. Age and Ageing 26:189–194

4 Life satisfaction

Jennifer C. Nitz

This chapter aims to:

- raise the awareness of readers to the needs of residents to obtain life satisfaction
- identify factors that can impact on attaining a liveable life style
- illustrate some examples of the physiotherapist's role in advocacy and attainment of residents' wishes.

Introduction

Happiness and contentment are a priority for life satisfaction. Residents living in an RACF might find that life satisfaction is related to both quality of care and quality of life. Kane (2001) identified 11 aspects of quality of life that require consideration if the resident is to feel happy and content with living in the RACF environment. Feeling safe and secure where people around the resident can be trusted can be considered by many older people to outweigh personal comfort in importance. Social interaction aspects including enjoyment, meaningful activity and the ability to develop a relationship with other residents or staff were other quality of life needs identified. Autonomy was seen to be very important for the resident in order to enable the individual to attain their maximal functional competence, both physical and mental. Dignity, privacy, individuality and spiritual wellbeing all relate to the autonomy allowed to the resident. Collectively these aspects of life should be integrated into mission statements of RACFs. The difficult task for the facility then comes when the individual differences that each resident and staff member brings to the RACF community need to be accounted for in developing the care programmes within the built environment available in the facility.

In order to achieve this ideal, Kane (2001) identified the need for a 'culture change' from a care approach based on hospital routine to more appreciation of residents as people and the satisfaction of the mind and soul as well as physical needs of the individual cared for. Inclusion of the resident and families in decision-making for care plans is a starting point. Allowing favourite pieces of furniture to be used as well as pictures and other decor items brought from home help in the deinstitutionalization of the RACF. Physiotherapists might be required to enable continued use of favourite furniture that is inappropriate in height, for example, by providing a safe method of raising height to assist with resident transfers as well as showing care staff how best to encourage independence or assist these transfers.

Most older people will at some stage need assistance with activities of daily living, basic nursing procedures such as wound dressings and supervision of medication administration. To the older person this aspect of care is of varying importance. Kane (2001) points out that some residents identify their care plans as 'instruments of terror' owing to lack of dignity, handling care, comfort and personal preferences. Furthermore, unless the social, intellectual and leisure needs are met 'life is not worth living' for residents. Depression is a very real problem for residents in RACFs and might be related to lack of attention to the basic needs for life satisfaction.

Paramount to happiness is being able to participate in leisure activities that we like such as reading, listening to the music we enjoy, choosing sport, theatrical and movie entertainment of our own liking and keeping company with people with whom we want to associate. Leisure pursuits that involve active participation and are chosen pastimes for many elderly people include sport such as lawn bowls, swimming and fishing, as well as cards, handcrafts and gardening. Cultural background and religious persuasion might also determine daily activity. All aspects of life have varying degrees of importance for all people and not to be able to continue a lifetime pursuit can lead to discontent, which might be expressed by mood disturbances and through uncooperative or disruptive behaviour. If the resident is unable or constrained in the ability to communicate this frustration and unhappiness, behavioural problems are more likely to be present.

Lack of privacy has been identified as a problem for residents (Ronnberg 1998). This lack of privacy or ability to be alone when desired can be a source of irritation for a resident who is unable to change his or her environment independently by moving to another room to get away from others or is unable to turn off the television or radio. In such circumstances frustration might be expressed by unsocial behaviour. Privacy should also be considered along with maintenance of dignity during care procedures, where adequate draping and screening from outside view is extremely important. Some of the older residents might not have undressed in front of their spouse, so can be quite traumatized by complete strangers undressing them during care activities. Respect for these sensibilities is vital if the resident is to feel safe and that the carer still respects them as a person.

Residential care has been considered to isolate people from the outside world (Ronnberg 1998). Boredom through lack of stimulation also causes restlessness and depression (Kane 2001). Residents who are blind or deaf need different sensory stimuli to prevent boredom. Similarly, residents who have acquired brain injuries that have affected sensory input in such a way that they have lost all reference to their surroundings and are unable to interpret where they are in the environment require a further variation in the stimulation approach chosen. These residents might benefit from increased touch and handling. This helps them to orientate with the environment, thereby reducing the continual, restless non-directional movement that can place them at risk of fall injury were they to wriggle out of bed or a chair. Davies (1994, p 57–58) discusses this problem and possible interventions that might be applied to relieve the aimless movement.

Most people identify the maintenance of autonomy over decisions relating to how they spend their waking hours and, when possible, activities undertaken as important for contentment. Such autonomy is often lost when older people move into a residential care facility where hospital-like routines are commonly followed by care staff (Schroll et al 1997). Physical and cognitive capabilities and the consequent level of dependency most often determines the amount of independence that a person retains regarding decisions about when to bathe, eat or go for a walk. If the resident requires assistance in some activity of daily living, medication administration or nursing procedure, care staff availability and time constraints enter the picture. The more dependent the resident the more their day is likely to be determined by staff routines. Conformity might be difficult for many new residents who have been autonomous up to RACF entry. The result of loss of control and autonomy might cause the resident to lack motivation, be passive during care activities and lose the capacity to learn new skills (Ronnberg 1998). To counteract this learned helplessness, the physiotherapist should work with the resident and care staff to ensure maximal functional independence is maintained, and also to ensure access to stimulating activities that the resident finds interesting. Discontent can arise if residents are not consulted regarding participation in activity programmes and are only assisted to attend those functions the staff member considers will interest the person. It is important to find out the resident's interests and facilitate integration into programmes appropriate for these interests run by the facility or outside in the community. The willingness of the carers to transport the resident to a venue in order for them to participate in an activity has been identified as a major determinant of how much social engagement is possible for dependent residents (Schroll et al 1997). The physiotherapist might need to encourage the care staff to assist individuals to achieve this activity interaction by identifying for the care staff the positive outcomes for the resident and the likely decline in physical and cognitive function in the resident if they are unable to access the activity.

Life satisfaction is such an individual state that there is no prescription that can be applied to suit all residents. The demographic make-up of the RACF population has to be considered when developing resources and educating carers. Once programmes are in place they need to be flexible as the population of the RACF changes with the turnover of residents. As a rule there will be some core factors that are common to varying proportions of the resident population that will need to be addressed by care staff in order to control behavioural problems and to ensure a better quality of life for residents and staff.

Factors that contribute to dissatisfaction with life

Environmental factors

Easy access to toilet facilities is very important for residents with continence problems. Kane (2001) suggests that toilets should be situated near the front door, communal activity and dining rooms and other places frequented by residents. Having to return long distances to their room to go to the toilet can cause episodes of incontinence that otherwise would be avoided. Mirrors also should be at wheelchair height so grooming can be undertaken independently. Light switches at an accessible height and remote controls for televisions and sound systems can all make life more comfortable for residents who are able to cope independently. By not providing these simple environmental facilities, the resident is forced to assume a level of helplessness that defies independence and ultimately causes increased disability and loss of quality of life. It also increases the workload for staff from both aspects.

Residents

Many residents will present with cognitive dysfunction. The cognitive dysfunction can be due to acquired brain injury or degenerative pathology such as stroke, closed head injury, multiple sclerosis, Parkinson's disease, Huntington's chorea, Creutzfeld–Jakob disease and Alzheimer's disease to name a few. In some RACFs there will be residents who have aged with low IQ in addition to multiple physical disabilities such as cerebral palsy, Down's syndrome, auditory loss and blindness. Many of these latter residents will have spent a considerable proportion of their life in care facilities. They can present with acquired disability from contractures and sensory deprivation not to mention pressure areas and nutritional problems. Irrespective of the presenting cognitive and physical problems, the aim of the carers should be to maximize quality of life. Where possible this should provide a living environment that ensures prevention of the additional disability often associated with immobility, poor nutritional intake, reduced respiratory function and lack of stimulation.

Cognitive function is dependent on cerebral oxygenation and glucose levels (Guyton 1991). Physiotherapists can enhance respiratory function through positioning the resident for sleeping and during the day such that chest movement and ventilation capacity is maximized. The safest position for taking sustenance should also be identified by the physiotherapist for each resident in order to prevent aspiration as well as to enhance enjoyment from eating. The reader is directed to the section on the immobile resident (Section 2) for further detail on these aspects of management.

A lower level of cognitive function is more likely to be correlated with a higher frequency of behavioural disturbance (Jagger & Lindesay 1997) and specifically disruptive vocalization (Burgio et al 2001). Between 10 and 30% of residents exhibit disruptive vocalization (DV) in any or all forms such as screaming, cursing, complaining, calling out for attention, perseveration and moaning (Burgio et al 2001). DV can occur continually or in bursts at various times during the day. Precursors related to circadian rhythm such as changes in body temperature and sleep–wake cycles or of an environmental nature such as lighting levels and care staff shift changes or busy times (Burgio et al 2001, Evans 1987) have been hypothesized to precipitate DV. Peaking of DV has been related to the 'sundowning syndrome', when other agitated behaviours such as wandering and confusion (Duckett 1993) are more frequent. DV is most disturbing for staff and other residents and might be considered a major factor affecting life satisfaction for all. There is, however, a strong correlation between agitation and other disruptive behaviours and medication, light exposure and sleep (Martin et al 2000).

We must acknowledge the importance of sleep and the disturbances to sleep that are encountered in RACFs. Depression, memory loss and confusion are also prevalent in residents. These problems worry the resident and can lead to stress-related behaviours or medical conditions such as gastric ulcers. Care planning and strategies for managing residents with cognition-related behaviour disorders depends on understanding aspects of sleep, depression and confusion that can be improved. Therefore these topics will be considered in more detail.

Sleep

Secondary insomnia is very common in residents and the elderly in general and is contributed to by intrinsic problems such as pain, incontinence problems, stress, depression, alcohol and tobacco abuse, caffeine, dementia and normal ageing. Many of the causes of insomnia present in elderly residents can be treated. Pain in particular can be better managed by a multidisciplinary team approach. The physiotherapist can offer many treatment interventions that can modulate pain from musculoskeletal and neural origin. The reader is referred to the chapter later in this text that addresses pain and its management (Chapter 15).

An extrinsic cause of sleep problems in residents is a noisy environment. Disruptive and noisy residents might contribute but so too can staff if they need to attend to a resident in a shared room during sleep hours. Unfortunately, the first avenue for sleep disorder management in the over 65-year-olds tends to be via prescription of benzodiazepines and hypnotic drugs. It is well documented that these drugs contribute to balance disorders and have been linked to falls (Adunsky & Hershkowitz 1993, Lord et al 1995, Nevitt et al 1989) and these falls often result in major injury such as fractured neck of femur. Neutel et al (1996) reported that the highest risk of a fall resulting in serious injury occurred within 15 days of commencing benzodiazepine medication. Benzodiazepines and hypnotic drugs have also been linked to changes in cognitive function, with confusion and memory impairment commonly found (Samuels & Evers 2002). Other less drastic side effects of these medications can be grogginess and daytime somnolence.

Table 4.1 *Conservative interventions to enhance sleep patterns*

Environment control
Ensure adequate warmth of the room and lightweight bedclothes to make bed mobility easier
Comfortable support from pillows of the desired height and a mattress designed to reduce pressure are mandatory. Sheepskins might also be used to protect bony prominences from excess pressure
Control noise by raising staff awareness and relocating disruptive residents
Consider lighting and provide easy access to night light switch rather than leaving the light on all night
Provide devices that give assistance to enable independence in bed mobility
Individual intervention
Encourage participation in physical and/or cognitive activities during the day that will lead to natural tiredness and desire for sleep
Discourage daytime napping
Encourage relaxation with relaxation techniques, massage, aromatherapy or a night-cap (hot milk or nip of alcohol)

Therefore logic should prevail and non-toxic modalities for assisting sleep such as relieving pain and discomfort should be attempted first. Conservative methods that might be used to achieve better sleep patterns in residents where there is no underlying concomitant problem such as pain are listed in Table 4.1. However, these ideas should be implemented as a general rule and in addition to addressing other symptoms.

Consideration should be given to the wishes of residents regarding lodging in an individual room or shared room where the facility provides a choice of accommodation. Loneliness at night, if unable to sleep, can be disturbing for residents. Just having another person nearby when awake at night might reduce the confusion that comes about when the resident has no immediate reference regarding what they should be doing or where they are (Milward 2001). Wandering can be a problem in residents with night-time confusion and this in turn is a causative factor in falls. In addition, it is important to be aware of REM sleep behaviour disorder and its association with nocturnal falls (Morfis et al 1997). In some instances this sleep behaviour disorder is responsible for violently aggressive behaviour that might lead to resident or carer injury (Portet & Touchon 2002). At other times the resident might act out a dream, and if this involves walking or running, the resident might get out of bed and consequently have a fall. Sleep studies might be indicated if falls risk is great or violent behaviour has occurred or when there is excessive daytime drowsiness. Another cause of daytime drowsiness and poor sleep is sleep apnoea.

Sleep apnoea

Sleep apnoea is most common in men who are obese and hypertensive and can be exacerbated by excessive alcohol ingestion. Sleep apnoea is also seen in people with myotonic dystrophy and other disorders affecting the oropharynx. During sleep, breathing ceases, most likely due to upper airway obstruction that can be contributed to by the resident lying supine to sleep. Spontaneous respiration returns after variable lengths of time and usually after a stronger inspiratory effort. The symptoms include daytime drowsiness, morning headaches and cardiac arrhythmias, which are caused by low arterial oxygen concentration due to the apnoeic periods. In residents with other cognitive problems, function can be further impaired by the presence of sleep apnoea. Treatment is dependent on diagnosis. Since residents can present with similar symptoms that are due to other causes, investigation for sleep apnoea is relatively uncommon in this population. When diagnosed, sleep apnoea is generally treated by weight loss, surgery or nasal continuous positive airways pressure (CPAP). The physiotherapist might be consulted regarding the use of CPAP. All these treatments aim to improve oxygenation and relieve the symptoms. Patients generally report feeling rested after a night's sleep, as having more energy and not having their usual headache. Cognitively, they may be brighter, able to concentrate and remember recent events better.

Depression

Schnelle et al (2001) found that the prevalence of depression among people in long-term care was underestimated owing to the care staff considering the symptoms as those associated with normal ageing. Between 30 and 75% of residents in nursing homes have some degree of depression (Ames 1993). Some of the factors contributing to depression have been identified as an awareness of imminence of death, loss of confidence and self-esteem, decreased opportunity for self-expression and the opportunity to cope with new challenges, reduced conversational opportunities, isolation and loneliness (Higgs et al 1998, Ronnberg 1998). A lack of fun and laughter is often present in RACFs as many are run on the same principles as hospital wards where light-heartedness is misplaced. However, if an RACF is to equate to a 'home' environment then fun times are essential. Laughter has been shown to improve the immune response and to generally relieve stress levels (Kamei et al 1997). Care staff should be encouraged to share funny stories and life experiences with the residents so all can have a good laugh. Participation in interactive programmes such as story-telling has been shown to reduce depression, improve spontaneous communication and generally improve quality of life (Ronnberg 1998). Similar improvements in quality of life have been demonstrated when residents participated in exercise and sensory stimulation programmes (Fiatarone 1994, Orsulic-Jeras et al 2000).

Confusion

Confusion is common among residents. The underlying cause of the confusion might be (early) dementia, a urinary tract or chest infection, dehydration, hypoglycaemia, medication related or chronic anaemia. All of these are common problems encountered in RAFCs and all except dementia are reversible by appropriate interventions if identified. Thus a confused resident should be assessed and not ignored owing to the care staff's assumption that the behaviour is due to the ageing process.

When confusion is due to an irreversible condition such as Alzheimer's disease or dementia of another cause, the resident often has retained some insight into their own behaviour and becomes worried about such things as forgetting appointments, people's names or to groom themselves properly, and where they are going or what they intended to do. Feil (1993) classified dementia into four stages. These were the period of malorientation, time confusion, repetitive motion and vegetation. Rarely are the stages clear but usually overlap. In order to assist family and carers to understand and cope with the odd behaviour and statements made by people with dementia validation therapy was developed to assist with communication (Feil 1993). Feil contends that using validation means showing empathy for the disorientated older person through understanding the stages of dementia, thereby rationalizing behaviours and allowing communication. This allows family members to put the behaviour into context by connecting it with life experiences of the elder; using the connection to validate and empathize with the elder might help coping with otherwise distressing situations. If successful management of the demented resident's behaviour is achieved through validation it is a well worthwhile approach to use in working for life satisfaction for resident, family and carers.

Communication

The inability to talk or understand the spoken word is common among residents. Hearing loss without additional pathology is the easiest communication difficulty to overcome if the resident can read. However, add visual impairment or illiteracy and more creative methods of communication need to be developed between the care staff and the resident. Mime or demonstration of the physical task the carer wishes the resident to perform or participate in generally results in an appropriate response. If the resident has a cognitive deficit or aphasia after a stroke, communication is more difficult and specific management strategies need to be incorporated in the care plan. Residents with expressive and/or receptive aphasia often become frustrated in their attempts to communicate. Ensuring a relaxed atmosphere that engenders a supportive and caring feeling between the resident and carer (Sundin & Jansson 2003) can achieve communication. Often there is no need for words if an empathetic relationship has developed between resident and carer who ultimately develops an anticipation of the resident's needs.

Various methods of communication have been developed for people without speech. Boards with pictorial representations of physical needs such as a drink, toilet, comb or toothbrush enable residents to attain some independence and autonomy regarding when activities relating to the pictured task occur. Computers have been programmed to communicate the thoughts of some disabled people to carers. Staff should ensure the resident is not denied access to the method of communication they use by inadvertently putting the communication board out of reach during care tasks and then not returning them to within reach.

A speech pathologist should be consulted when communication difficulties arise with new or old residents so that the most effective method of communication is achieved. Life satisfaction is drastically affected when isolation occurs through inability to communicate.

Sexuality

Sexuality and intimacy are most important aspects contributing to life satisfaction. There are many myths and misconceptions regarding sexuality in older people and specifically those elders who reside in RACFs. Sexual expression and intimacy do not decline with ageing. More commonly any decline is related to medication, illness, loss of a life-long partner, lack of opportunity, or social expectations and culture (Kaye 1993). For residents many of these situations are pertinent. However, institutionalization should not preclude the development and continuation of a relationship between residents. Unfortunately, not all RACFs cater for couples by providing double rooms, nor do they always provide privacy and support for partners who are separated by the care needs of one. Care staff should be aware that sexual activity is normal throughout life and should not look on older residents as being abnormal or depraved if they participate in sexual activity (Kaye 1993). All people feel the need for caring, sharing, loving and intimacy. These emotions and actions are reciprocal between people and do not necessarily involve a sexual relationship. Therefore care staff and residents incorporate many of these aspects in day-to-day interactions where privacy, trust and respect are probably more likely words used to describe the relationship. It is interesting to note that Kane (2001) did not identify sexuality as a major determinant of life satisfaction and the needs of people in long-term care. Nor was the topic identified overtly or discreetly in the study by Chou et al (2002) that investigated resident satisfaction in RACFs.

Establishing a relationship with other residents was found by Lee et al (2002) to be a challenge for new residents and cultural considerations might interfere. Kaye (1993) identified the need to define the 'rules' for new residents so that self-determination could determine interpersonal wishes.

On occasion when dementia or confusion is present in a resident, sexually overt behaviours are found. Such actions might be related to the need to urinate and an inability to communicate that need in any other way. Similarly, undressing in public might indicate the person is too hot. On the other hand, 'patting a carer on the bottom' might be construed as uninhibited sexual behaviour between an elderly male resident and female carer when in reality the action was meant to be one of appreciation for care received. There is the situation when such an action is the result of disinhibited behaviour and appropriate behaviour modification intervention is indicated.

The paucity of research that addresses sexuality in the elderly residing in aged care indicates the need to raise awareness of this aspect of life satisfaction with providers of RACFs as well as care staff. Incorporation of items related to sexuality and intimacy in quality of life questionnaires and evaluations of care seems highly appropriate.

Interventions that might enhance life satisfaction

We would all love to live in utopia and to be able to provide an RACF that approached this ideal. The Eden Alternative is one example of a philosophy that embraces the search for improvement in RACFs. It aims at eliminating loneliness, helplessness and boredom by modifying the social and physical environment. The core concept is to see the environment as a habitat for human beings rather than facilities for the frail and elderly. The Eden Alternative uses companion animals and gives residents the opportunity to give meaningful care to other living creatures. (For more information go to www.edenalt.com.) Some ideas that might be useful suggestions for enhancing life satisfaction for residents are listed in Table 4.2 to enable the reader to work towards this goal.

Table 4.2 *Suggestions for enhancing life satisfaction for residents*

Built environment
Heated swimming pool and spa will encourage increased activity or therapy possibilities
Landscaped gardens with seats, shade, contemplation areas, fish-ponds and water features
Ready access to toilets with disabled access
Gymnasium and community recreation rooms
Bistro area where residents can have coffee or an alcoholic beverage while socializing
Provision of a designated hairdresser room with hair washing basin, mirrors and hair drier
Provision of a dedicated room or building where residents can fulfil their religious or spiritual needs
Provision of double room for couples
Activity variety
Provision of computers with internet access so residents can contact friends and family by email as well as access the World Wide Web
Build up a facility borrowing library with large print books, magazines, films on video and music compact discs
A garden area with raised garden beds where residents can plant annuals or vegetables and look after the crop is most relaxing for residents who love gardening
A woodwork shop where residents can make toys or furniture (under supervision if needed) is also possible
Regular exercise classes, relaxation training and brain-teasing sessions such as debating or 'trivial pursuit'

Social activities
Barbecue area for residents to have family events as well as resident gatherings
Regular outings to theatre, cinema and sporting events on the wheelchair accessible facility bus
Encourage involvement of family and friends with care planning and visiting as well as taking the resident out on day excursions
Resident committees can be encouraged and given responsibility for arranging outings, visits by entertainment groups, and publication of a facility newsletter if the resident demographics includes cognitively capable older people

Caring
A cat or a dog can provide companionship for residents who are used to having a pet
A small aviary or fish tank can also be conducive to relaxation and can encourage communication among residents
Regular hairdresser attendance at the facility
Carers to take *time* to listen and talk with residents and their families and friends
Encourage volunteer groups to visit residents to talk, teach new skills such as how to use a computer, play contract bridge or bonsai a tree. The list could be as long as lateral thinking allows
Manicures, pedicures or facials can be very soothing interventions that many residents enjoy and want to continue to receive
Enable couples to stay together when in residential care
Understand and accommodate in a tasteful manner sexuality needs of residents, especially if young or living in a stable relationship

Conclusion

Life satisfaction should be the ultimate goal of physiotherapy management with residents living in RACFs. This goal should be achieved through a clear understanding of the issues involved and consultation with individual residents to establish their aspirations and needs.

Summary

- Life satisfaction relies on both quality of care and quality of life.
- Safety, trust, comfort, happiness, contentment, social interaction and autonomy are all important considerations in determining life satisfaction.
- Dignity, privacy, individuality and spiritual factors all play an integral part in a resident's perception of satisfaction in their life.
- The most important features of life satisfaction will depend on that particular resident. Life satisfaction is individual – different things will be important to different people!

- Individual consideration (or assessment) is of great importance. The involvement of the resident and their family in decision-making should be a priority wherever feasible.
- Participation in chosen leisure activities and outings should be made possible.
- Diversional therapists and activities officers have an integral part to play in ensuring stimulation through a wide range of activities, outings and concerts.
- This chapter examined areas which may contribute to dissatisfaction with life such as: environmental factors; other residents; poor sleep and sleep apnoea; depression; confusion; poor communication; and sexuality issues.
- Intervention ideas have been suggested which may be considered for use in practice (Table 4.2).

References

Adunsky A, Hershkowitz M 1993 The role of psychotropic drugs in the elderly with hip fractures. Clinical Rehabilitation 7:135–138

Ames D 1993 Depressive disorders among elderly people in long-term institutional care. Australian and New Zealand Journal of Psychiatry 27:379–391

Burgio L D, Scilley K, Hardin M, Hsu C 2001 Temporal patterns of disruptive vocalization in elderly nursing home residents. International Journal of Geriatric Psychiatry 16:378–386

Burney-Puckett M 1996 Sundown syndrome: etiology and management. Journal of Psychological Nursing 34:40–43

Chou S-C, Boldy D P, Lee A H 2002 Resident satisfaction and its components in residential aged care. The Gerontologist 42(2):188–198

Davies P M 1994 Starting again: early rehabilitation after traumatic brain injury or other severe brain lesion. Berlin, Springer-Verlag, p 57–58

Duckett S 1993 Managing the sundowning patient. Journal of Rehabilitation 59(1):24–29

Evans L K 1987 Sundown syndrome in institutionalized elderly. Journal of the American Geriatrics Society 35:101–108

Feil N 1993 The validation breakthrough: simple techniques for communicating with people with Alzheimer's-type dementia. Maclennan & Petty, Sydney

Fiatarone M A 1994 Exercise training and nutritional supplementation for physical frailty in very elderly people. New England Journal of Medicine 330: 1769–1774

Guyton A C 1991 Textbook of medical physiology, 8th edn. W B Saunders, Philadelphia, p 679–684

Higgs P F D, MacDonald L D, MacDonald J S, Ward M C 1998 Home from home: residents' opinion of nursing homes and long stay wards. Age and Ageing 27(2):199–206

Jagger C, Lindesay J 1997 Residential care for elderly people: the prevalence of cognitive impairment and behavioural problems. Age and Ageing 26(6):475–481

Kamei T, Kumano H, Masumura S 1997 Changes in immunoregulatory cells associated with psychological stress and humor. Perceptual and Motor Skills 84:1296–1298

Kane R A 2001 Long-term care and a good quality of life: Bringing them closer together. The Gerontologist 41(3):293–302

Kaye R A 1993 Sexuality in later years. Ageing and Society 13:415–426

Lee D T F, Woo J, Mackenzie A E 2002 The cultural context of adjusting to nursing home life: Chinese elders' perspectives. The Gerontologist 42(5):667–675

Lord S R, Anstey K J, Williams P, Ward J A 1995 Psychoactive medication use, sensori-motor function and falls in older women. British Journal of Clinical Pharmacology 39:227–234

Martin J, Marler M, Shochat T, Ancoli-Israel S 2000 Circadian rhythms of agitation in institutionalized patients with Alzheimer's disease. Chronobiology International 17(3):405–418

Milward D V 2001 Lonely nights in long-term care. Age and Ageing 30:271–272

Morfis L, Schwartz R S, Cistulli P A 1997 REM sleep behaviour disorder: a treatable cause of falls in elderly people. Age and Ageing 26:43–44

Neutel C I, Hirdes J P, Maxwell C J, Patten S B 1996 New evidence on benzodiazepine use and falls: the time factor. Age and Ageing 25:273–278

Nevitt M C, Cummings S R, Kidd S, Black D 1989 Risk factors for recurrent nonsyncopal falls. JAMA 261:2663–2668

Orsulic-Jeras S, Schneider N M, Camp C J 2000 Special feature: Montessori-based activities for long-term care residents with dementia. Topics in Geriatric Rehabilitation 16(1):78–89

Portet F, Touchon J 2002 REM sleep behavioural disorder. Revue Neurologique 158(11):1049–1056

Ronnberg L 1998 Quality of life in nursing-home residents: an intervention study of the effect of mental stimulation through an audiovisual programme. Age and Ageing 27(3):393–398

Samuels S C, Evers M M 2002 Delirium: pragmatic guidance for managing a common confounding, and sometimes lethal condition. Geriatrics 57:33–38

Schnelle J F, Wood S, Schnelle E R, Simmons S F 2001 Measurement sensitivity and the minimum data set depression quality indicator. The Gerontologist 41(3):401–405

Schroll M, Jonsson P V, Mor V, Berg K, Sherwood S 1997 An international study of social engagement among nursing home residents. Age and Ageing 26(6):S55–S60

Sundin K, Jansson L 2003 'Understanding and being understood' as a creative caring phenomenon – in care of patients with stroke and aphasia. Journal of Clinical Nursing 12(1):107–116

SECTION 2 CARE OF THE IMMOBILE OR BARELY MOBILE RESIDENT

5 The complexity of the immobile or barely mobile resident

Jennifer C. Nitz

This chapter aims to:

- identify residents at risk of succumbing to complications of immobility
- identify the consequences of immobility
- discuss the implementation of management using a clinical reasoning process that incorporates evidence-based practice as well as identifying where evidence is lacking and the need for clinical studies
- stress at all times the quality of life of the resident with respect to rationale for suggested interventions that could be incorporated into care plans.

Introduction

The information contained in Section 2 is of pivotal importance to the care of immobile or barely mobile residents. These residents will be encountered in centres providing homes for people who are highly dependent owing to the severity or multiplicity of their structural or functional disabilities. It is very difficult to implement care plans for these very dependent residents if the carer has little or no understanding of the whys and wherefores regarding instructions. Lack of this aspect of knowledge in carers has been identified as one of the main reasons for non-compliance with care plan instructions and the consequent quality of life issues that arise for residents. We therefore aim to present a very complex problem situation in a cause, effect, consequence and prevention model.

The resident

The extremely frail elderly resident who is unable to move or change position efficiently is typical of a large proportion of people in aged care facilities. There are, however, some younger adults residing in RACFs as a result of acquired disability.

There are five major categories of resident with limited mobility:

1. residents who are able to communicate their need to change position but need assistance to change position and with activities of daily living (ADLs), e.g. tetraplegics

2. residents who can move independently and might need some assistance with ADLs, e.g. bilateral lower limb amputees
3. residents who can move independently and be independent in ADLs but cannot verbally communicate, e.g. cerebrovascular accident (CVA) with expressive aphasia
4. residents who are unable to communicate their need to change position and need assistance to change position and with ADLs, e.g. acquired brain injury or end-stage dementia
5. residents who lack safety awareness while retaining independent movement and ADLs but may or may not be able to communicate reliably, e.g. CVA or dementia.

For each of these categories of resident there is a different degree of assistance required from care staff. Often the care staff will need to anticipate when the resident will need help to move or maintain safety. Such anticipation cannot be regimented into a care plan but will be determined by the vagaries of the resident and the ability of the care staff to identify when intervention is pertinent. This situation is especially important when dementia or anosognosia prevents the resident from appreciating the potential for falling and supervision or assistance is needed to ensure safety when moving. Caring for a resident who has intact cognition and is able to communicate their needs clearly is easy but a relatively rare occurrence in aged care. The effect of medication as well as emotional and behavioural states such as depression also need to be considered. Physiotherapists also have to assess whether the cause of immobility is reversible or not. It is possible that immobility has been precipitated, for example, by medication usage to control wandering in a person with dementia or voluntarily through fear of falling prior to RACF admission. Such situations should be identified at the admission assessment and an appropriate intervention initiated so that the potential for improved quality of life through some independence in ADLs is maximized for the resident.

Factors contributing to immobility

It is often the utter frailty of the resident that has rendered them immobile. No one cause is usually identified but a multitude of causes that have contributed. In most instances immobility has been acquired in later life but some residents will have congenital or acquired disability from birth or early in life. These residents might not be very elderly but will present with many of the physiological and pathological problems of frail elders. Residents with severe cerebral palsy, intellectual and physical impairment might present in this fashion. Other not so old residents might include people with acquired brain or high cervical spinal cord injury, multiple sclerosis, Alzheimer's disease, motor neuron disease, severe arthritis and cancer. Then there are the elderly who have multiple systemic pathology, stroke, dementia, Parkinson's disease or all of the above. All of these groups of residents will have reduced mobility and most will eventually become immobile towards the end of life. It is therefore important to maintain the ability to move or assist with transfers or bed mobility for as long as possible. To this end, all residents should be encouraged to participate in functional activities.

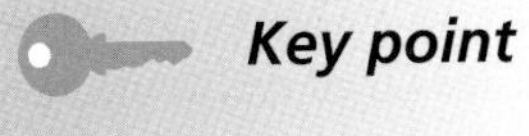
Key point

All residents should be encouraged to participate in care activities and to do as much as possible for themselves. 'Hands off' can be more caring and beneficial than all the help in the world.

Some residents will lose social skills because they are reliant on others to move them from one venue to another in order to participate in activities. Interaction and communication will be affected by this situation, with the result that potential to participate in physically and mentally stimulating activities will be decreased and this will have an impact on motivation to make the most of life. Where possible, residents should be assessed to determine potential to mobilize independently or with assistance in using a wheelchair. Many younger residents would benefit from specialized seating consultations and provision of electric powered or manual wheelchairs. Unfortunately in many facilities there are no wheelchairs available for residents to use for independent mobility since the RACF has to purchase such wheelchairs and funding is generally insufficient. Residents are required to purchase their own wheelchair. Often the most inappropriate wheelchair is chosen through ignorance and because of price. The outcome then is discomfort, injury to the resident when performing transfers and at the other extreme, unavailability as the staff have borrowed it to move another resident.

Depression often accompanies chronic illness or disability and is relatively common in older people (Jorm et al 2000). It can aggravate the degree of immobility found in a resident due to the apathy and lack of interest in life that are symptoms of the condition. Depression should be identified and treated so that functional potential is maximized. Unfortunately immobility can be a result of polypharmacy or poor excretion of drugs with sedative effects. If sedation is suspected as the cause of decreased arousal, medical evaluation of the drug regime should be sought. Inertia and depression due to thyroid disease can be treated in many cases and should be suspected in some residents (Finucane & Anderson 1996).

Another more sinister cause of acquired immobility has been emerging with the advent of the 'no lift' policy in manual handling of residents. Many residents have been deemed hoist transfers because of an acute episode such as a respiratory tract infection that has affected balance or strength and this change in care plan had been made to prevent a fall or injury to a carer during assisted transfers. In most cases this debility can be reversed with the instigation of a judicious exercise programme developed by the physiotherapist. Similar situations occur when a resident puts on weight and independent transferring ability declines to a point where assistance from a carer is needed. In this situation the size of the resident might be considered a risk factor for carer injury and hoist transfers commenced. A better management would be for the physiotherapist and dietitian to assess the resident and instigate an appropriate exercise and eating programme that the resident can undertake that aims to strengthen, reduce weight and maintain independence. Decline in ability is reversible in many cases, especially those involving younger, less frail residents, and should be considered thus. Incorporation of the resident and their families in all phases of development of an intervention designed to retain independence should always occur. This enables the resident to retain autonomy and enhances compliance.

Implications of immobility

When you go to the theatre or watch the cricket or a football match you do not sit in one spot without moving. You wriggle, move the position of your legs by crossing and uncrossing them, lean your trunk forwards, twist in your seat and even stand up to see more clearly. Why do you think you move so much? Consider the situation if you could not perform any of these movements. You would feel stiff, get a numb or sore bottom, lose interest in the entertainment and become focused on your discomfort and generally become grumpy. This is exactly what happens every day to many residents who are left sitting out in a chair all morning or afternoon. These residents are often given 'entertainment' by positioning them in front of the television. Furthermore, if they ask to be moved or put in a different chair, they might be considered a bother and left to sit in discomfort in wet pants for even longer. So it is no wonder they try to stand up and fall over, or cry out and become disruptive to other residents.

Therefore the most obvious outcomes of immobility are physical discomfort and sensory and emotional deprivation. This often leads to the need for increased pain relief. Feelings of hopelessness and lack of worth can ensue that may progress to depression. In many situations behavioural problems or aggression can present and these might be managed inappropriately with sedation or restraint, both of which further aggravate the problem of immobility. Each resident should be evaluated and appropriate diversions supplied. Find out from the relatives what the individual likes. Talking books and classical music provided through headphones might fix the behaviour problem in the intellectually inclined resident who had previously been 'forced' to endure contemporary music and children's television shows. Sometimes residents will find dictating their life stories fulfilling and provision of a Dictaphone might provide hours of relief by enabling this activity.

> *Speaking generally, all parts of the body which have a function, if used in moderation and exercised in labours to which each is accustomed, become thereby healthy and well developed, and age slowly; but if left unused and left idle, they become liable to disease, defective in growth, and age quickly.*
>
> Hippocrates

Physiological problems associated with immobility include circulatory stasis, decreased ventilation and hypoxia, decreased gut motility and constipation, urinary drainage problems and decline in the ability to integrate movement and sensory input, thus increasing balance problems. These residents get very little vestibular stimulation owing to the reclined positions in bed and chair that are interchanged throughout the day. It is no wonder that hoist transfers, which can involve swift movements in many planes of movement, can cause the resident to cry out and become agitated through fear and confusion.

If we analyse resident responses and behaviours using a clinical reasoning process it is often obvious what is causing discomfort and by extending the reasoning, solutions should be sought and implemented in order to improve quality of life for the resident.

Consequences and complications arising from immobility

The visible evidence of immobility that includes pressure areas, skin maceration and venous ulcers are only a few of the complications arising from not being able to move independently. Many residents have the potential for venous stasis and deep vein thrombosis (DVT) formation due to inefficient cardiac and muscle pumps. However, cancer is a common diagnosis and alone can increase the potential for DVT development. The reader is referred to Chapter 3 devoted to resident injuries where circulatory and pressure aspects were addressed.

The not so obvious complications that might affect the immobile resident can also contribute to system decline and are possibly lethal.

Swallowing problems and inability to guard the airway are not solved by nasogastric tube or PEG (percutaneous endoscopic gastrostomy) feeding except to maintain nutrition and hydration of the resident. Saliva is still secreted and if not swallowed or dribbled is likely to be aspirated into the lungs. This can lead to hypoxia from repeated chest infections or pneumonia. Even when this scenario is not present, respiratory function is diminished by the habitual reclined position care staff favour for the immobile resident. Ventilation is impaired when reclining in 'geri-chairs' (seating is discussed in detail in Chapter 7). The supine position is similar to the reclined sitting-out position and it has been shown that such a position causes an increase in the functional residual capacity as well as a decrease in tidal volume (Vitacca et al 1996). This position also results in the inhibition of diaphragm movement and a change to the uniformity of inspired gas and pulmonary gas flow distribution for healthy subjects. Therefore the effect this position has on the lungs of frail elderly people who already demonstrate structural changes such as kyphosis, reduction in alveolar volume, reduced compliance and altered gas exchange due to the ageing process (Webster & Kadah 1991) needs to be considered. In the frail elderly there is a reduced cardiac output that further limits tissue oxygenation. Cumulatively these lowered oxygen levels might lead to reduction in cognition and arousal, delayed wound healing, and delirium (Samuels & Evers 2002).

When the ability for independent movement is lost, joints and muscles lose the ability to change position. The joint capsule becomes tight and muscles can no longer lengthen sufficiently to allow full joint range of movement. Muscle weakness and spasticity that limit the amount of movement available are other factors that might contribute to joint contracture (Farmer & James 2001). However, physiotherapists must remember that muscle, neural and vascular tissue has also shortened. Entrapment of peripheral nerves might have occurred and this is often complicated by adhesion formation, thereby causing neuromechanosensitivity (Butler 2000). Injudicious stretching during passive movement by untrained carers can cause pain from tissue tears or increase in neural tension from entrapment or adhesion. The pain resulting from these outcomes can increase the loss of range of movement and exacerbate the disability imposed by the contractures. When range of movement is lost, difficulties arise in finding sitting positions that are supported and comfortable for the resident and variations on a theme of lying are adopted to 'sit out' the resident. Personal care becomes difficult when hip adduction and shoulder adduction contractures prevent the perineum and axillae from being washed and dried well. The hands of some residents with increased tone in the upper limb also pose problems for personal hygiene. Skin maceration occurs in these areas due to sweating and incontinence, and ulceration is common. Ultimately this can lead to a lethal outcome from infection.

Not moving also leads to sensory deprivation. Vestibular, proprioception, touch, pressure, hearing and visual input is lacking and this leads to integrative problems such as perceptual dysfunction, visual conflict and allodynia. Many residents also have vision and hearing loss, while others have decrease in touch, pressure and thermal sensation that can further interfere with the integration of sensory input. Ultimately the resident might react to these altered perceptions with disruptive behaviour such as crying out as most sensations become quite frightening and uncomfortable to endure. The physiotherapist should be able to identify residents who are at risk of developing or who already suffer these problems and assist the carers with strategies to reduce the resident's discomfort.

Vision and hearing loss can lead to isolation of the resident. Together they can contribute to an inability to communicate with care staff or other residents and so reduce the opportunities for entertainment and interactive activities. The consequences of immobility are summarized in Table 5.1.

The barely mobile resident

The barely mobile resident is one who might only be able to help the carer roll them. Others might be able to help when moving from lying to sitting or with a standing transfer from bed to chair and possibly taking a few steps. Assisting when bathing, dressing, drinking or eating might also be possible. These little abilities can easily be lost if the resident is not encouraged to continue to participate in care activities. Care staff often discourage participation for reasons such as time constraints or even a

Table 5.1 *Consequences of immobility*

Problem	Implication
Injury to the skin	Maceration, tear, pressure, ulcer, infection
Reduced respiratory capacity	Decreased air entry, decreased oxygenation, increased functional residual capacity, decreased cough, increased retention of secretions
Swallowing problems	Decreased guarding of airway, increased potential for aspiration of saliva or food
Inability to move	Joint contractures are acquired, fear of movement develops, pain on movement occurs, difficulty in hygiene and care activities
Pain	Altered perception of sensory input might cause the resident to perceive the feeling of movement or touch as pain
Sensory deprivation	Reduced visual and auditory stimulation, decreased and/or habitual vestibular stimulation, decreased touch, altered perception of sensory inputs
Decline in communication ability	Inability to make eye contact, project voice, see person they are talking to, observe facial expressions and emotion in others
Bladder and bowel problems	Increased residual volumes and likelihood of urinary tract infection. Constipation and discomfort from bloating that often accompanies aperient use. Incontinence increases the potential for skin irritation, infection and pressure areas
Reduced quality of life	Depression, apathy and loss of worth as a person

misguided sense of the role a carer should take, so that everything is done for the resident rather than enabling the resident to assist. Part of the role of the physiotherapist is to educate the care staff regarding the disabling effect the practice of 'helping too much' has on the resident's retention of functional motor ability. Considerable discussion is generally needed with carers to ensure the resident retains their rights to continue performing functional motor tasks. The common argument put forward by the care staff is that the carer does not have the time to wait for the resident to perform the activity as they take a long time and carers have limited time to devote to that individual. Negotiating time management strategies can sometimes alleviate the workload situation but there needs to be considerable willingness to change usual practice before this approach is successful. This aspect has a huge impact on life satisfaction issues for the resident.

The physiotherapist can organize the provision of assistive devices such as bed poles or overhead rings or a low bed that allows the feet to touch the floor for a standing or slide board transfer to facilitate resident participation. Self-esteem is enhanced when a resident can achieve some independence. It encourages a less passive acceptance and more desire to participate in activities that will enhance quality of life. By practising a functional task, the resident can improve the level of proficiency and possibly reduce the need for assistance from care staff. This approach can assist with reducing the workload of carers.

Enabling the resident who can weight-bear to stand up from a raised bed with the assistance of two carers and a walk belt and thus assist in performing a standing transfer might be evaluated and implemented if the physiotherapist considers it safe. Retention of the ability to weight-bear can have far-reaching benefits for the resident.

Thus the barely mobile resident should be fully assessed by the physiotherapist and encouraged to keep active by participation in restorative or maintenance exercise programmes specifically designed for that resident. Team conferences can ensure medications are not contributing to immobility and diversional programmes should be utilized to improve or maintain cognitive function and sensory stimulation and integration. Those residents who have some degree of physical dependency but retain cognitive capacity should be given special assistance to maintain their capabilities so that they can stay in low care situations for as long as possible.

The potentially mobile resident

Assumptions of permanency of immobility can be made for residents entering the RACF from acute hospital care. It is relatively common for people who have suffered a stroke and have considerable sensorimotor or perceptual deficit to be listed for RACFs before any recovery has occurred or if recovery is slow. Many of these residents will improve with appropriate physiotherapeutic intervention to facilitate movement recovery and functional task ability. Often depression overlies the physical presentation in people after a stroke and it is not until this inertia is overcome that positive progress towards recovery can be made. The physiotherapist should always fully assess the new stroke resident and instigate appropriate treatment so that potential is maximized. Advice to the staff regarding management of specific problems presenting in the individual resident is also important. Such an example would be the resident with a stroke presenting as a 'pusher' (Ashburn 1995). Most carers would automatically try to hold the resident upright but would not be aware that pushing against the side to which the resident is leaning exacerbates the problem. In these cases the carers should be taught to use a structured environment that enables the resident to use sensory and verbal cues to move away from the direction to which they 'push'. It is only the repeated experience of moving into this space that normalizes the sensory and motor integration; this ultimately allows confidence in interpretation of sensory input and leads to safer movement (Pedersen et al 1996).

Strategies for preventing complications arising from immobility

The initial care plan meeting should involve the resident, the family, physiotherapist, carers, medical officer and pharmacist. All aspects of the admission assessments will be discussed, with identification of the main problems relating to care needs considered. At the same time, the goals and aspirations of the new resident should be incorporated in the care plan. All members of the team must realize that the care plan that eventuates at this initial meeting remains flexible. It should reflect the individual differences possessed by the resident and his or her family and potential for change in the condition and functional abilities of the resident. Remember the important components that contribute to life satisfaction. These considerations should not be denied to residents who are terminally ill or in a vegetative state from brain injury just because it is easier to follow protocols rather than comply with stated desires and needs.

An extremely simple way of increasing the resident's ability to move independently is to provide assisting devices. Work with the resident. If given the potential to solve a personal problem of mobility many residents, young or old, will be encouraged to do more. In other words, the resident is shown respect and there is value placed on their opinion and ideas. Self-esteem immediately rises. They might have devised individual methods of undertaking a task that is not 'usual practice'. The role of the physiotherapist in these instances might be to ensure safety is preserved in the new environment of the RACF or to suggest a more efficient method of achieving the same independence in the task. We should be careful not to ridicule innovative though unsafe methods the resident has devised.

When potential for functional improvement is evident the physiotherapist must immediately instigate a programme that is most effective in restoring function. Goal-oriented task practice (Dean et al 2000) is probably the most useful approach in these circumstances. It allows the resident, family and carers to see the meaning of the task being practised in relation to self-care, communication and functional independence.

If the resident is not able to improve their functional status, the responsibility of the carers is to prevent complications. Thus the safest, most comfortable and supportive as well as stimulating environment should be provided to ensure quality of life to the end. Therefore pain and incontinence need consideration in addition to the furniture and environment to fulfil these needs. The succeeding chapters will look at these aspects in considerable detail.

The tragic outcomes of cost cutting and ignorance

Insufficient staff can lead to complaints that there is insufficient time available to assist with mobility. The most common instance where care staff can assist with maintenance of mobility is in helping residents walk to meals. Accompanying the resident to provide direction when the ability to find the venue is lost or to ensure safety if balance is a problem is the care task that is considered too time-consuming as resident walking pace is very slow. Thus to speed up the process residents are placed in wheelchairs and sped from their room to the dining room. A novel solution that would assist with such a problem would be to team up cognitively capable residents who can mobilize independently with residents who get lost and encourage them to help by performing the guide role. Of course this only works if there are residents with the capability to assist. On the other hand, the carer might ask the disorientated mobile resident to accompany him or her while assisting the resident with poor balance. Thus two residents are delivered to the dining room and time is saved. Simple time-saving strategies might need to be identified for staff, with suitable resident combinations also identified by the physiotherapist.

Unfortunately, if all residents are treated in the same manner without regard for their individual abilities and personal preferences, they will soon assume the same non-responsive immobile persona. Lack of willingness to change the care approach, on the grounds that it is too hard and time-consuming to do so, should not be acceptable for residents, families or RACF management. The argument that the change might cost more and no funds are available should not be acceptable. Inflexibility born of ignorance can be overcome by judicious discussion, problem-solving sessions and utilization of the skills the physiotherapist has in education and negotiation to assist care staff and management to change practices in order to improve life satisfaction for everybody.

Summary

- Frail, fully dependent, immobile residents require special attention within RACFs. Because of their condition, complex problems often arise which require a preventative, educational approach to management.
- Communication, cognition and safety are key factors that influence the management of immobile residents. Physiotherapists and other staff need to use a great deal of anticipation in order to prevent poor or risky situations and therefore avoid negative consequences.
- Assessment initially needs to establish whether the resident's immobility is reversible. If this may be possible, treatment should target mobility as a priority in order to prevent the cascade of negative factors associated with the inability to move and walk.
- Many factors may contribute to immobility. One of the most preventable features is 'learned disuse', or 'learned helplessness' caused by staff assisting a resident too much. It is crucial that staff learn to encourage the resident to do as much as possible for themselves – 'hands off', unless necessary.
- The implications of immobility are vast. They include physical and emotional problems, and discomfort. The consequences

of this can be increased pain, morbidity and mortality due to many problems (see Table 5.1).

- Good management is essential and does not just include pressure area care alone. Therapeutic exercise to prevent soft tissue shortening and joint contractures, respiratory exercise, vestibular stimulation, diversional therapy and ongoing review are all important.
- Swallowing ability and appropriate positioning or techniques for assisting with meals should be documented by the physiotherapist (in association with the speech therapist), whenever concern regarding a particular resident is raised.
- 'No lift' policies are important in terms of workplace health and safety. The decision to use mechanical lifters with a resident is not usually an easy one, but physiotherapists need to remember to review their decisions in light of new abilities. Residents may improve and no longer require hoist transfers after acute illnesses or periods of deterioration.

References

Ashburn A 1995 Behavioural deficits associated with the 'pusher' syndrome. Proceedings of World Congress of Physiotherapists, Washington DC, p 819

Butler D S 2000 The sensitive nervous system. Noigroup Publications, Adelaide

Dean C, Richards C, Malouin F 2000 Task-related circuit training improves the performance of locomotor tasks in chronic stroke: a randomised, controlled pilot trial. Archives of Physical Medicine and Rehabilitation 81:409–417

Farmer S E, James M 2001 Contractures in orthopaedic and neurological conditions: a review of causes and treatment. Disability and Rehabilitation 23(13):549–558

Finucane P, Anderson C 1996 Thyroid disease in older patients: diagnosis and treatment. Current Therapeutics 4:72–79

Jorm A F, Grayson D, Creasey H, Waite L, Broe G A 2000 Long-term benzodiazepine use by elderly people living in the community. Australian and New Zealand Journal of Public Health 24(1):7–10

Pedersen P M, Wandel A, Jorgensen H S et al 1996 Ipsilateral pushing in stroke: incidence, relation to neuropsychological symptoms, and impact on rehabilitation. The Copenhagen Stroke Study. Archives of Physical Medicine and Rehabilitation 77(1):25–28

Rappl L, Jones D A 2000 Seating evaluation: special problems and interventions for older adults. Topics in Geriatric Rehabilitation 16(2):63–71

Samuels S C, Evers M M 2002 Delirium: pragmatic guidance for managing a common confounding, and sometimes lethal condition. Geriatrics 57:33–38

Vitacca M, Clini E, Spassini W et al 1996 Does the supine position worsen respiratory function in elderly subjects? Gerontology 42:46–53

Webster J R, Kadah H 1991 Unique aspects of respiratory disease in the aged. Geriatrics 46(7):31–43

6 Managing problems encountered in immobile or barely mobile residents

Jennifer C. Nitz

This chapter aims to:

- identify why and when movement is important for residents unable to move themselves
- discuss methods of maintaining movement potential by maintenance of joint range, control of abnormal tone and prevention of deformities
- discuss the factors that might change from time to time that could impact on ability to maintain physical performance in residents
- raise the carer's awareness of the potential for resident or carer injury when assisting movement
- discuss maximizing respiratory function through preventative intervention and treatment of acute or chronic chest conditions.

Introduction

There are a number of problems that the physiotherapist and carers encounter in residents who are immobile or barely mobile. These problems are related to the medical conditions presenting in the resident as well as problems that have been acquired through immobility. In the previous chapter the consequences of immobility were identified. Now methods of managing these problems are discussed using clinical reasoning and evidence-based arguments. In many instances the physiotherapist relies on care staff to assist with implementation of an intervention programme as part of the care plan. Carers often ask physiotherapists why they should be asked to assist residents to move or to perform passive movements of limbs. In many instances these questions are posed because of a care plan order and the carer's perception that compliance is a waste of time or an imposition upon an already tight schedule. Unfortunately, the need for untrained carers to implement physiotherapeutic intervention programmes stems from cost cutting by managements and the lack of understanding that these interventions require continual reassessment and adaptation during application in order to accommodate to the responses gained from the resident. This skill is only provided by physiotherapists and is the reason why response to intervention is better if the treatment is undertaken by them. Quality of care is determined by the quality of service.

The fully dependent resident

The life expectancy for residents who are fully dependent for all care depends on the reason for immobility. The resident might be in a vegetative state from an acquired brain injury. In these instances the age and presence of co-morbidities often determine length of survival. Or the resident might have suffered a high spinal cord injury. In this instance the potential for communication and cognition is normal and the person is trapped in their body. Often these residents are young and their life expectancy might be a further 50 years. At the other end of the spectrum the fully dependent state might only last hours or a few days, as might be the case for some cancer sufferers. In all instances the rights of the resident must be respected. They and their families should expect and receive the highest standard of care. The residents are still individuals and must have assessments that identify their own problems, and care plans that set goals that fit their needs and wishes, not some outdated and inappropriate protocol that was originally designed to treat the 'fully dependent resident'.

Problems likely to be encountered in the fully dependent resident can vary widely. All have immobility and the need to rely on others for movement, eating, drinking, hygiene and control of continence. When movement is not undertaken, tissues and joints lose their extensibility and contractures form (Johnson et al 1992). Some of these residents also will have lost skin sensation and are therefore at greater risk of trauma from friction, pressure and shear forces. Communication might be possible with some residents but difficult, variable or impossible with others. Other problems might include joint damage, abnormal muscle tone, oedema, poor respiratory function and pain. Ultimately many of these problems can be alleviated to some extent through maintaining movement ability either with the individual's volition or with full assistance. There are three levels of movement.

- *Active* movement describes the movement that a resident can initiate and control independently.
- *Assisted active* movement utilizes some effort to initiate and control movement on the part of the resident, with the carer assisting performance so that a complete movement is possible.
- *Passive* movement describes the situation where all movement is performed by the carer for the resident.

The importance of maintaining movement ability

Movement of body parts may occur from volition on the part of the individual or involuntary activation of motor activity due to central nervous system pathology, or it is imposed on the body by an outside force such as gravity. Once the resident loses the ability to voluntarily control or initiate movement and has lost postural stability, potential for safe independence in activities of daily living is lost. Additionally the resident acquires an increased risk of developing co-morbidities that might be life-threatening as they are now reliant on carers for prevention. Table 6.1 identifies the consequence of immobility and the possible implications for the resident and the carers.

Remedial measures that might be taken to limit the development of co-morbidities from immobility commonly include passive movement of limbs. Passive movements appear to the observer to require little skill. This is not so. The use of passive movements of body parts to prevent shortening of soft tissues, maintain joint range of movement and provide sensory stimuli requires extensive knowledge in the areas of anatomy, the pathologies of ageing and abnormal tone if injury is to be avoided.

Passive movement

Why is there the need for anatomical knowledge when passively moving a limb? Most joints are complex and allow for more than one plane of movement. Flexion and extension of a joint is commonly seen by unskilled carers as the only direction that needs to be addressed when passive movements are performed, thereby neglecting abduction and adduction, rotation and glides. Carers without physiotherapy training do not generally possess sufficient anatomical or kinesiological knowledge to incorporate the complex interaction between adjacent joints that allows movements such as arm elevation above the head to occur. Stiffness in the vertebral joints through lack of trunk movement also impacts on costovertebral joints and respiratory function, scapular mobility and upper limb function.

Passive movements should move the joints through the available range of movement in a reciprocal fashion. Repeated rhythmical movement assists with improving blood supply to the muscles, lubricates joints and slides neural and vascular tissue inside the fascial sheaths. This increases the extensibility of the tissues and enables slightly more movement to occur with repetition. Changing the length of muscle with passive movements also stimulates the muscle spindles (Lewis & Byblow 2002, Seiss et al 2002) and Golgi tendon organs as well as joint mechanoreceptors, thereby increasing proprioceptive input. In addition the manual handling of the body facilitates touch and pressure nerve endings in the skin. The combined sensory inputs produce considerable central nervous system stimulation (Radovanic et al 2002). Thus these sensory stimuli are vital for preventing situations of decreased sensorimotor integration that contribute to sensory deprivation and an agitated frightened resident. Residents who might benefit from passive movements include those who are fully dependent and those who are unable to move a limb or limbs through full range independently such as after a stroke or spinal cord injury.

Table 6.1
Consequences of immobility

Consequences of immobility	Implications for residents
Shortening of soft tissues including muscle, neurovascular bundles and joint structures	Pain and loss of range of movement
Altered perception of movement	Fear and reduced desire to move
Loss of joint range of movement in the:	
Hip and shoulder joint	Difficulty in maintaining perineal and axillary hygiene and dressing
Hand	Skin breakdown from trapped moisture Untrimmed fingernails growing into the flesh
Hip, knee and ankle	Lower limb joint range loss can make provision of appropriate seating difficult and expensive to obtain
Inability to relieve pressure	Increased potential for skin trauma and ulcer development
Decreased sensory stimulation	Loss of efficiency of sensorimotor integration causing further decline in postural stability, muscle strength and potential to assist in physical activities Greater likelihood of adverse reactions to movement, especially during hoisted transfers when sudden vestibular stimulation might cause fear and anxiety because of inability to integrate the sensory input Allodynia might present owing to altered sensory input
Any painful stimulus such as a pressure ulcer, sore joint, full bladder or bowel	Exaggerates increased tone
Accelerated loss of bone mineral density and worsening of osteoporosis	The resident becomes more susceptible to bone fracture from trivial trauma such as unskilled passive movements of limbs affected by spasticity
Inefficient muscle pump	Dependency oedema
Decreased options for mobility if the resident does not possess a wheelchair	Reduced possibility for communication, participation in entertainment activities and for excursions outside the RACF
Increased isolation	Increased depression, decreased motivation and decline in cognitive function
Decreased bladder and bowel function	Lack of movement can reduce gut motility and cause constipation or gut obstruction Bladder drainage is limited

Precautions and contraindications for passive movement

When passive movements are performed by an operator on the resident the aim is generally to maintain length of soft tissues and range of joints. To this end movement might be limited to a single joint or to multiple joints and the surrounding soft tissues. The more complex the movement produced the less control the operator has over the movement and there is a greater risk of unintentional injury. Thus if the physiotherapist is instructing unskilled carers in the art of passive movement it is advisable to keep the movements simple and localized to a small area.

Residents who might benefit from passive movements often have medical conditions that present with problems that increase the risk of injury during passive movement application. The physiotherapist should be the person who determines suitability for having passive movements applied by persons other than trained physiotherapists. A thorough assessment incorporating an understanding of the past medical history in the context of the presenting problems in the resident should allow the physiotherapist to make a clinically reasoned decision regarding whether passive movements are indicated. From this process the physiotherapist will determine who should apply them and any precautions that need to be taken during application. All this reasoning process must be entered in the resident's file with specific reference to rationale for contraindications to application or when caution and specific care must be taken. Table 6.2 lists the conditions and the problems that indicate that passive movements are contraindicated or that extreme care must be taken during application.

Nurses in general do not have the knowledge needed to make informed decisions regarding passive movement prescription. Care should be taken to ensure that nursing procedures for the management of immobile residents do not include passive limb movement as a routine entry. Such routine practices risk causing injury to residents and might open the facility to litigation.

Once the decision is made that passive movements are appropriate for the individual resident, those movements that are suitable for the resident should be entered in the care plan and the person who is to apply the technique identified.

The following section discusses the rationale and possible applications of passive movements for residents.

Where to start encouraging movement or applying passive movements

Head and neck movement

Many residents will retain the ability to move their head and they should be encouraged to move as often as possible. Carers can draw the resident's attention to interesting objects so that they are stimulated to turn their head and look. Residents should also be encouraged to turn their heads and talk to other residents. Head movement not only maintains joint range but also assists in increasing vestibular stimulation and the integration of vision and vestibular input with proprioception from the neck joints and muscles. Some residents will need assistance to move to the limits of range, and in these cases gentle assistance should be given to enter that range. Care should be taken not to hold extremes of range as vertebrobasilar insufficiency is very common in the older person. The speed of movement should also be moderated so as to be tolerated by the person. Some residents will be unable to move their own head.

Table 6.2
Contraindications and precautions for application of passive movements

Condition	Rationale for contraindication or caution
Osteoporosis Elderly residents Connective tissue diseases (RA, SLE) Steroid drug use (organ transplant, COPD, CTD) SCI, ABI, MS and other non-ambulant residents	Potential for pathological fracture is great. Force applied at the end of range might cause fracture. Rotational forces are most likely to cause fracture of long bones and vertebrae. *Caution* should be used at all times
Cancer and possibility for bone metastases	Any forced movements might cause a pathological fracture. *Contraindicated* for non-physiotherapy staff
Joint instability RA, Charcot joint, polio Hip or knee joint replacement Girdlestone's procedure	Lack of capsular and ligament support prevents accurate 'feel' of end of joint range and the correct plane of movement thus trauma to structures is likely. *Caution* is needed
Pain	Pain from any cause indicates movement is *contraindicated* until the cause is identified and treated
Abnormal muscle tone Spasticity (SCI, MS, stroke, TBI) Rigidity (Parkinson's disease, CP) Athetosis (CP) Flaccidity (polio, peripheral nerve lesion, diabetic neuropathy, muscular dystrophy)	As many of the conditions that present in older people and lead to increased tone or decreased tone also cause limited mobility, these residents will be most likely to present with osteoporosis and/or joint instability that require *caution* when considering passive movement application
Rheumatoid arthritis	The neck vertebrae of people with RA can be very unstable between many segments thus increasing the potential for spinal cord injury. *Passive neck movement is contraindicated*

SLE, systemic lupus erythematosus; RA, rheumatoid arthritis; COPD, chronic obstructive pulmonary disease; CTD, connective tissue disease; SCI, spinal cord injury; ABI, acquired brain injury; MS, multiple sclerosis; CP, cerebral palsy; TBI, traumatic brain injury.

Sometimes this is due to an increase in muscle tone that is limiting all or some movement directions. The presence of medical conditions such as rheumatoid disease must be identified before any passive movements of the head and neck are initiated for the reasons identified in Table 6.2.

Trunk movement

Gentle rotational movements between the upper and lower trunk applied while the resident is lying on the side will assist in maintaining rib movement range as well as reducing joint stiffness that might be contributing to the resident's pain. Trunk-on-trunk rotation can also be gained by gently rocking the bent lower limbs from side to side while the resident is lying in supine. The speed of movement should be slow with care taken not to force into extra range at the available movement extremes. Force can precipitate fracture of vertebrae and femurs affected by osteoporosis. Encouragement to participate in the movements should also be mandatory for residents able to cooperate and produce some muscle activity. If the ability of the resident to assist with trunk rotation is improved, they are more able to assist with rolling from side to side and less effort is then needed from the carer. The movement also may increase comfort for the resident by improving joint nutrition and flexibility throughout the skeletal system. Discomfort is often brought about by prolonged periods with little movement in beds or chairs.

Spasticity affecting neck and trunk musculature also can be reduced to some extent with the application of slow rhythmical rotational movements.

Scapula movement

The movement of the scapula around the rib cage might be limited by joint stiffness or muscle tightness. The muscle tightness can be due to habitual posture and adaptive shortening of muscles such as the pectorals and parts of serratus anterior. An increased thoracic kyphosis due to osteoporotic collapse of vertebrae will precipitate this postural adaptation. Generally the opposing muscle groups will then be maintained in a lengthened position induced by the posture and any contractile ability will be inhibited, which increases the postural deformity.

Increased muscle tone from central nervous system pathology commonly affects the muscles that elevate and retract the scapula and internally rotate the glenohumeral joint. These muscles include the pectoral, teres major, subscapularis, rhomboid and latissumus dorsi muscles (Bohannon et al 1986, Mayer et al 1997, Van Langenberghe & Hogan 1988). Tightness in these muscles may cause limitation of scapular movement into depression, protraction and lateral rotation and may also limit glenohumeral joint movements of flexion, abduction and external rotation. These movements are necessary to direct the glenoid cavity upwards and allow full glenohumeral movements that enable elevation of the arm above the head.

The side lying position is the best for the resident when scapular movements are being performed. It is important to support the weight of the arm while moving the scapula. This might be done on pillows or by the person applying the movement. The scapula is grasped by both hands, one placed near the glenohumeral joint the other inferiorly on the medial border. These hand positions allow the operator to control the movement well. When applying the passive movement the operator should be cognizant of the need to move around the curve of the rib cage and not grind the scapula across the ribs during the movement, as this could be uncomfortable for the resident. Movements can also be combined. Moving the scapula in the two diagonal patterns of movement is recommended. One pattern combines retraction with elevation then movement towards protraction and depression and the second pattern protraction and elevation combined followed by movement towards retraction and depression. The principle of combining movement components was emphasized by the proprioceptive neuromuscular facilitation philosophy (Adler et al 1993).

Upper limb movement

Any passive movement that involves elevation of the arm above the head should incorporate scapular movement. Thus the operator should move the arm with one hand while ensuring appropriate scapular positioning with the other. This is a complex skill that needs coordination between the hands and knowledge of scapulohumeral rhythm. Maximal range of movement is more easily obtained if the operator holds the humerus close to the glenohumeral joint in the axilla. This hold allows incorporation of external rotation of the humerus with humeral flexion so that impingement of the greater tubercle of the humerus and rotator cuff does not occur under the acromial process (Tyson & Chissim 2002). If these aspects of movement are not undertaken, injury will occur and pain and further loss of joint range will eventuate. Adherence to these principles is advised when handling residents who have paralysis of the arm such as occurs after a stroke.

Loss of external rotation of the glenohumeral joint has been identified as a contributing factor for shoulder pain in a number of pathologies including tetraplegia from spinal cord injury (Salisbury et al 2003) and stroke (Bohannon et al 1986, Joynt 1992, Zorowitz et al 1995). The latissimus dorsi muscle plays an important part in limiting trunk-on-trunk rotation, trunk flexion, scapular protraction and abduction and glenohumeral external rotation, abduction and flexion (Nitz 1982). Thus when moving any of the body parts addressed so far, the influence of tightness in this large muscle should be considered and special attention paid to maintaining length and associated joint ranges of movement.

The elbow and superior radio-ulnar joint

Combining elbow flexion with supination and extension with pronation of the forearm allows movement of joint structures as well as maximum lengthening of the muscles crossing the joints. It also utilizes the normal muscle synergy combinations, thus enhancing the sensorimotor effect. Commonly the biceps, brachialis and brachioradialis and forearm pronators as well as long wrist and finger and thumb flexors are affected by

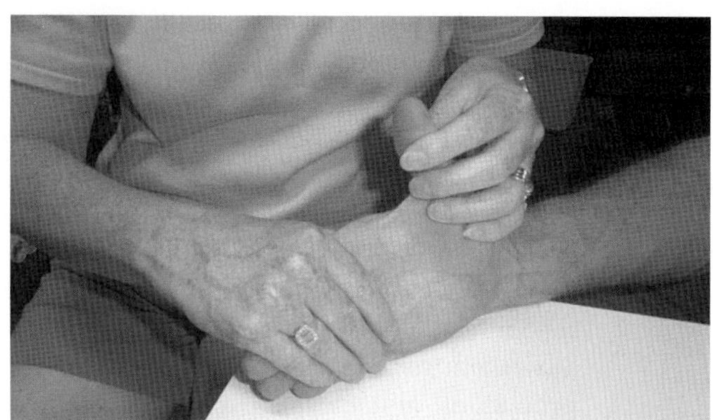

Figure 6.1 *Correct method of handling the thumb for passive movement application.*

spasticity (Mayer et al 1997). Slow rhythmical movement of the limb in this manner provides the additional advantage of reducing this spasticity.

Wrist and hand movements

Gentle wrist movements might be incorporated into the elbow movement. However, in the presence of tight muscles, loss of muscle length often prevents the combining of these passive movements. Wrist movements should include flexion, extension, radial and ulnar deviation. The tenodesis effect of enabling finger extension with the wrist in flexion might be a useful method of maintaining finger joint extension range when shortness and/or spasticity is present in flexor digitorum superficialis and flexor digitorum profundus muscles (Mayer et al 1997). Carpometacarpal glides will help maintain the ability of the hand to 'cup' so that thumb opposition remains effective and hand function is retained. It is equally important to open out the hand so it can be flattened on a surface so it can be used as a prop to assist with sitting balance or for stabilizing an object. Spasticity commonly affects the thenar muscles of the thumb (Mayer et al 1997). Passive movements of the thumb should be undertaken carefully, with the operator grasping the first metacarpal during opposition, extension, abduction, flexion and adduction movements. Otherwise, if the phalanges are held, abnormal stresses might be imparted to the metacarpophalangeal (MCP) joint causing trauma. Figure 6.1 shows the correct method of handling the thumb for passive movement application and Figure 6.2 shows the effect of poor handling. Movements of the MCP joints should include flexion and extension combined with finger flexion or with the fingers in extension. Abduction and adduction movement should also be undertaken with the MCP joints in extension. If the MCP joints cannot be extended, these movements should not be done because anatomically abduction and adduction are not possible in the flexed MCP joint.

Lower limb movements

Specific attention should be given to maintaining hip abduction and external rotation range so that perineal hygiene can be easily attended to. Before any large limb movements are carried out, gentle hip rotations with the limb supported flat on the bed help to reduce stiffness of arthritic joints and improve the result of subsequent movements. The speed of

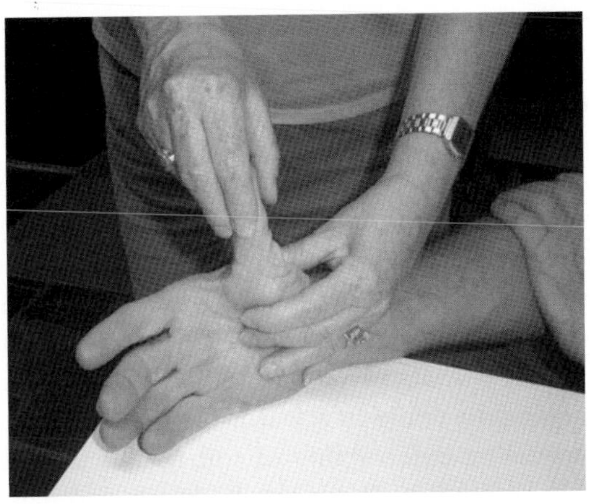

Figure 6.2
The effect of poor handling.

passive rotation mobilizations will be determined by the presence of increased tone from central nervous system pathology but slow movements still are effective. This procedure can still be done if there is a hip flexion contracture. Support the leg on pillows then gently and slowly rock the femur to obtain the rotations. Always make sure the heel is not rubbing on the sheet and being damaged by friction during this manoeuvre. Passive movement of the hip is contraindicated when protrusio acetabuli or severe osteoporosis is known to be present in the femoral neck. Never force a movement. After a few rotations, gentle hip abduction and adduction, flexion and extension should be undertaken. Internal and external rotation plus hip abduction and adduction with the hip being held in a flexed position might be considered. Caution is advised especially when a hip replacement is present. These movements will help reduce spasticity in the affected muscles including hip adductors, hamstrings and hip flexors (Mayer et al 1997).

Knee joint movement might be obtained most easily when the resident is sitting in a chair or by supporting the hip in some flexion then moving the shank. Again gentle slow rotation of the tibia on the femur when the knee is in about 60 degrees of flexion will help maintain cartilage health and hamstring length. Combining hip extension with knee flexion is also necessary to stretch the quadriceps muscle where spasticity and tightness is common (Mayer et al 1997).

It is extremely important to maintain the plantigrade position of the foot. Ankle dorsiflexion movements that stretch soleus performed with the knee flexed will allow this. Calf stretches that are applied with the knee in extension certainly maintain gastrocnemius muscle and neurovascular bundle length, but possible problems caused by applying passive dorsiflexion movement in this position include pain from neural tension, muscle or tendon tears or posterior knee joint capsule injury. Passive movements that stretch muscles such as gastrocnemius and tibialis anterior with long tendons have been shown to maximally lengthen the muscle-tendon units (Herbert et al 2002). With the response to stretch focused in this region extra care should be exercised during application, as it is known that changes in this tissue due to ageing might increase the risk of tears. The reader is referred to Chapter 1, where the age-related changes to tissues were identified.

Maintenance of the length of the longitudinal ligaments of the feet can help reduce the possibility of varus deformities that can interfere with footwear in younger disabled residents. Gentle distraction of the calcaneus from the anterior foot structures can help.

Passive movements can be applied when the resident is on the bed, sitting in a chair or in the bath. Many residents respond well to gentle movement while in a warm bath. Some advantages include the warmth increasing extensibility of soft tissues as well as general relaxation and pain reduction. The warm bath can also make the passive movements a pleasurable sensory experience that might have a calming effect for agitated residents. In some instances the warmth of the bath might reduce muscle tone.

Many residents suffer medical conditions that have resulted in abnormal tone. It is therefore appropriate to consider management procedures for coping with abnormal tone other than passive movement.

Managing the resident with abnormal tone

Spasticity

Spasticity presents in well-recognized synergic patterns. When spasticity is due to conditions such as stroke, multiple sclerosis (MS) and spinal cord injury, the forces acting on joints and muscles determine the prevailing patterns. In both the upper and lower limbs, gravity produces a distracting force and is imposed on a limb that is dependent and not bearing any weight. This force will stretch muscles and result in a flexion abduction and externally rotated posture of the hip with the knee flexed in the lower limb. In the upper limb, the elbow is flexed, shoulder adducted and internally rotated, the forearm pronated and the wrist and hand flexed. These flexion synergies are perpetuated if continually stimulated by the effect of gravity or a noxious stimulus. In other residents with atherothrombotic brain infarct (ABI), extensor synergies of the upper or lower limbs might predominate. In the lower limbs, knee extension, equinovarus and great toe extension accompany hip extension, adduction and internal rotation. The upper limb extensor synergy includes shoulder extension, adduction, internal rotation, elbow extension, pronation and wrist and finger flexion. Variations of these spastic synergic presentations are found. Factors that facilitate the abnormal tone include gravitational pull, head position, pressure under the ball of the foot, or on the toes, pain and irritating stimuli such as tight bedclothes, socks, shoes and unrelieved pressure. Less obvious causes include a full bladder (possibly due to a blocked catheter) or a full bowel or wind, abdominal pathology commonly includes diverticulitis, gut obstruction, gall bladder or renal stones or bile duct or ureter obstruction. Differential diagnosis of medical or surgical conditions is the realm of the doctor but the physiotherapist should be able to determine aggravating causes of the spasticity and instigate management practices that help the resident and carers to lead a satisfactory life. Any change in the presentation of spasticity or an increase in isolated muscle spasm should be investigated, with all possible aggravating factors considered. Often the solution is simple. For example, the unexplained increase in spasms in the lower limbs of a resident with complete spinal cord injury might be due to new shoes that are too tight across the toes and causing pressure injury. In this instance the noxious stimulus from unrelieved pressure mediates the flexor withdrawal response, which is a spinal reflex (Bannister 1978). Inspection of the skin of the feet will show redness or even skin breakdown in the area of irritation and changing the shoes easily solves the problem.

When spasticity interferes with the life satisfaction of the resident by causing pain, disturbing sleep and causing major difficulties for carers, the physiotherapist and doctor might discuss treatment options with the resident and other team members. At this meeting clear goals for relieving spasticity need to be identified and the methods of measuring the outcome of the interventions determined (Barnes 1998, Pierson 1997). Some of the goals are very simple and pertain to increasing the ease with which carers can attend to hygiene, control continence, dress or transfer the resident. The potential for carer injury should also be considered as a reason for instigating additional spasticity control. The muscle spasms experienced by residents with spinal cord injury are often so strong that they might cause the resident to 'jack-knife' during a hoisted or slide board assisted transfer or when seated in their wheelchair. If the carer tried to 'catch' the resident to prevent a fall, personal injury might be sustained. Prescription of oral anti-spastic medication is usually the first management choice. Many of these medications cause drowsiness or in some instances are liver toxic, so the lowest effective dose is preferred (Barnes 1998). The physiotherapist might be required to monitor the response to medication through applying a suitable outcome measurement so that titration of the most effective dose is achieved easily.

More recently control of annoying local muscle spasm has been achieved through injection with botulinum toxin into individual muscles that have particularly troublesome spasms (Ward 2002). In some very severe cases intrathecal medication delivered at a continual rate via a pump might be indicated to control spasms (Barnes 1998). Residents might also benefit from phenol injection into selected peripheral nerves. This blocks the neural excitation of the muscle and stops the spasms. It can also cause sensory loss, damage to other local tissues and pain (Barnes 1998).

Adjunct management initiated by the physiotherapist or occupational therapist such as special positioning, seating and splinting or casting is useful. Bed and seating considerations are addressed in the following chapter, which includes quite complex discussion of furniture components and rationale for choosing specific chairs and attachments.

Orthotic devices such as static splints or serial casts have been used to prevent contracture development or to lengthen tissues when spasticity is present (Barnes 1998). It is likely that both biomechanical and neurophysiological mechanisms are contributing to the gaining or maintenance of tissue length (Lannin et al 2003). Most therapists agree that the use of orthotics is not indicated when active movement is present. Thus residents who are immobile and at risk of developing contractures from habitual postures and/or spasticity of muscle groups might benefit from the use of orthotics for co-morbidity prevention. It is very important to stress that movement must still be provided for the resident. An orthosis does not negate this activity. However, some residents come to the facility with established contractures. The cause of the contracture must be established so that the most appropriate method of overcoming the problem can be chosen. When spasticity is a major contributor anti-spastic medication needs to be considered so that the adjunct treatment using orthotics can have the best chance of being effective. Lengthening of soft tissues and joint structures will involve stretch being applied. This is often painful and if spasticity is present the noxious stimulus will increase the spasm. This will increase pressure between the skin and orthotic interface and the possibility of tissue damage. Therefore any splinting should be delayed until spasm is controlled. If this control is unsatisfactory with oral mediation, botulinum toxin injection might be deemed appropriate.

The most troublesome and potentially the most harmful contractures are those affecting the hand, where the fingers and thumb are clenched in a fist and there is the potential for maceration, infection and skin breakdown (Wilton 1997). Spacers placed between the fingers and palm are used to prevent this problem. Wilton (1997) recommends that the spacer is placed adjacent to the proximal and middle phalanges so that the amount of flexion at the MCP and proximal interphalangeal (PIP) joints is controlled. Adding more rigid materials to the centre of the rolled spacer might increase range. Ideally the spacer should be washable so that odour from sweat is removed. The spacer should be removed daily so that the hands can be washed and thoroughly dried and passive movements undertaken to assist with gaining more range and comfort. Inflatable plastic spacers are another way of providing this type of stretch in the hand.

Serial casting might be considered to increase knee or elbow joint range of movement. It is advisable for a physiotherapist, occupational therapist or orthotist skilled in their application and conversant with the problems specific to the older person to apply these casts. Skin trauma from excessive interface pressure is a high risk and the consequences of this eventuality should be considered fully before deciding to use this technique to gain range or when deciding to use any splint to maintain range in the presence of spasticity.

Other interventions with relatively short-lasting effect include cold or heat application. Cold in the form of ice packs or ice baths has been utilized by physiotherapists for reducing muscle spasm so that facilitation of normal movement is possible (Price et al 1993). Tone might be reduced somewhat for up to one hour but then gradually returns. In two of the subjects in the study by Price et al (1993) spasticity was aggravated by the application of ice. However, ice treatments are generally contraindicated for older people owing to the prevalence of obstructive arterial disease (OAD). Since over 80% of residents in RACFs have been identified as having OAD (Paris et al 1988), only the occasional resident with MS might be suitable for this method of reducing tone. The physiotherapist is cautioned that although young the resident with MS might have circulation problems and should be assessed for signs of arterial and venous insufficiency and autonomic dysfunction prior to introducing this treatment.

Gentle warmth is possibly more appropriate and can be combined with passive movement application in a bath for more effect. Stronger heat treatments including hot packs are not recommended because of the need for efficient circulation responses as were needed for cold tolerance. Also the presence of skin sensory loss is common in the residents with muscle spasms and so contraindicates their use.

Electrical stimulation has also been used to reduce spasticity and enhance the potential for motor activation of opposing muscle groups in people after stroke (Alfieri 1982). This concept of functional electrical stimulation (FES) has been utilized by physiotherapists for motor retraining in many neurological conditions. There has been very little use for specifically reducing muscle tone without the added advantage of stimulating contraction of opposing muscles. The proposed neurophysiological mechanism that inhibits spasticity in the antagonists to the muscles being stimulated is the stimulation of Golgi tendon organs in these antagonists as a result of the contraction of the stimulated muscles (Alfieri 1982). This principle has been shown to reduce spasticity when applied in both the upper and lower limbs (Alfieri 1982, Seib et al 1994) and is well worth trying as the stimulation can be applied using the burst mode available on many TENS units.

Measurement of response to intervention should be an integral part of spasticity treatment. Although there are some scales that measure spasticity such as the Ashworth Scale (Bohannon et al 1986), they lack meaning when considering the stated goal for using anti-spastic medication or adjunct therapies. Pierson (1997) recommends that functional improvement be measured. Depending on the ability of the resident the functional measure chosen might include many items such as the Functional Independence Measure (Rankin 1993) or the Clinical Outcomes Variable Scale (Seaby & Torrance 1989). In other situations where the resident is immobile and the goal of treatments is to make it easier for carers to provide hygiene assistance, carer satisfaction might be the better measure.

Rigidity

Rigidity and akinesia are major problems for residents with Parkinson's disease and other conditions affecting the extrapyramidal system. Medication is the main method of controlling the movement disorder of Parkinson's disease. It is vitally important for the dose to be adjusted so that maximal benefit is obtained from the lowest dose. Carers must be aware of the need to provide medication on time. It is also recommended that the early morning dose be taken one hour before the resident is expected to start the activities of the day. This allows time for the medication to reach its maximal effect on movement control (Morris et al 1995). When the resident is able to participate in movement, but is affected by 'freezing', a number of strategies might be used to control movement. The resident should be encouraged to rehearse the movement in their mind and break the sequence of movements into simple steps before commencing the task. While performing the task, the resident should concentrate fully on the movement. It is not recommended that more that one task is undertaken at any time. For example, the resident should concentrate on rolling over in bed and not talking to the carer at the same time. Sometimes visual or auditory cues can be useful in assisting initiation of a movement such as a step. When a carer needs to help initiate movement, gently rocking the resident's weight to each side of the buttocks, or forwards and backwards, can help initiate movement (Morris et al 1995).

Flaccidity

Flaccidity or low muscle tone is found in residents who have muscular dystrophy or peripheral neuropathy such as post-polio or Guillain–Barré syndrome. The major consequence of flaccidity is the inability to protect joints from injury from abnormal movement or positioning and the difficulty in controlling body position during hoisted transfers and when sitting upright. Particular care should be taken during passive movement application. Also the sling chosen for a hoist transfer must be very supportive as the flaccid resident will easily slide out of the support if the size or application of the sling does not match the resident's needs. The physiotherapist should identify the most appropriate sling to use with hoisting and ensure that carers are aware of the potential dangers if the sling is not applied carefully on every occasion.

Managing oedema

Peripheral oedema is relatively common in older people and is generally multifactorial in origin (Smith 1996). Because it is often mild or not causing particular distress, diagnosis of the causative factors and initiation of management procedures is often overlooked. Haemodynamic factors play a major role in the development of peripheral oedema, with cardiac and muscle pump inefficiency the most common. Other contributing factors include renal failure (Menon et al 2001), liver failure (Forrest et al 1996), deep venous thrombosis, critical limb ischaemia (Khiabani et al 2000a), low serum albumin (Khiabani et al 2000b, Waterlow 1984), calcium channel blocker medication (Borrild 1997) or non-steroidal anti-inflammatory drugs, proximal lymphadenopathy or disruption of proximal lymphatic vessels (Berlin et al 1999, Uher et al 2000) and orthostatic oedema from dependency (Streeten 1975). Thus it is important to determine which factors are contributing to the peripheral oedema that presents in the resident as certain management methods will be contraindicated in some instances. Although often present in the lower limbs, peripheral oedema can be present in the hands and upper limbs as well as in dependent parts of the body. When the oedema is determined to be due to fluid retention that is associated with renal and liver failure, hypertension or chronic heart failure, management is by reduction of the fluid overload (Anand & Florea 2001, Forrest et al 1996, Menon et al 2001). Medication change might be considered when medication is thought to be contributing to the presentation. A previous history of surgery or radiotherapy for the treatment of cancer will often identify lymphoedema as the cause of swelling. In these instances complex regional lymphatic drainage consisting of massage, compression bandaging, active exercise and skin care is indicated to decrease the swelling, control pain and improve functional capacity (Mason 1993). Compression therapy using manual compression, intermittent compression pumps, bandaging, compression stockings or sleeves can be very effective in reducing the swelling (Berlin et al 1999). Adding muscle pumping exercise enhances the effect of these interventions (Simons et al 1996). However, many of the immobile residents with swelling are unable to perform these exercises effectively. Assisted active or passive movement of the limbs will have some compressive effect on the venous pump systems and assist with oedema clearance when added to manual or pump compression, bandaging or compression garments. Segers et al (2002) found that the pressure in the chambers of multi-chambered pressure cuffs used for sequential pressure therapy did not conform to the manufacturer-predicted pressures. They cautioned that pressures should be less than 30 mmHg as tissue damage was likely if this upper limit were used. When swelling in the legs has been determined to be caused by venous stasis, compression stockings have been useful in improving the venous haemodynamics but mainly when the person was still able to mobilize (Ibegbuna et al 2003). In residents who are immobile and also have fragile skin, application of compression stockings might cause additional skin trauma that ulcerates. Therefore this method of controlling oedema due to venous insufficiency is not an appropriate choice.

The physiotherapist is urged to use caution if recommending elevation of the feet to control lower limb oedema. Possible problems other than causing further circulation problems include the possibility of acquiring a footdrop and injury to the skin on the calf due to pressure from the legrest. Alternation between elevation and dependency is important so that plantigrade ankle range can be maintained and the calf pressure can be relieved. When the legs are elevated it is important to support the thigh as well as the lower leg so that the knees are not stressed.

When peripheral oedema is present in a limb with chronic arterial insufficiency, microscopic changes such as wide gaps between cells in the capillary walls have been demonstrated (Anvar et al 2000). This structural change prevents any oedema control method from being effective and if, for example, compression or elevation was applied it might precipitate more tissue damage and pain.

Hand oedema is often seen in residents who have suffered a stroke and have developed a complex regional pain syndrome (CRPS) or shoulder-hand syndrome. Roy et al (1995) found 57% of their group of 76 patients with stroke had signs of CRPS. CRPS has been reported as appearing between the second and fourth month post stroke and has been associated with spasticity (Braus et al 1994). It was also suggested by Braus et al (1994), on the basis of post-mortem findings, that peripheral nerve injuries were responsible for CRPS appearing. How these injuries came about remains controversial. Possible causes include direct internal or external trauma to a flaccid and/or insensate upper limb (Corrigan & Maitland 1995). Another possibility is that there was direct damage to the central components of the autonomic nervous system at the time of stroke. It would appear that trauma is not the only contributing cause of CRPS in the stroke patient. A correlation was also found between CRPS and severe paralysis, spasticity and glenohumeral subluxation (Braus et al 1994). In addition to a swollen hand, the resident will have pain on passive movements of the limb, reduced or absent voluntary movement in the limb and obvious arterial blood flow changes. Gentle massage comprising effleurage stroking can assist with drainage of the swelling. Encouragement of active or assisted active movement augments the effect of massage (Uher et al 2000). However, Geurts et al (2000) debate whether any method of management is superior or even effective in treating this problem after stroke.

Considerations relating to the barely mobile resident

The resident who falls into this category is one who is at major risk of losing what little mobility remains. These residents might be able to stand with the assistance of carers, wall bars or with a standing hoist (Fig. 6.3). The benefits gained from weight-bearing through the legs - the visual, vestibular and somatosensory stimulation, muscle contraction and joint movement not to mention the satisfaction of being able to achieve this level of function - should not be underestimated. Furthermore, the maintenance or improvement in this level of function should be a major aim for the resident, physiotherapist and carers. That these residents are at risk of falling must also be acknowledged. This risk is due to the physical ability level but also increased when cognitive deterioration is present. If the resident can understand that they should wait for assistance before trying to stand then safety is not a major problem. However, if the resident cannot remember to wait for assistance or is impulsive, then sustaining a fall while trying to stand is most likely. This situation is most disturbing for the carers as any injuries sustained might be seen to reflect on their competency. In this situation a team meeting should be called that includes all stakeholders and a solution decided on that is then entered in the care plan for the resident.

Interventions that might improve functional ability are similar to those used by more mobile residents and are discussed in the following chapters.

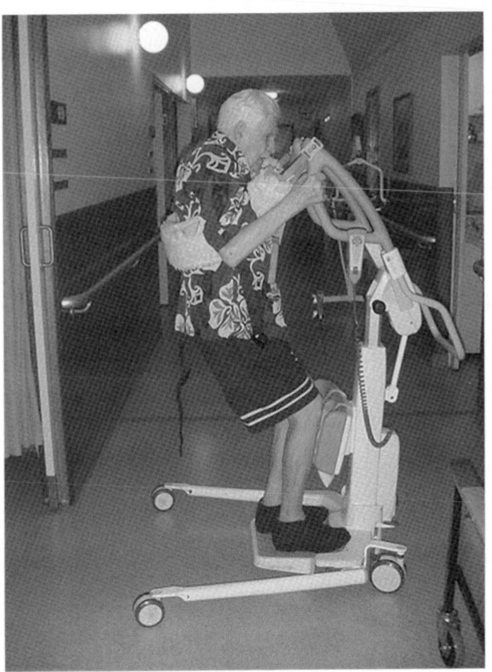

Figure 6.3
Standing hoist in use.

As a rule, barely mobile residents need more experienced people to assist with an exercise programme so that the input is individually tailored to their problems and the response to intervention can be continually monitored for effect. Any adverse responses can then be identified and the intervention immediately modified. Thus physiotherapists are the most appropriate people to provide treatment for this category of resident.

Factors that can affect performance

Decline in physical ability might occur due to an acute episode or insidiously over time. Some causes of fluctuating or acute change in performance ability are identified in Table 6.3. An acute change in ability might put both resident and carer at risk of injury if simple evaluation of resident competency is not checked at each transfer.

The important consideration in determining the management of the changed physical functional level of the resident in these circumstances is whether the problem causing the change is identifiable and whether it is reversible to an extent that will enable the resident to regain the loss. For this reason changes to care plans should be flexible, and appropriate intervention from the physiotherapist should be instigated once the medical management has controlled the condition. The physiotherapist will usually work closely with the doctor as the medication dosage is titrated to suit the individual resident. For example, the physiotherapist's role when the resident with Parkinson's disease is having their medication adjusted is to measure the effect on function and the duration of this effect so that timing of medication and dose can be optimal.

Table 6.3
Factors that can change the ability of residents to perform at their usual level of participation in activities of daily living

Causes of change in physical ability	Consequence of change in ability
Acute neurological insult, e.g. transient ischaemic attack or stroke	Loss of motor and/or sensory function – increased risk of falling
Acute infection, e.g. chest, urinary tract, cellulitis or septicaemia	Increased muscle weakness and confusion
Cardiac insult, e.g. myocardial infarction, chronic heart failure	Confusion, muscle weakness and shortness of breath
Fluctuation in performance associated with:	
Medication dose, e.g. Parkinson's disease	'Freezing'
Fatigue	Inability to weight-bear in afternoon
Muscle spasm	Too stiff or knees 'give way'; often related to timing of medication
Change in medication	Decreased level of arousal Increased confusion Lethargy Decreased motor planning Decreased strength
Pain	Decreased strength, avoidance of weight-bearing through the painful limb or knees 'give way'
Peripheral oedema from decreased efficiency of the cardiac or muscle pump, cellulitis, lymphoedema, medication or low serum albumin	If severe, oedema in the feet and lower legs can interfere with the ability of the resident to dorsiflex the feet, which makes stand transfers more difficult, increases the amount of assistance needed from the carer to move to standing, and reduces the sensory input from the feet and efficiency of muscle function, thereby reducing balance ability

How to decide when full hoist is necessary for transfers

In many circumstances it is easy to decide that a resident requires full hoisting for transfers. These residents will include those who are unable to communicate or physically participate in a transfer. Residents who are in the late stages of dementia or in a vegetative state from ABI might be examples. Other residents might be unable to physically stand or weight-bear such as those with bilateral lower limb amputation, spinal cord injury or other severe neurological dysfunction.

Progression of medical conditions or acquisition of new pathology generally precipitates the progression to full hoist. These residents might have previously been using a standing hoist, pulling to stand at a wall bar or depending on assistance from carers to stand for transfer. The most important deciding factor will be inability to continue to transfer with safety for the resident or the carer. Safety will be compromised when:

- lower limb weakness has progressed to the point where the resident is unable to weight-bear or to take weight reliably
- a flexor withdrawal response is stimulated by weight being taken through the balls of the feet because a plantigrade position is no longer possible for the resident
- the resident has become too heavy
- joint stability has declined to the point where trauma is occurring during the stand
- the resident can no longer use a standing hoist as they slip through the support
- shoulder or knee pain, arthritis and/or lack of range of movement prevents the use of the standing hoist
- multiple factors have contributed to decline in ability.

Some residents will have been independent or requiring some assistance with slide seated transfers. This ability might be lost when upper limb pain, reduced strength or loss of range of movement interferes with using the upper limbs to effect the transfer. Every effort should be made to solve the problem by changing the point of weight-bearing from the hands and wrists to the forearms but often this is not successful and full hoisting is the only solution. Assessment of joints, muscle function and identification of the cause of loss by the physiotherapist might enable specific treatment interventions to be undertaken to preserve independence but in the elderly disabled resident this is often only a temporary reprieve.

When confusion compounds the increased difficulty in transferring safely, full hoist might be used for transfers but in the absence of staff supervision some of these residents might try to stand. In these circumstances restraints have been employed to prevent injury.

Restraints

Residents who are at risk of falling, wandering off or inflicting self-injury owing to their physical frailty and/or cognitive dysfunction pose a major problem for carers who are responsible for their safety. In many countries restraints are employed to prevent movement that might lead to injury. Their use is controlled by ethical and legal issues that have led to formal legislation regarding usage and who is allowed to direct restraint implementation and determine type of restraint (Ljunggren et al 1997). However, there is much controversy surrounding restraint use, which has arisen from the adverse occurrences that have been recorded during usage. These complications include increased agitation, pressure areas, skin tears and bruising, sedation and cognitive decline, strangulation and death (Shorr et al 2002). Restraints can be physical in the form of belts, straps attached to the trunk or limbs or pharmaceutical in the form of sedatives or tranquillizers. Chair design can be such that it prevents egress and so has a restraining effect on independent mobility (Rappl & Jones 2000). Unfortunately, injuries still occur during restraint use. Confused residents are most likely to struggle free and fall or be injured by the restraints (Ljunggren et al 1997, Shorr et al 2002). Thus the argument that staff numbers are insufficient to ensure resident safety and so restraint is necessary is not supported by evidence of incident decline when restraints are used. Change in the approach to caring for these at-risk residents might reduce the number of injuries. Problem-based solutions address the underlying reasons for the activity undertaken by the resident that precipitated the fall.

Maintaining or maximizing respiratory function

All residents will be affected by age-related decline in respiratory function. The ability to maintain normal oxygen levels is reduced further by poor posture or position. Intrinsic differences specific to the resident such as obesity or chronic lung pathology will also affect respiratory function. Thus it is important to control for these effects in order to maximize functional and/or cognitive potential.

The habitual positions for the immobile resident in lying or reclined sitting have been compared to the upright sitting position. This has shown that recumbent or reclined positions reduce forced vital capacity, forced expiratory volume at one second, peak expiratory flow rate, dynamic lung compliance and tidal volume but increase the respiratory rate to tidal volume ratio (Vitacca et al 1996). The study by Nitz et al (2004) supported these findings by showing that in frail immobile residents the reclined sitting position led to poorer oxygen saturation than when positioned in upright sitting. Maintenance of optimal oxygenation is desirable so that cognitive state is not further compromised. Therefore when 'sitting out', these frail immobile residents would benefit from being positioned in a more upright posture in the chair. If the resident is very obese the more upright position is also preferred, as Ferretti et al (2001) demonstrated that the supine position significantly affected the expiratory flow rate and contributed to dyspnoea.

It is important that the posture of the resident is optimal in the upright sitting position. The resident needs to be able to sustain an erect spinal posture, and not collapse into a kyphotic hunched posture that will compress the abdomen and chest, in order to obtain the benefit of the position. Tilting the chair in space through 25 degrees, as discussed in the next chapter, can alleviate this problem while maintaining the benefits of improved respiratory function.

Other intrinsic factors encountered in the residents relate to the level of fitness or habitual activity. Residents who have been immobile or restricted in mobility for any length of time will have reduced respiratory function and will be at greater risk of acquiring problems related to poor ventilation. Those residents with chronic lung pathologies have an even greater risk of infection and hypoxaemia-related disorders. However, mild to moderate chronic airways disease where the older person can maintain relatively normal blood oxygen levels has not been implicated in cognitive decline (Incalzi et al 2002) if the person is still mobile and living in the community. Therefore maintaining mobility in the resident with chronic lung disease should be a primary aim for physiotherapists. At all times residents should be encouraged to participate in the discussion and decision process that determines the medical, pharmaceutical and physiotherapy management of their condition. This active participation will encourage more active self-participation in all aspects of management of their condition and enhance quality of life (Oliver 2001). Even when the resident is no longer able to perform activities of daily living independently, they should be encouraged to participate to the best of their ability by helping to perform rolling or dressing activities, for example. The physiotherapist should observe the manner in which residents with advanced lung disease perform activities. In a number of cases bad habits will have been acquired such as breath holding while moving. This habit reduces the oxygen delivery levels during a time of oxygen demand from the muscles and increases the perceived exertion and dyspnoea with the attendant prolongation of recovery time. Simply pointing out the habit and the detrimental effect on ability to function might be beneficial.

Some residents might also need specific interventions that aim at improving ventilation and assist with secretion removal. Prior to commencing any active treatment for airway clearance or to improve ventilation, the resident should be assisted into the best position for attaining the desired response. This might be the upright sitting position. Ensure that the upper limbs are supported, thereby controlling accessory muscle activity and reducing the work of breathing. Many of these residents will also have pain, neuromuscular disorders, a weak cough and abnormal airways so might benefit from airway clearance techniques such as autogenic drainage and active cycle of breathing (Hardy & Anderson 1996). When the resident is unable to participate in airway clearance techniques such as when confused due to a chest infection, facilitation of movement such as rolling or just changing position might stimulate a cough. On the rare occasion when osteoporosis is not a problem, stretch facilitation applied to the chest wall will assist in increasing ventilation volumes (Adler et al 1993, Nitz & Burke 2002) and address the problems of atelectasis and retention of secretions. Passive movement of the upper limb can assist with increasing inspiratory volumes when the resident is unable to participate with treatment. When the physiotherapist has access to equipment that might be used to assist with secretion removal, these might be used after due consideration of indications and contraindications for use. One simple and low cost piece of equipment is a bubble blowing kit. If the resident can cooperate, encouragement to blow bubbles will increase tidal volumes and increase the ability to remove secretions or limit atelectasis.

The physiotherapist should also ensure that supplementary oxygen or delivery of medication by nebulization is being undertaken safely and appropriately. Carers might not understand that increasing the flow rate and therefore the oxygen concentration being delivered to a resident with chronic airflow limitation should not be done if the resident is short of breath. Similarly oxygen should not be used to drive the nebulizer when delivering medication to these residents, as the flow rate needed to produce nebulization is much higher than that used to deliver 24 or 28% oxygen – the likely safe limit for these residents. Medical air or a compressor pump is recommended instead.

Conclusion

The immobile or barely mobile resident poses a major challenge for physiotherapists and carers, who need to work together to maintain comfort and prevent the complications of immobility whilst encouraging continued social interaction. In this chapter we have looked at the importance of maintaining movement and methods of assisting the resident to achieve this, as well as methods of controlling abnormal muscle tone, peripheral oedema and maximizing respiratory function. When to decide that a resident needs full hoisting for transfers and the use of restraints has also been discussed.

Summary

- Maintenance of movement through assisted standing, passive or assisted active movement is vital in order to prevent co-morbidities associated with immobility.
- Control of spasticity with medication and physiotherapeutic modalities enhances resident comfort and function.
- Rigidity associated with Parkinson's disease and extra-pyramidal pathology can be managed to a degree with medication and motor control strategies.
- Hypotonicity needs to be managed with appropriate support from chairs and poses special problems during transfers.
- Peripheral oedema seen in residents has many aetiologies and the causes must be determined before using elevation or other physiotherapeutic modalities for management.
- Often the decision to use a hoist (standing or full) with a resident is a difficult one. There are many factors that must be taken into account but the primary decision is based on safety and the ability of a resident to weight-bear.

- Standing hoist use relies on weight-bearing ability, a degree of joint stability, cooperation and the ability to maintain an erect posture. Shoulder or knee joint pain, deformity or limitation can inhibit the use of a standing hoist.
- Method of toileting and continence must be considered as the use of a full hoist with a resident requiring or requesting frequent toileting does have major implications for nursing management.
- Restraint use is a contentious issue and in some areas is prohibited. Where restraints are in use, sound rationale should be the basis of choice regarding type, time, application and monitoring. Restraints used poorly can cause injury, and even death. It is imperative to control their use as they can lull carers into a false sense of security regarding accidents. The use of restraints does not remove the necessity for regular position changes, pressure area care and toileting requirements.
- Exercises, positioning and stimulation all contribute to maintaining respiratory function. This is clearly important in optimizing functional and cognitive potential.

References

Adler S S, Beckers D, Buck M 1993 PNF in practice: an illustrated guide. Springer-Verlag, Berlin

Alfieri V 1982 Electrical treatment of spasticity. Scandinavian Journal of Rehabilitation Medicine 14:177–182

Anand I S, Florea V G 2001 Diuretics in chronic heart failure – benefits and hazards. European Heart Journal Supplements 3:G8–G18

Anvar M D, Khiabani H Z, Nesland J M, Stranden E, Kroese A J 2000 Vascular and stromal features in the skin of the lower limb in patients with chronic critical limb ischaemia (CLI) and oedema. European Journal of Vascular and Endovascular Surgery 20(2):125–131

Bannister R 1978 Brain's clinical neurology, 5th edn. Oxford University Press, New York, p 307

Barnes M P 1998 Management of spasticity. Age and Ageing 27(2):239–246

Berlin E, Gjores J E, Ivarsson C et al 1999 Post-mastectomy lymphoedema – treatment and a five-year follow-up study. International Angiology 18(4):294–298

Bohannon R W, Larkin P A, Smith M B, Horton M G 1986 Shoulder pain in hemiplegia: statistical relationship with five variables. Archives of Physical Medicine and Rehabilitation 67(8):514–516

Borrild N J 1997 Patients' experiences of antihypertensive drugs in routine use: results of a Danish general practice survey. Blood Pressure Suppl 1:23–25

Braus D, Krauss J, Strobel J 1994 The shoulder hand syndrome after stroke: a prospective clinical trial. Annals of Neurology 36(5):728–733

Corrigan B, Maitland G D 1995 Practical orthopaedic medicine. Butterworth Heinemann, Oxford

Ferretti A, Giampiccolo P, Cavalli A, Milic-Emili J, Tantucci C 2001 Expiratory flow limitation and orthopnoea in massively obese subjects. Chest 119(5):1401-1408

Forrest E H, Jalan R, Hayes P C 1996 Review article: renal circulatory changes in cirrhosis: pathogenesis and therapeutic prospects. Alimentary Pharmacology and Therapeutics 10(3):219–231

Geurts A C, Visschers B A J T, van Limbeek J, Ribbers G M 2000 Systematic review of aetiology and treatment of post-stroke hand oedema and shoulder-hand syndrome. Scandinavian Journal of Rehabilitation Medicine 32:4–10

Hardy K A, Anderson B D 1996 Noninvasive clearance of airway secretions. Respiratory Care Clinics of North America 2(2):323–345

Herbert R D, Mosely A M, Butler J E, Gandevia S C 2002 Change in length of relaxed muscle fascicules and tendons with knee and ankle movement in humans. Journal of Physiology 539(2):637–645

Ibegbuna V, Delis K T, Nicolaides A N, Aina O 2003 Effect of elastic compression stockings on venous hemodynamics during walking. Journal of Vascular Surgery 37(2):420–425

Incalzi R A, Bellia V, Maggi S et al 2002 Mild to moderate chronic airways disease does not carry an excess risk of cognitive dysfunction. Aging Clinical and Experimental Research 14(5):395–401

Johnson E R, Fowler W M, Lieberman J S 1992 Contractures in neuromuscular disease. Archives of Physical Medicine and Rehabilitation 73(9): 809–810

Joynt R L 1992 The source of shoulder pain in hemiplegia. Archives of Physical Medicine and Rehabilitation 73(5):409–413

Khiabani H Z, Anvar M D, Kroese A J, Stranden E 2000a The role of veno-arteriolar reflex (VAR) in the pathogenesis of peripheral oedema in patients with chronic critical limb ischaemia (CLI). Annales of Chirurgiae et Gynaecologiae 89(2):93–98

Khiabani H Z, Anvar M D, Kroese A J, Stranden E 2000b Transcapillary forces and the development of oedema in the lower limb of patients with chronic critical limb ischaemia (CLI). European Journal of Vascular and Endovascular Surgery 19(6):598–604

Lannin N A, Horsley S A, Herbert R, McCluskey A, Cusick A 2003 Splinting the hand in the functional position after brain impairment: a randomized, controlled trial. Archives of Physical Medicine and Rehabilitation 84(2):297–302

Lewis G N, Byblow W D 2002 Modulations in corticomotor excitability during passive upper-limb movement: is there a cortical influence? Brain Research 943(2):263–275

Ljunggren G, Phillips C D, Sgdari A 1997 Comparisons of restraint use in nursing homes in eight countries. Age and Ageing 26(6):S43–S48

Mason M 1993 The treatment of lymphoedema by complex physical therapy. Australian Journal of Physiotherapy 39(1):41–45

Mayer N H, Esquenazi A, Childers M K 1997 Common patterns of clinical motor dysfunction. Muscle and Nerve Suppl 6:S21–S35

Menon M K, Naimark D M, Bargman J M, Vas S I, Oreopoulos D G 2001 Long-term blood pressure control in a cohort of peritoneal dialysis patients and its association with residual renal function. Nephrology, Dialysis Transplant 16(11):2207–2213

Morris M, Iansek R, Kirkwood B 1995 Moving ahead with Parkinson's. Kingston Centre, Australia

Nitz J C 1982 Latissimus dorsi: the muscle often neglected when spasticity is present. Australian Journal of Physiotherapy 28(6):22–24

Nitz J C, Burke B 2002 Facilitation of respiration in myotonic dystrophy. Physiotherapy Research International 7(4):228–238

Nitz J C, Steer M E, Hourigan S R 2004 A study of two sitting positions in frail, elderly, non-mobile and totally dependent residents of aged care facilities. (in preparation)

Oliver S M 2001 Living with failing lungs: the doctor–patient relationship. Family Practice 18(4):430–439

Paris B E, Libow L S, Halperin J L, Mulvihill M N 1988 The prevalence and one-year outcome of limb arterial obstructive disease in a nursing home population. Journal of the American Geriatrics Society 36:607–612

Pierson S H 1997 Outcome measures in spasticity management. Muscle and Nerve Suppl 6:S36–S48

Price R, Lehmann J F, Boswell-Bessette S, Burleigh A, de Lateur B J 1993 Influence of cryotherapy on spasticity at the human ankle. Archives of Physical Medicine and Rehabilitation 74(3):300–304

Radovanovic S, Korotkov A, Ljubisavljic M et al 2002 Comparison of brain activity during different types of proprioceptive inputs: a positron emission tomography study. Experimental Brain Research 143(3):275–285

Rankin A 1993 The functional independence measure. Physiotherapy 79(12):184

Rappl L, Jones D A 2000 Seating evaluation: special problems and interventions for older adults. Topics in Geriatric Rehabilitation 16(2):63–72

Roy C W, Sands M R, Hill L D, Harrison A, Marshall S 1995 The effect of shoulder pain on outcome of acute hemiplegia. Clinical Rehabilitation 9:21–27

Salisbury S K, Low Choy N L, Nitz J C 2003 Shoulder pain, range of movement and functional motor skills after acute tetraplegia. Archives of Physical Medicine and Rehabilitation 84(10):1480–1485

Seaby L, Torrance G 1989 Reliability of a physiotherapy functional assessment used in a rehabilitation setting. Physiotherapy Canada 41:264–271

Segers P, Belgrado J P, Leduc O, Verdonck P 2002 Excessive pressure in multichambered cuffs used for sequential compression therapy. Physical Therapy 82(10):1000–1008

Seib T P, Price R, Reyes M R, Lehmann J F 1994 A quantitative measurement of spasticity: effect of cutaneous electrical stimulation. Archives of Physical Medicine and Rehabilitation 75(7):746–750

Seiss E, Hesse C W, Drane S et al 2002 Proprioception-related evoked potentials: origin and sensitivity to movement parameters. NeuroImage 17(1):461–468

Shorr R I, Guillen M K, Rosenblatt L C et al 2002 Restraint use, restraint orders, and the risk of falls in hospitalized patients. Journal of the American Geriatrics Society 50(3):526–529

Simons P, Smith P C, Lees W R, McGrouther D A 1996 Venous pumps of the hand – their clinical importance. Journal of Hand Surgery – British and European Volume 21B(5):595–599

Smith E 1996 A survey of peripheral oedema in elderly patients admitted to a geriatric ward. British Journal of Clinical Practice 50(1):20–21

Streeten D H 1975 The role of posture in idiopathic oedema. South African Medical Journal 49(13): 462–464

Tyson S F, Chissim C 2002 The immediate effect of handling technique on range of movement in the hemiplegic shoulder. Clinical Rehabilitation 16(2): 137–140

Uher E M, Vacariu G, Schneider B, Fialka V 2000 Comparison of manual lymph drainage with exercise therapy in the complex regional pain syndrome 1. A randomised controlled trial. Wiener Klinische Wochenschrift 112(3):133–137

Van Langenberghe H V K, Hogan B M 1988 Degree of pain and grade of shoulder subluxation in the painful hemiplegic shoulder. Scandinavian Journal of Rehabilitation Medicine 20:161–166

Vitacca M, Clini E, Spassini W et al 1996 Does the supine position worsen respiratory function in elderly subjects? Gerontology 42(1):46–53

Ward A B 2002 A summary of spasticity management – a treatment algorithm. European Journal of Neurology 9(Suppl 1):48–52

Waterlow J C 1984 Kwashiorkor revisited: the pathogenesis of oedema in kwashiorkor and its significance. Transactions of the Royal Society of Tropical Medicine and Hygiene 78(4):436–441

Wilton J C 1997 Hand splinting. Principles of design and fabrication. W B Saunders, London, p 186–187

Zorowitz R D, Hughes M B, Idank D, Ikai T, Johnson M V 1995 Shoulder pain and subluxation after stroke: correlation or coincidence? American Journal of Occupational Therapy 50(3):194–201

7 What about beds and chairs?

Jennifer C. Nitz

This chapter aims to:

- identify the desirable features of beds and bed equipment that benefit residents and carers
- discuss devices that improve comfort and prevent or minimize injury to the resident whilst in bed
- identify the desirable features in chairs and identify how individual differences and needs are catered for by the design
- discuss the advantages of the seated position for eating, communication and mobilizing.

Introduction

Immobile or barely mobile residents will spend the whole 24 hours of the day either in their bed or sitting in a chair of some design. Over 60% of older adults living in residential aged care have difficulty transferring in and out of bed or a chair (Alexander et al 1997). It is therefore vitally important that these items of furniture are chosen appropriately so that they maximize the remaining function of the resident and do not contribute to co-morbidity problems.

Beds

As a general rule the beds supplied in RACFs are single. Only a few residences provide double beds for couples or allow new residents to bring their own beds from home. RACFs that accommodate low care residents could easily allow any bed that the resident prefers, as many of these residents have the potential to be independent in bed mobility and transfers. Their need for care is more likely due to cognitive impairment or the need for supervision and assistance in bathing and dressing. Thus specific features needed on beds in RACFs mainly apply to those housing more dependent high care residents.

The bed features can be divided into those relating to the resident and those for the carer. Table 7.1 lists these features.

Mattresses

Mattresses should be firm and supportive so that optimal posture can be maintained. Waterproof coverings that are commonly used to protect

Table 7.1 *Resident and carer based bed needs*

Resident	Carer
Ability to lower the bed to allow the feet to easily touch the floor for safe sitting balance and transfers to standing or a wheelchair. Low bed height might also minimize injury in the case of a fall from the bed	Ability to raise the bed for more ergonomic posture during care tasks,cleaning and linen changes
Ability to elevate the head of the bed for relief of breathlessness or to read or watch television more comfortably. It also assists those residents who take meals in bed	An elevating bed head enables easier attainment of an upright posture for drinking and feeding
Easy addition of assisting devices such as bed poles, overhead ring, bed rails, bed ladder or bed rope. These should be detached if not needed as any addition increases the chance of injury to the resident from bumps or scrapes	Wheels with efficient brakes to allow movement of the bed in an emergency and to ensure safe manual handling
Space under the bed for motors to drive ripple mattresses and still allow the bed to be low enough for independent seated transfers	Electronic controls are better than manual wind-up controls, which can pose an injury risk for the lumbar spine when the carer stoops to wind the control and from bumps and knocks on the protruding winding handle

them from damage due to incontinence can affect the supportive potential of the mattress. These plastic covers also increase the possibility for skin damage by trapping moisture. The combination of shear forces, pressure and moisture that is acidic have been identified as potent factors in the development of pressure ulcers (Taler 2000). Rather than protecting the mattress the focus should be on protecting the resident. A number of absorbent draw sheets or two-way stretch waterproof covers are available that act to draw moisture away from the skin while providing mattress protection. Using these sheets with incontinence protective clothing is a suitable though fairly expensive solution.

Many mattresses used to relieve pressure and assist in the fight against pressure ulcers are so soft and squashy that the bed occupant requires considerable strength and ability to sit up in order to move laterally in the bed and turn over. Thus if such a mattress is used, the resident might lose independence in bed mobility if weakness or level of disability is severe enough. In such cases the pressure-relieving mattress might have been considered because the resident had muscle paralysis or severe arthritis and was at increased risk of pressure ulcer formation. But a more appropriate choice might have been to provide sheepskins to relieve pressure under bony parts and to encourage the resident to change his or her position regularly at night in order to preserve independence. This is an example of disablement versus enablement and illustrates that blindly following a protocol for pressure ulcer prevention does not usually take individual differences or self-determination into account.

Pressure ulcer and injury protective devices

Most protective devices are used to relieve pressure from pressure-intolerant areas such as the heels including the Achilles tendons, elbows and ears. They are made from various materials such as sheepskin, and silicon gel. In all situations efficient function of the device is dependent on correct application and regular checks to ensure the device has not been dislodged during care procedures or by muscle spasm in a paralysed resident.

Bed cradles are useful for keeping the weight of the bedclothes from the feet. This weight relief is not only needed to prevent the mechanical effect on the feet that might lead to plantarflexion deformities, it is also desirable when the resident has a peripheral neuropathy in the lower limbs. Peripheral neuropathies can present with hyperaesthesia that makes any touch on the skin in the neuropathic area intolerable owing to the noxious sensations it causes. Removal of any such noxious stimulus will enhance comfort, in some instances reduce muscle spasm and enable better sleep.

Some very restless residents with acquired brain injury that results in uncontrolled or uncoordinated limb movements might be at risk of injury due to striking the bed rails. In these situations a cheap and effective solution is to cover the bed rails with recycled padded quilts (Fig. 7.1).

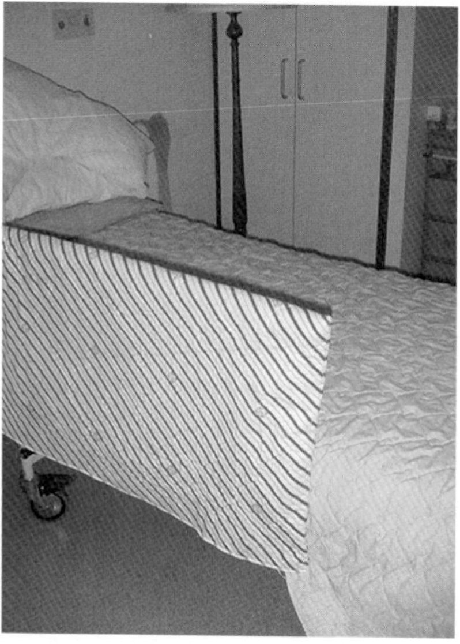

Figure 7.1
Bed rail protectors in situ.

Chairs

Residents can in some situations bring a favourite chair from home. Often these chairs are comfortable and enable the new resident to retain a familiar object that links them tangibly and through memories back to the community. When a resident has to give up all their possessions on entering an RACF, there is likely to be greater stress surrounding the move.

Chairs occupied by residents often need to provide more than a comfortable place to sit. They might be required to give support to the body and head when muscles are paralysed, assist in the control of muscle spasm and prevent muscle contractures as well as enable easy access and egress. Furthermore, the chair might need to provide support to enable communication and social interaction, increase personal independence to perform activities of daily living and assist with mobility. Thus function is paramount and since the residents demonstrate many different needs a variety of chairs should be available to meet these individual needs. Physiotherapists often need to be proactive in this regard by consulting with and providing documentation to support chair choice to RACF managements when new furniture is being bought. They will also assist families to invest in wheelchairs or lounge chairs that suit the individual need of the resident who is a family member.

Choosing a chair

In many instances the purchase of chairs for residents in RACFs has been undertaken by interior designers or architects, who as a rule do not understand the importance of fitting the chair to the user and their individual needs. Pedersen (2000) comments that long-term care facilities tend to buy wheelchairs and lounge chairs in bulk, thereby taking advantage of discount prices. This practice allows few if any choice of size or feature options such as removable footrests. Only rarely will a chair be suitable for a resident without considerable modification. When choosing the chair, size dimensions, the extent of support needed, flexibility to accommodate joint range loss, how the resident will transfer in and out of the chair and potential for independent mobility whilst seated all require consideration. Only when these aspects are provided should upholstery material and colour be chosen. The material used in the upholstery is important, as the skin-to-upholstery interface is a site of trauma in many frail older people. The upholstery should ideally be soft and pliable, not hold moisture and not stick to the skin (Rappl & Jones 2000).

A comprehensive assessment of the physical and functional status should be undertaken for each individual needing specific seating. This will ensure that all support, protection and social requirements can be considered. However, the cost of the ideal chair or wheelchair can be prohibitive so some compromise might have to be made. In these situations, the pros and cons of various aspects of the chair should be discussed with the resident and their family and the best option purchased. Specific note should be made of the physical and pathological aspects identified in Table 7.2.

All chairs have a seat and backrest. Additional features include armrests, tray-tables, swing-away and removable and/or elevating legrests and

Table 7.2 *Assessment aspects essential for chair prescription*

Aspect	Rationale
Skin	Poor or absent sensation will increase risk of pressure areas Poor circulation increases risk of injury and pressure areas Scar tissue can increase risk of shear force injury
Posture	Older people often have increased thoracic kyphosis and decreased lumbar lordosis. Determine if deformity is fixed or flexible and if the resident can actively straighten the spine. The chosen chair should limit progression of the deformity
Joint range of movement (ROM)	Available hip ROM will determine seat-to-backrest angle Tight hamstrings will influence leg elevation potential Reduced shoulder ROM will influence the height of armrests and wheel access for residents using manual wheelchairs
Neuromuscular status	Increased muscle tone due to acquired brain injury or spinal cord injury can be controlled to some extent by positioning Tone can be increased by poor head and body position, discomfort, increased pressure causing skin trauma and anxiety caused by fear of falling and lack of sensory input Residents with low tone or muscular dystrophy need support to protect them against the effect of gravity on posture
Respiratory function	Residents with chronic respiratory disease might need a wheelchair for ambulation that allows the upper limb to be supported while the trunk is in the forward leaning position, as this position enhances ventilation capacity Other residents who have poor muscle function and find it difficult to maintain the upright position against gravity might need a well-supported, slightly reclined position to maximize ventilation capacity
Communication and eating	Eye contact is vital for communication. Inability to raise the head due to thoracic kyphosis, muscle weakness or vertebrobasilar insufficiency should be noted and a slightly reclined position adopted, preferably using a 'tilt-in-space' option (maximum tilt 25 degrees). Note that the head also needs support if reclining This position is also optimal for eating and drinking

Aspect	Rationale
Mobility	If the resident is independently mobile or walks with assistance then access and egress are an issue with respect to seat height, depth, armrest access, foot room under the front of the chair and whether or not the resident is cognitively safe to mobilize independently If the resident uses his or her feet to propel the chair, the seat height and under-chair obstructions are important considerations for minimizing leg trauma and increasing efficiency Residents who use manual wheelchairs need to have the method of transfer considered to ensure safety from leg trauma, sit-to-stand efficiency, slide board position, need for armrest or legrest removal or hoist access. They also need to have wheel access considered, push posture, upper limb function and ventilation capacity optimized Residents who use motorized wheelchairs for independent mobility often use a hoist for transfers, so the chair can be slightly higher and/or 'tilt-in-space' to enhance communication, eating, ventilation and function. A confounding problem arises when transfers are performed using a standing hoist. In these instances the seat of the motorized wheelchair is often too high and there is difficulty in positioning the bottom far enough back on the seat. In these cases a lower seat height should be prescribed

wheels. Thus chairs can be adapted to offer assisted or independent mobility. These components of chairs will be discussed in detail as they are of considerable importance when matching the chair to the individual needs of the resident. One aspect that might be useful to consider is whether the residents using particular chairs are ambulant or not. Ambulant residents need chairs that they can get up from without too much difficulty. 'Geri-chairs' or recliners do not allow the feet to be positioned close to the front of the chair, as is needed to stand up, because of interference from the folded legrests that extend during the recline mode. Therefore 'geri-chairs' might prevent independent egress from the chair or increase the risk of a fall during egress. This safety issue should be carefully explained to residents, family and carers so that appropriate choices can be made regarding chair usage (Pedersen 2000).

Seat

The depth and width dimensions of the seat will determine the ease of access and egress as well as the ability of the backrest to provide support. Ideally, the seat should be no deeper than the measurement from the

Table 7.3 *Problems caused by inappropriate seat dimensions*

Measurement	Consequence
Seat too deep	Inability to position the buttocks to the rear of the seat and still place the feet in the correct position on the floor for egress The buttocks will be too far forward on the seat and this necessitates leaning the trunk back to use the backrest, thereby tilting the pelvis posteriorly and leading to shortening of the hip extensor muscles. This position also negates any lumbar spine support incorporated in the backrest and facilitates more thoracic and lumbar kyphosis
Seat too shallow	Less surface area for weight-bearing through the buttocks and back of thighs, which could increase the possibility of excess pressure on the ischial tuberosities and sacrum. This is accentuated if the backrest is at an incorrect angle to the seat
Seat too wide	Reduces lateral support from armrests in maintaining sitting balance and when used to assist with balance on access and egress for ambulation
Seat too narrow	Inability to sit down without potential trauma to the outer thighs Increases heat retention and skin rash Increased difficulty in positioning slings and gaining access for adjusting clothing during transfers and care needs

posterior of the buttocks to a point about 7 cm from the popliteal fossa. The width should be 5 cm wider than the spread of the resident's bottom and thighs when seated. Table 7.3 identifies the problems induced by seat dimensions that are too big or small.

Seat cushions

Some chairs provide pressure relief cushions as the usual seat cushion. In the case of wheelchairs, a pressure relief cushion is generally placed on top of a sling upholstery seat. Each of these situations needs to be taken into account when the height of the armrests is considered.

Immobile residents who are unable to relieve the pressure from their ischia and coccyx efficiently, reliably and independently should use a cushion specifically designed to reduce point pressures under bony prominences and spread the load evenly over the pressure-tolerant soft tissues of the buttocks and posterior thighs. However, carers should be warned that using cushions such as these does not preclude the need to assist movement to enable pressure relief every couple of hours. Ridges of clothing trapped between the skin and the cushion will still cause tissue damage if no movement occurs. An additional problem encountered in some elderly residents is the presence of a cystocele or rectocele that protrudes below the ischia and therefore takes the brunt of pressure when the person is sitting. Should this be the case, special cushions that can be contoured to accommodate for the deformity and still spread pressure on surrounding pressure-tolerant areas should be used so as to prevent tissue injury and necrosis. Contouring can be achieved with air-filled compartments, silicon gel, foam inserts or cut-outs. Often the determining factor for choosing one over another is the financial cost to the resident. However, the physical suffering imposed by not endeavouring to prevent pressure and shear injury must also enter the equation.

Some chairs utilized by older residents have water cushions for pressure relief. Like waterbeds they can be very cold and so can increase the possibility of the user becoming hypothermic in the colder months or in air-conditioned RACFs. They also promote the fetal position and reduce the potential for active movements, as they are too soft.

Seat-to-floor height

It is easiest to rise from a chair if the seat-to-floor height is equivalent to knee-to-floor height (Alexander et al 1996, Sweeney & Clarke 1991). If the seat is lower, the occupant needs to use faster and larger trunk movements to stand (Alexander et al 1996) and needs increased leg strength and range of motion in all lower limb joints. This puts them at greater risk of losing control and suffering a fall due to compromised stability (Nitz 2000). Raised seat heights are supposed to make egress easier for older people and those with weakness and arthritis. Alexander et al (1996) found that unimpaired elders preferred knee height chairs to high chairs. Older people using higher chairs were more fearful standing up from these chairs than from knee high chairs, possibly due to having to scoot the buttocks forwards and reach down to the floor. This task is essentially unstable and the concern expressed by the older people in the study by Alexander et al is quite understandable. This problem arises in addition to difficulties the elderly face in assuming a safe elimination position by installation of raised toilet pedestals. Provision of foot stools only addresses the ability to assume a good elimination position. Foot stools become a safety issue for residents when accessing the toilet by introducing an obstacle in the area.

Backrest height

Most backrests are too high for residents as the chairs are designed using 'normal' anthropometric measurements that do not take into account 'shrinkage' due to loss of disc height, osteoporosis and vertebral crush fractures. The backrest also should provide support that assists by keeping the pelvis in a neutral tilt. Consequently contours of standard backrests tend not to equate to the older spinal curves and often accentuate thoracic kyphoses and forward head position. Any potential for head support is thus negated and well-meaning care staff often compound the problem by filling the gaps with pillows that further push the head and trunk into more flexion. The result of this is less ventilation capacity, communication ability and discomfort, which can lead to agitation and calling for help if the resident is demented or unable to move into a more comfortable position.

Lateral support of the trunk is desirable for a number of residents who have neurological or musculoskeletal conditions that affect the ability to perceive or maintain the vertical position. In these instances the width of the backrest needs to be close to the shoulder and hip width of the occupant. Little if any support is provided if the backrest is too wide or too narrow. Changing the contours of the backrest with foam inserts cut to the shape of the resident is a cost-effective method of alleviating this problem.

Choosing the correct seat-to-backrest angle is also vital for addressing the support needs of the resident.

Seat-to-backrest angle

The ideal seat-to-back angle is around 95 degrees (Alexander et al 1996). Sweeney & Clarke (1991) proposed that the most appropriate support was provided to the occupant of the chair if the whole chair was tilted back 6 degrees, thus providing the chair tilt of around 100 degrees found by Alexander et al (1996) to be most comfortable for older adults. Unfortunately the negative aspect of posteriorly angling the seat is that egress is made more difficult. Older people find it more difficult to move to the front of the seat to prepare for standing up, and if reduced hip flexion range is present the forward lean of the trunk achieved by flexing at the hips is inhibited, thus making egress less efficient and safe. In these circumstances the seat should be kept horizontal to the floor and at a height that does not exceed knee height while inclining the back around 5 degrees.

Reduced range of movement at the hip can be encountered in many elderly residents. Arthritis, joint arthroplasty and muscle contractures are common causes. Other less common findings include heterotrophic ossification or joint arthrodesis. Ultimately further loss of range in the joints is undesirable so where possible the limbs and trunk should be supported in a comfortable position that encourages optimal joint position for hygiene and function. Foam wedges, 'bean bags' and correctly fitting chair dimensions can assist with maintaining range.

Increased extensor tone in the trunk and lower limbs can lead to the resident sliding forwards and out of the chair. Generally, if the hips can be kept flexed to around 90 degrees by the seat-to-backrest angle this will control the slide. However, the bottom must be kept at the back of the seat so that the support provided by the chair keeps the hips at this angle. If the buttocks are positioned forwards on the seat or the occupant has slid forwards due to slippery clothing, control will be lost. Also, if the head is allowed to flex forwards, this can stimulate an extensor response in the trunk and hips that slides the occupant forwards in the seat. Using the 'tilt-in-space' idea can control these responses. Good foot support with the feet in the plantigrade position assists in maintaining control. If the pressure through the feet acts through the balls of the feet an extensor response or clonus might be facilitated and forward slippage can occur. Thus combining good postural support, position in space and a seat cushion to maintain comfort and relieve pressure is essential to prevent the resident sliding out of the chair and suffering injury.

There are times when loss of flexion range at the hips prevents these measures from controlling the forward slip. If the loss is unilateral the seat cushion might be split between the right and left sides under the thighs so that the more extended hip is positioned in as much flexion as is available and the other hip flexed to 90 degrees. Thus the seat-to-back angle is essentially around 90 degrees and is then 'tilted-in-space' to an angle of around 25 degrees to the upright. A tilt of 25 degrees to the vertical still allows for maximal function. It also reduces shear forces at the interface between the body and cushion to almost zero, thereby reducing the risk of tissue injury. On the other hand, if the seat-to-back angle is opened to 115 degrees the shear forces increase by 25% (Hobson 1992).

Footrests and legrests

In order to maintain the potential for a resident to stand and walk the ankles and feet should be able to achieve a plantigrade position. Therefore lounge chairs should have a seat height that allows the feet to be positioned flat on the floor without having to adjust the position of the buttocks while still providing postural support. If the chair occupant is no longer ambulant, plantigrade feet are still needed to assist with maintaining a stable sitting position. This enables more efficient manual wheelchair propulsion, control of spasticity and prevention of falls from the toilet. The increased stability of the feet on the footplates afforded by the plantigrade position also helps prevent the feet falling off the footrests during activities such as showering and outings and thus prevent foot and leg trauma from bumps or scrapes. The consequence of injuries to the feet and lower limbs in frail residents, especially when arterial insufficiency is present, can be as drastic as amputation and death and at the very least pain and sleep loss.

The height of the footrests should be related to knee height so that the seat of the chair can support the posterior thighs and distribute the weight over a larger support surface. If the footrests are too low, excessive pressure might be applied to the popliteal area, causing discomfort and potential tissue damage. If the footrests are too high, more pressure is transferred to the ischial tuberosities, coccyx and sacrum and this can increase the risk of pressure ulcer formation in these pressure-intolerant areas. In Figure 7.2 we see a resident whose lower limbs and feet have been elevated without due support and with added pressure being placed on the calves. Positioning such as this can lead to poor outcomes such as foot drop, ankle contractures, calf deep vein thrombosis, impaired circulation and discomfort.

Armrest height and size

The armrests should be at a height that allows the occupant to rest their forearms without having to slump to the side or forwards or for the shoulders to be hunched whilst receiving the support. The individual differences encountered in different residents' body sizes means that the correct height will rarely be found in chairs shared by residents. Chairs belonging to individuals should be fitted to provide this degree of support.

Other considerations relate to the chairs used by residents who walk independently with or without an aid or need assistance from carers to transfer

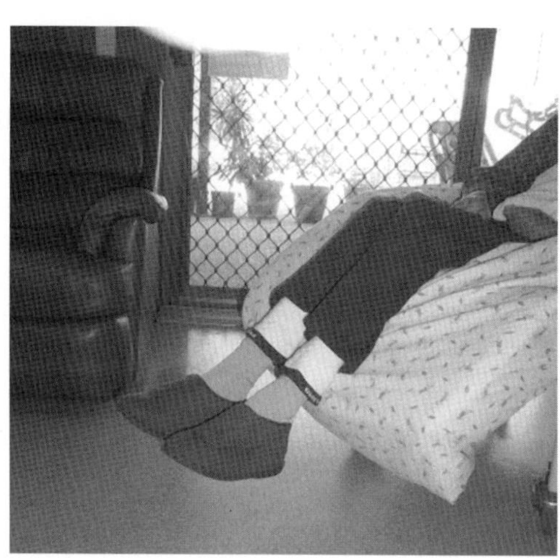

Figure 7.2
Poor leg positioning.

to and from standing safely. In these instances the chair armrests should extend to the front of the chair seat so that good leverage can be gained from the resident to control the transfer. This help from the chair also reduces the physical assistance the carer needs to provide. Thus the resident maintains strength and stability and the carer is at less risk of injury during the task.

Full seat depth armrests also allow the option of a desktop to be attached. This addition helps reduce the fear of falling forward out of the chair. It also provides a surface to prop the forearms to achieve the supported forward lean position useful for occupants who suffer shortness of breath as well as a place to put a communication board for residents who are unable to speak. Desktops also allow independent access to a water bottle with a straw, and support for a book or remote control for entertainment and for meals. This provides self-determination and independence with some basic activities for residents ageing with high cervical level spinal cord injuries or with conditions such as motor neuron disease, multiple sclerosis or cerebral palsy.

In some circumstances the armrests can be shorter (desk arms) to allow closer table access. This set-up might be found on a wheelchair when the occupant transfers using a hoist or slide board. In these cases removable armrests are also desirable wheelchair attributes. Another useful addition is the flip-down armrests found on some lounge chairs. These might assist in hoist or lateral slide transfers using a slide board and slide sheet with the resident in sitting or supine lying.

The armrests should be padded to prevent pressure areas should the occupant use them for support in order to remain upright. Chairs that the resident transfers to and from by standing should provide armrests that afford firm support and also reduce the risk of the hands slipping during the transfer to increase safety.

Recliners or 'geri-chairs'

These are often chosen for residents as they provide variable seat-to-backrest angles with a built-in elevating legrest and as such are presumed to be the best option. Other designs only provide the leg elevation option, water cushion seat and no ability to change the seat–backrest angle. These 'geri chairs' are favoured by care staff as they decrease the work of the carer and allow the resident to be pushed around as they are on wheels. They also enable elevation of the legs to control ankle oedema and are perceived to provide comfort, pressure area prevention and control of the effects of abnormal tone. However, Rappl & Jones (2000) consider 'geri-chairs' or the fully reclined chair position to be a restraint. They also consider that this use of the chairs should only be a last resort decision by caregivers owing to the disabling result for the older person. The supposed benefits of using such chairs, listed above, are now discussed in more detail, so that readers can draw their own conclusions from the arguments given.

Elevation of the feet and legs to prevent ankle oedema

Dependency is rarely the only cause of the foot and leg oedema encountered in residents and so mandatory elevation of the legs of non-mobile residents when 'sitting out' has little support from clinical rationale. Some of the factors that preclude leg elevation without a considerable transfer of weight-bearing surfaces from the buttocks and thighs to the sacrum are: shortened posterior and lateral thigh muscles especially the hamstrings, adductor longus, tensor fasciae latae, gracilis, neurovascular bundle and joint capsule of the knee (Pedersen 2000). Stretch of these shortened tissues can lead to pain felt locally and from pain referred distally or proximally and emanating from the neural tissue on stretch. When the range of movement is insufficient to fulfil the needs of the chair-to-legrest angle, an undesirable increase in pressure applied to the calves or heels will also ensue. The discomfort so caused might lead to the resident sliding the buttocks forward in the seat to relieve the pain and pressure. If this occurs then any support of the lower back curves that had been provided by the chair is lost. Thus the resident is likely to assume a flexed posture that in turn will affect gut motility, respiration, circulation and cause joint and muscle pain. The change in weight-bearing surfaces will also increase the risk of pressure ulcer development on the sacrum, spinous processes, Achilles tendons or heels of the feet.

Perceived comfort

Many of the residents positioned in 'geri-chairs' for comfort would benefit from being positioned in upright well-supporting lounge chairs. This is especially so when contractures of soft tissues and the hip and knee joints prevent the resident assuming the reclined positions with legs elevated. Thus, comfort is rarely achieved for a resident placed in a 'geri-chair' unless they have full range of movement available and are able to change position independently.

Pressure area prevention

Some aspects relating to the manufacture of 'geri-chairs' have pressure-relieving properties. However, the frail immobile resident will still need to be assisted to change position frequently to achieve this goal through the chair. Many of the arguments cited previously support the proposal that the 'geri-chair' does not prevent pressure ulcer formation.

Control of spasticity

The most distressing result of hypertonicity for care staff is the resident who continually slides the buttocks to the front of the chair seat and on to the floor. These residents often have acquired brain injury from various injuries or pathologies and in many instances cannot communicate. Therefore gaining cooperation for maintaining a particular seated position is unlikely to succeed.

There are a number of factors that might contribute to the facilitation of increased tone in these residents. Noxious stimuli such as pain from a pressure ulcer, full bladder or constipation can increase tone in people with central nervous system pathologies (Bannister 1978). Just feeling stiff and aching will induce movement to relieve the discomfort in unaffected people so can be the reason for residents with neurological conditions to wriggle also. The movement, however, occurs in the only way possible and that is through combinations of movement that are representative of spastic synergies. These synergic patterns might be symmetrical or asymmetrical, thus accounting for the difficulty in maintaining the position first achieved on being placed in the chair. The first requirement when finding the right chair for the resident with a neurological problem that presents with muscle hypertonicity is to undertake a thorough assessment. This assessment should describe the distribution and presentation of the hypertonus. Factors that aggravate the tone such as head or hip position, the presence of pressure ulcers, sore joints or muscles must be identified so that the chair does not compound the problem. Once these aspects have been addressed, then any loss of limb range of movement resulting from the hypertonicity can be considered. The presentation of muscle spasticity (flexor or extensor) will determine the loss of range and therefore the specific requirements of a chair. In some cases the chair seat configuration might assist in controlling unwanted responses. In general this control is achieved by keeping the pelvis in a position of neutral tilt that maintains slight lumbar lordosis and the normal thoracic kyphosis and normal cervical position. This position enables good weight distribution between the buttocks, thighs and feet and thereby increases the potential for the resident to function at their maximal potential for upper limb movement and for communication (Pedersen 2000). The physiotherapist might consider the introduction of a movement programme that aims to regain lumbar mobility so that the optimal pelvic position can be obtained for residents who are very stiff around the hips and pelvic area. Some strategies that might be employed were discussed in the previous chapter.

The reclining 'geri-chair' obviously does not support the pelvis in the desired position to control the tonal response. It acts as a restraint and might stop the resident from sliding out of the chair but it is also likely to increase the hypertonicity problem and the acquisition of limb contractures through the constant stimulation or reinforcement of the spastic patterns of movement. Independence and function in activities of daily living will also be decreased. Thus the ideal chair for a resident with these problems is one that controls the pelvic position and supports the feet, back and head as well as optimizing function.

The other distressing presentation for carers is the resident who 'jack-knifes' out of their chair. This is most common in the spinal injured resident. A strap around the chest fastened to the backrest is usually necessary to control these spasms as anti-spastic medication does not always prevent their occurrence. This strap should not be considered a restraint as the context of usage is to enhance functional capacity and possible independence if the resident is mobilizing in an electric powered wheelchair.

Advantages of a good chair

The aim of specifically supplying equipment and/or furniture should be to maximize function. The factors that are advantageous to this are many and each item varies in importance depending on the needs of the individual using the chair. Thus the advantages of a good chair include the provision of the following.

- Easy access and egress that is provided by the seat height being at knee height. This means chairs of varying heights or adjustable leg lengths should be available in any facility so tall and short residents are catered for. Armrests that extend to the front of the chair seat enhance safety during these transfers in addition to assisting the movement by making the forward trunk lean safer. The result of providing chairs that make standing up easy is that residents maintain independent or assisted mobility for longer even if the sit-to-stand transfer is only used to assist with hygiene needs.
- Maximization of communication and social interaction occurs when the resident is sitting upright and able to see the person talking with them.
- Optimal postural support through adequate control of pelvic position and the spinal curves or support of spinal deformities so as to reduce the progression of deformity can control the onset of pain.
- Good support assists in obtaining and maintaining postural stability which in turn improves the ability to use the upper limbs and retain maximal functional ability.
- Comfort is provided through good support. When residents are comfortable they will be less agitated and more able to participate in physical care and social activities (Rappl & Jones 2000).
- When the chair enables the resident to assume the upright position safely, vestibular input and integration is improved. This reduces the tendency for the resident to push into extension and lessens the likelihood of the resident falling backwards when standing during care activities or when being assisted to mobilize (Nitz 2000).
- Maintains verticality and possibly visuospatial normality.
- To enable adequate nutritional and fluid intake the resident needs to be positioned upright (Steele et al 1997). Unless this position is used there is a danger of the resident aspirating fluids and developing aspiration pneumonia.
- The upright position maximizes respiratory function, especially when the spinal curvature is well supported. This improves the potential for

cerebral oxygenation, thus controlling agitation and aggression that might result from cerebral hypoxia (Nitz 2000).

Concluding comments

The chair design that suits most requirements is one that has a seat-to-back angle of no more than 95 degrees. The chair should support the pelvis in a position that allows slight lumbar lordosis, and also the spinal curves, length of the thighs and the feet in a plantigrade position on the floor or footplate. Upper limb support from armrests should not elevate the shoulders and cause the occupant to slouch or lean laterally to gain support. Adding a 'tilt-in-space' element to this configuration enables improved forwards stability for residents who have difficulty in maintaining the upright position due to weakness or conscious control. A backwards tilt also changes the direction of gravitation forces acting on the thoracic spine of the resident who has a progressive kyphotic deformity due to vertebral collapse caused by osteoporosis. The 'tilt-in-space' option can also control muscle tone by maintaining pressure and touch through the feet and thighs and keeping the head position in neutral flexion–extension. It also allows the resident to rest out of bed. However, where possible the resident should be put on the bed for a rest if staffing numbers allow. This enables the limbs to be straightened and moved to reduce joint stiffness and discomfort but also to relieve pressure from the seated weight-bearing surfaces. Recently a new chair design has become available that allows the backrest to be lowered flat and the legrests to be elevated so that the occupant can lie flat. This option allows the limbs to be straightened out and the resident nursed side-to-side for maintenance of joint range and pressure relief while using the chair. A change of scenery is possible for immobile residents by using these chairs as they also have wheels for easy relocation. These chairs also have drop-down sides that allow slide transfers from bed to chair or from bed-bath to chair so hoisting can be eliminated.

Summary

- It is imperative to evaluate furniture and ensure it is appropriate for the given resident. Good equipment prescription helps to optimize resident function and assists in preventing likely co-morbidities and injuries.
- Both residents' and carers' needs should be taken into account when deciding upon suitable beds.
- Numerous devices are available to help with injury prevention including pressure-relieving cushions, bed cradles and padded bed rail protectors.
- Appropriate chair choice is based on good rationale, and all components of the chair must be considered to match the individual. Desired outcomes often relate to comfort, tone control, posture, joint positioning and functional outcomes.
- The advantages of a correctly fitted chair are numerous.

References

Alexander N B, Koester D J, Grunawalt J A 1996 Chair design affects how older adults rise from a chair. Journal of the American Geriatrics Society 44:356-362

Alexander N B, Schultz A B, Ashton-Miller J A, Gross M, Giordani B 1997 Muscle strength and rising from a chair in older adults. Muscle and Nerve Suppl 5:S56-S59

Hobson D A 1992 Comparative effects of posture on pressure and shear at the body-seat interface. Journal of Rehabilitation Research and Development 29:21-31

Nitz J C 2000 The seating dilemma in aged care. Australian Journal of Physiotherapy 46:53-58

Pedersen J P 2000 Functional impact of seating modifications for older adults: an occupational therapist perspective. Topics in Geriatric Rehabilitation 16(2):73-83

Rappl L, Jones D A 2000 Seating evaluation: special problems and interventions for older adults. Topics in Geriatric Rehabilitation 16(2):63-72

Steele C M, Greenwood C, Ens I, Robertson C, Seidman-Carlson R 1997 Mealtime difficulties in a home for the aged: not just dysphagia. Dysphagia 12:43-50

Sweeney G M, Clarke A K 1991 Selecting easy chairs for people with arthritis and low back pain. Physiotherapy 77:509-511

Taler G 2002 What do prevalence studies of pressure ulcers in nursing homes really tell us? Journal of the American Geriatrics Society 50:773-774

SECTION 3 THE CHALLENGE OF THE MOBILE RESIDENT

8 The profile of the mobile resident and how to protect such residents from falls

Jennifer C. Nitz and Susan R. Hourigan

This chapter aims to:

- identify the abilities and potential problems of residents who are mobile
- discuss the needs of these residents to maintain safe mobility and reduce the potential for losing functional capacity or being injured by a fall.

Introduction

There is rarely a resident in an RACF who has no limitations at all to mobility. At some time or another most residents will have suffered some injury or illness or have other issues which make their mobility limited and their functional performance variable. Most mobile residents will require the use of a mobility aid for support and/or confidence, and at the very least the physiotherapist should ensure proper use and maintenance of this equipment.

The most obvious issues which spring to mind for mobile residents are balance, falls prevention and relevant exercise prescription. Other issues relate to mobility aids, and principles of assessment and treatment (clinical reasoning). As balance and falls prevention are such topical issues we have designed a chapter to deal with this subject individually; see Chapter 9.

This chapter therefore will profile the mobile resident and identify their needs in order to remain safe and mobile. The mobile resident includes any person who can manage to walk with or without physical assistance from carers and/or walking aids. The distance that the resident can walk might only be a few metres although some residents will be able to walk many kilometres. Cognitive function and physical disability are the main determining factors for safe ambulation. These residents might be housed in low care or high care facilities depending on the amount of assistance or supervision that is required to achieve a safe standard of living. When transferring, these residents will not rely on mechanical devices, although they might need some assistance from a carer to rise from a low chair and to walk short distances.

It is imperative to conduct a full assessment of the resident in order to decide what, if any, will be the treatment ideals and to determine goals. A thorough assessment will also allow the therapist to prescribe a relevant exercise programme in order to maintain the resident's mobility, independent function and quality of life for as long as possible. Perhaps the most important issue related to quality of life is that of independent function and ambulation – it is the key factor which enables residents to make their own decisions and to go where they please. This self-determination enables them to bring themselves to activities of choice or remove themselves from unwanted places, people or situations. It is often the key to maintaining dignity, privacy and happiness.

The profile of functional capacity of mobile residents

Some residents will be independently mobile in all environments but require supervision due to problems with orientation and the potential to become lost. At the other extreme are residents able to walk a short distance with the support of up to two carers and a walking aid. The importance of maintaining or gaining even the lowest level of mobility cannot be overstressed. It might represent the difference between being able to visit family for celebrations, including being able to access the toilet while on the visit, and being unable to leave the RACF. Thus the possible levels of mobility encountered in residents in low or high care might be described by five major categories in our Mobility Dependency Scale (Table 8.1).

The physiotherapist has a responsibility to ensure that the resident remains safe when mobilizing. All residents are at risk of suffering a fall.

Table 8.1 *The Mobility Dependency Scale*

Level	Degree of dependency
4	*Fully dependent (barely mobile but can take up to 10 steps).* Requires two carers possibly using a walking belt and walking aid, e.g. multiple infarcts
3	*Moderately dependent.* Requires two carers using a walking belt for safety, e.g. Parkinson's disease Requires one carer ± using a walking belt and walking aid, e.g. stroke
2	*Minimally dependent (stand-by supervision, some assistance to rise from a chair or for orientation).* Requires a walking belt and carer assistance for safety, e.g. frail older person
1	*Semi-independent (uses an aid and needs environmental modification).* Independent with walking aid, e.g. diabetic amputee. Supervision to overcome disorientation but no physical assistance required, e.g. dementia
0	*Fully independent.* Independent with or without walking aid and not requiring supervision, e.g. global aphasia and little physical restriction post-stroke

Even the most seemingly capable resident is at risk as in many instances they have age related balance decline or have cognitive dysfunction that interferes with their ability to move safely in the environment.

The role of the physiotherapist is to maintain or maximize function and this generally entails regular assessment of functional capacity and balance ability and the prescription of an exercise programme. The findings from the assessment should also be used to identify for the resident and the carers any specific problem such as visual perceptual, motor planning dysfunction or loss of muscle strength that might be putting the resident at increased risk of a fall. A careful explanation needs to be given so that all parties understand the mechanism that increases the risk.

Protection from falls

The resident is never totally protected from suffering a fall but the risk of an injurious fall might be reduced if some adjustment to current practice is made. All over the world RACFs have some form of falls prevention programme in place but residents still suffer falls at an alarming rate. We believe that the content of these programmes is essentially correct and theoretically should reduce the prevalence of falls. However, it is the lack of explanation given to residents and carers regarding the whys and wherefores of the components of the falls prevention programme that leads, through ignorance, to choices being made that reduce compliance.

In the following pages we will explain some of the items included in falls prevention programmes. We will identify factors that increase the likelihood of falls and examine related problems encountered in older people that are due to ageing and acquired pathologies. Enabling all parties to understand the clinical reasoning behind the components of falls prevention programmes will make it more logical to comply with recommendations. Most falls prevention programmes are multifaceted and include components such as environmental adaptations, resident assessment and exercise interventions, education and information to residents and staff and consultation on medication and assistive devices (Becker et al 2003). Even if fall prevention programmes are comprehensive and cover all these aspects, their effectiveness is only as good as the completeness of the coverage of all risk factors for falling as well as the understanding of how the risk factors interact with the older person. Carers, family members and residents all need to understand how the individual will be affected by the risk if strategies to control or avoid these risk factors are to be fully exploited. Thus any educational package must include explanations of cause and effect so that informed decisions, warnings or directions can be made or given by all concerned. The following information is provided to enable readers to understand the mechanics and interpretation of risk assessment findings.

Risk assessment

The assessment of falls risk must include environmental influences, those attributable to the carer, assistive equipment and the intrinsic risk factors found in the resident. A number of processes can then be put in place to reduce the risk but the human factor associated with the potential for minor to catastrophic change in residents or carers must not be discounted.

Environmental falls risk assessment

Changes to depth perception, visual acuity in low contrast situations as well as edge perception difficulties (Lord & Dayhew 2001, Tinetti 2001) that are normal ageing changes will be amplified in some environmental situations. These influences might be limited if changed by refurbishment or if the carer interprets the visually conflicting situation and reassures the resident regarding the interpretation of the environmental situation. The independently mobile resident will not be able to benefit from carer interpretive information and so will still be at major risk in some visually confounding situations.

Small rooms with a number of pieces of furniture reduce the area in which the residents and carers can manipulate walking aids and safely turn to reach the bed or a chair. Poor depth perception or visual field losses put residents at risk of a fall. Items of personal equipment or shoes left lying around increase the risk of tripping. Furthermore, a carer cannot efficiently assist a resident to walk if they are stepping over or around furniture or clutter on the floor and are themselves at risk of a fall. Corridors and common areas must be kept clear of clutter so independently mobile residents are not put at risk.

Furniture can pose major risk factors for falling. The beds used by residents contribute a number of potential fall precipitators. Side rails are often raised bilaterally in the belief that the resident will be protected from a fall from the bed. When the resident is cognitively able, raised side rails might serve as a reminder to call for assistance when getting up or to enable independent rolling during the night by providing a solid point to pull on when rolling and security from rolling out of bed. However, if the resident has some cognitive deficit the rails might only be seen as a barrier to climb over and so cause a fall from a greater height resulting in injury or death from becoming wedged between the rails (Capezuti et al 2002). Great care should be exercised when using bed rails to 'protect' the resident from a fall and each case must be evaluated individually taking all aspects of the resident's physical and mental status into account. If safety is ultimately compromised putting the mattress on the floor for the resident to sleep on will eliminate the potential for a fall, although it makes nursing more difficult.

Some falls from bed can be related to the height of the bed from the floor. If the bed is too high and the resident is unable to easily reach the floor with their feet after swinging their legs over the side of the bed, stability is lost and a fall might follow. Similarly, if the resident has to slide the bottom forwards to the edge of the bed before their feet touch the floor, stability might be lost and a fall ensue. Therefore the bed should be lowered to chair height so that the feet easily touch the floor for egress. New beds can usually be lowered to about 50 cm above the floor. This is still higher than most dining room chairs (45 cm) so will still pose the problems outlined previously but not to as great an extent as some of the older design of beds.

Care must be taken to apply all the brakes on the bed wheels so that the bed does not 'run away' from the resident during a transfer in or out of bed. This aspect is also very important for preventing carer injury at any time when the carer is helping a resident who is in bed. Often the thighs of the carer are leant against the bed for extra support and stability during the task. If the bed moves at any time serious back, neck or other injuries are likely to be suffered. Similarly, if a standing or full hoist is used to transfer a resident, the brakes should be applied during any procedure when the equipment is stationary. This ensures added stability and safety.

Floor materials can pose major problems for mobile residents. They should be non-shiny and non-slip. Floors that are shiny even if not slippery will change the gait of all people walking on the surface. The perception that the floor is slippery will slow the cadence, reduce the step length, broaden the base and in so doing might raise the strength demands by reducing the effective use of momentum for forward propulsion. This might interfere with postural stability and balance enough to increase the risk of a fall.

Carpet can become worn and patchy, causing variability in height of the pile. In some places carpet tiles are used so that heavy wear areas can be controlled. However, the edges of carpet squares or carpet of variable height pile can cause the resident to trip when they have difficulty in lifting their feet when walking.

Colour changes or floor-covering changes between rooms or corridors can lead to visual conflict and increase the potential for a fall. All older people have some degree of acuity loss, age-related macular degeneration or cataracts that reduce the efficiency of their vision and are put at increased risk of a fall by misinterpreting what they are seeing. On the other hand, colour contrast between chair upholstery and floor coverings can enhance the ability of the resident to see the edge of the chair and therefore be able to transfer from standing to sitting with more safety than if the colours of the decor blended.

Shadows falling across corridors due to sunlight streaming through windows can produce such light and dark effects that residents with problems of visual conflict might perceive this light effect as a step up or step down. This might cause hesitation or the resident might try to negotiate a step only to cause a fall through losing balance.

The *outside environment* also can pose a major fall risk. Automatically opening doors are useful to prevent the problem of losing balance while trying to pull or push open heavy doors. However, automatically opening doors can also affect postural stability through the effect of the movement of the door through the visual field and the stimulation of the vestibular optic reflex changing postural muscle activity. Care should be taken to ensure the doorway is not visually confounding and the door runners are not causing hesitation or obstruction.

Paving material that is not slippery when wet should be chosen. Small pavers that might become uneven or poorly maintained should be avoided so that trips and falls are averted. The same should be said for ramps. They should be at the correct incline (readers are encouraged to consult the Building Standards for their part of the world to find the legislated requirements) and have solid railings. Outside communal areas where residents might congregate for social occasions or for time with families should be protected from the sun, rain and wind. Being able to spend time outdoors is important for vitamin D synthesis, so should be made possible for the resident. If a grassed area is accessible it should be very flat and kept mown short. Thick, though manicured lawns are quite unsafe for residents with poor balance as the proprioceptive input from the lower limbs is confounded and more reliance on vision and vestibular input is demanded. Muscles also need to be stronger and reaction time faster to maintain balance on thick grass. Many residents enjoy gardening and if raised beds accessed by a suitable pathway are available, then provision of a safe area such as this where they can potter is very calming and good exercise. Two heights of raised garden bed are advisable. Garden beds should be at chair height for those residents who garden from a wheelchair and higher for the walking gardeners. Garden paths should always be swept clean as dropped leaves and flower petals can be very slippery if damp. Other hazards include gutters and stormwater grates, so where possible alternative solutions to removal of water that keep the ground flat and non-slippery should be employed.

Resident equipment risk factors

Walking aids

Very few residents will walk without the benefit of an assistive device. These walking aids fall into two major categories, those with wheels and those without, and all have some inherent safety issue that relates to efficient maintenance of the equipment. *Wheeled* devices might have solid tyres or pneumatic inner tubes. If pneumatic tyres are used then they should always have equal pressure in the tubes, otherwise they become unstable and can tip the resident off balance and thus precipitate a fall. All wheeled devices need to have some braking mechanism so that the resident can control the speed of progression. Many have bicycle-type brakes that require the resident to have reasonably strong hand grip and speed of coordination as well as sufficient cognitive ability to apply the brakes to enable safe function. If these requirements are not present in the resident then safety becomes a major issue. Other wheeled walking frames utilize the application of downward pressure on the handles to engage the brakes. This is quite useful if the resident loses balance in a forward direction, which will apply the brakes. Still other wheeled assistive devices have no brakes at all and are only safe for use by residents with good balance or with maximal assistance being given to the resident by carers who then control the movement of the walking aid. Wheeled walking aids can be very useful but also can introduce additional safety considerations, so all assistive devices should be evaluated for level of maintenance as well as appropriateness of prescription for the resident, and the physiotherapist is the professional most able to perform this task.

Walking sticks or canes, whether they are single-point or four-point, are generally fitted with rubber stoppers on the feet. When the treads on these stoppers become worn, they are liable to slip on the floor and cause the user to have a fall. Therefore the stoppers should always be checked for sufficient tread and the stopper replaced if it is showing wear.

The height of the walking assistive device must be correct so that it can provide the appropriate level of support. Walking aids that are too high or too short will affect the posture of the user and contribute to instability and might precipitate a fall.

Shoes

Painful feet, foot deformity and inability to put on one's own shoes can be reasons for wearing no shoes or ill-fitting shoes or slippers when walking. Painful or deformed feet alone can increase the risk of a fall (Menz & Lord 1999) but if a supportive, well-fitted shoe is worn the risk of falling should not be increased. On the other hand, if the resident wears shoes that are too big because of trying to accommodate deformities or are poorly secured to the feet, the risk of tripping on the shoes or walking out of the shoe and tripping is increased. This mechanical risk is added to by slow and inefficient balance reactions. Slipping due to decreased friction between the shoes and the support surface is another problem attributable to footwear that can precipitate a fall. Menz et al (2001) showed that no shoe could be considered safe from slipping on wet surfaces. The dynamic coefficient of friction at the shoe–surface interface was different between types of shoe, application of a textured or leather sole and different heel geometry, but there was still need to control manufacturing standards for casual footwear to enhance safety, especially for older people.

Even if the shoes are supportive and secure on the feet, heel soles that are unevenly worn can produce postural instability that might contribute to a fall. Care should therefore be taken to ensure that excessive sole wear is repaired or new shoes bought so that the resident is not put in danger from this cause.

Long or trailing clothing

Many older people lose height due to osteoporosis or weight from disease or illness and as a consequence can find it difficult to obtain clothing that is short or small enough that it does not trail on the floor and pose a tripping hazard. In some cases, the resident does not consider trailing clothing as a fall risk and this hazard should be identified and a solution such as raising the hemline or tying the dressing gown cord implemented.

Glasses

Poor vision has been identified as a major contributing factor for falls. Many residents have vision deficits that will benefit from wearing glasses that improve acuity and stereoscopic vision, as this will enhance the ability of the resident to judge distance and distinguish visually confounding situations. Thus by encouraging residents to use their glasses appropriately, safety when mobilizing might be enhanced. Carers should be aware that some residents might need to be reminded to put their glasses on when dressing as well as having them cleaned so that the lenses are fully functional.

Lord et al (2002) showed that multifocal glasses increased the potential for falling in older people with depth perception and edged contrast sensitivity deficiencies as they blurred the visual field when the person walked. This came about when the visual line coincided with the change in lens focal length. It is recommended that older people use separate reading and distance glasses rather than multifocals to reduce the potential for this cause of falling.

Hearing aids

Hearing loss has been linked to instability and increased potential to suffer a fall in nursing home residents (Bumin et al 2002). Hearing and sound location ability is vital for safety in congested areas and to prevent the resident from being startled by a person or vehicle suddenly appearing in the visual field. If balance is poor these situations might precipitate a fall. Using a hearing aid or bilateral hearing aids might improve hearing to an extent that reduces the risk of a fall and so all staff should encourage this practice. Often residents lack the fine manual skills needed to replace the batteries in hearing aids and this task then falls to the carers or does not get done, so residents discontinue hearing aid use, thus putting themselves at risk of a fall. Carers should be ready and able to assist with hearing aid battery replacement and application to residents. Regular education sessions provided by an audiologist to residents, their families and carers might increase confidence in using and assisting residents to use hearing aids, thereby improving safety and reducing the risk of a fall.

Education regarding procedures for prolonging battery life by turning off the hearing aid or opening the battery case to save the charge might assist in reducing the need for maintenance and frequent battery change. This in turn will reduce frustration from a useless aid and improve resident safety and quality of life.

Resident intrinsic risk factors

More than three co-morbidities or in some cases the presence of specific medical conditions such as stroke, Parkinson's disease, arthritis, depression and dementia are all identified, intrinsic resident risk factors for falls (Tinetti et al 1988). Muscle weakness and pain have also been included as contributing factors.

Postural hypotension can be a major cause of falls in the elderly. It might be related to medication or the actual pathology that the resident presents with such as Shy–Drager syndrome. On the other hand, it might be due only to the effect of ageing on the sympathetic nervous system, heart and cardiac output. A thorough physical examination by the medical practitioner and consultation with the pharmacist should help identify the factors that are contributing to the hypotension so that if possible some remedial action can be undertaken. If there is no treatment then all carers and the resident must be made aware of the risk of a fall due to postural hypotension and of steps that might be taken to reduce this risk, such as pausing after moving from lying to sitting and after standing up.

Another risk factor common in the elderly is vertebrobasilar insufficiency (VBI). Many older people have extreme thoracic kyphoses that require them to extend their upper cervical spine to see where they are going when walking. This position might cause dizziness or loss of consciousness if sustained so residents and carers should be warned of the risk associated with this movement. A similar situation of sustained upper cervical extension is assumed if the resident has to look up to the carer to talk. This is another reason why the carer should always get down to the same level as the resident when conversing.

The physiotherapist will also perform a full functional and balance assessment that should identify physical fall risk factors. These assessments are discussed in Chapter 2 and also in more detail in the next chapter, which deals with balance exclusively.

Medications and the problem of polypharmacy have been identified as major contributors to increased risk of a fall. All the medications taken by the resident including those prescribed by the doctor and those bought over the counter should be identified, as four or more medications increase the likelihood of recurrent falls (Leipzig et al 1999, Yip & Cumming 1994). Sedatives, psychotropic drugs and opioid analgesics are specific medications that have been shown to increase the risk of a fall (Neutel et al 1996, Weiner et al 1998). Other drugs that might contribute to a fall are: antihypertensives, antiarrhythmics, anti-Parkinson's disease drugs and hypoglycaemic agents (Yip & Cumming 1994). In addition, drug interactions are common in the elderly and a pharmacist is the person best suited to identify the presence of potential drug interactions in a resident. Another problem encountered in older people is the change in half-life and excretion of many drugs owing to liver and renal dysfunction.

The physiotherapist's role in protecting residents from a fall

Primarily physiotherapists will perform the most efficient physical examination to determine the physical factors that contribute to increased risk of falling. In collaboration with the nursing staff they will determine the level of assistance or supervision required during activities of daily living and for special situations such as walking in the garden. The physiotherapist will identify physical problems that might be improved in function with an exercise intervention programme that specifically targets these problems, thereby improving the physical function and safety of the resident. Assessment and treatment of balance problems are covered in detail in the following chapter. Thus the physiotherapist has an important role in identifying the resident who is at risk of falling. Physiotherapists are also responsible for monitoring the status of residents and noting changes that might indicate more assistance or intervention is required as the resident ages or acquires further disabilities, as might occur should they suffer a stroke.

Physiotherapists should also be involved in conferences to determine the contributions to falls risk from medication or personal equipment, especially when intervention is needed and the team needs to decide on a mode of action with the consent and cooperation of the resident and their family. Therefore it is usually important to include the resident and/or family member in this conference.

Physiotherapists are usually responsible for the manual handling training of carers and as such have an ideal situation to educate the carers about the risk factors for falls during these sessions. Manual handling is intimately related to falls prevention as it considers the risks for the resident as well as the carer. Explaining when to be most vigilant when walking a resident and why this is important will increase carers' compliance with instructions as relevancy is emphasized. This enables the logical reasoning behind the instructions to be considered by both carers and residents and so enhances willingness from all participants to apply the instruction.

The physiotherapist's role in educating staff regarding safe patient handling

Patient handling refers to the moving or 'handling' of people. The tasks involved are those activities which require the use of force exerted by a carer to hold, support, transfer (lift, lower, carry, push, pull, slide), or restrain a person at the workplace.

'No lift' policies aim to protect both residents and staff members by ensuring that the manual lifting of residents is eliminated in all but exceptional or life-threatening circumstances (Royal College of Nursing 1996). Such policies require that residents who are able to assist are encouraged to do so, whereas mechanical devices such as hoists are used for those residents who are unable to assist in order to minimize the strain on the worker and lessen the likelihood of injury to the resident.

It is the physiotherapist's responsibility to individually assess residents' mobility and ability to transfer on admission and as regularly as is necessary. The physiotherapist is the professional staff member most appropriately trained to undertake this assessment. The assessment will attempt to ascertain the resident's rehabilitation needs and their ability to participate whilst always considering the needs of other staff members. The aim is to protect both workers' health and residents' health, and the goal is primarily to protect both parties. The contribution provided by the physiotherapist is discussed in detail in Chapter 2.

Safe patient handling systems are introduced to facilitate a safe environment, as mentioned previously. Other goals of a patient handling 'no lift' system which should be focused upon include reducing the numbers of injuries and injury severity, complying with organizational policy, meeting union imperatives, complying with workplace health and safety legislation, assisting with quality improvement systems, increasing the skills and knowledge of staff members and improving patient care. With these goals in mind it is easy to realize the extreme importance of safe patient handling. It is also easy to realize that this job requires an enormous amount of organizational skill, educational prowess and the ability to assess and teach on the part of the physiotherapist in the RACF. Developing and continuing patient handling programmes is arguably the biggest responsibility an RACF physiotherapist has.

Workplace health and safety legislation requires both employers and workers to meet various obligations. The RACF must ensure the health and safety of workers by providing equipment, space and training to employees. Workers must ensure they follow instructions given in relation to manual tasks and not wilfully place themselves or another's health or safety at risk. Staff members must follow instructions given in training programmes and use patient handling equipment that is provided by the facility. Carers need to check the resident mobility plan which is designed after assessment by the physiotherapist, communicate with the resident and other staff involved, refer to senior staff for assistance if required, and be responsible for reporting risks within the workplace.

A risk management system must be developed. This should ensure equipment maintenance requirements are met and any problems are reported in a timely and efficient manner. Incident and accident reports should be formalized in order to enable statistics to be recorded and risk management strategies to be developed and refined. Staff should be empowered to be involved in processes which contribute to maintaining best practice in the area of resident care, health and safety management and quality improvement strategies. Figure 8.1 shows how the risk management process is continuous.

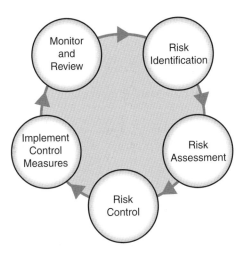

Figure 8.1 *The risk management process.*

The individual resident's risk assessment is part of the initial and ongoing physiotherapy review. This assessment and the development of the residents' mobility plans are the first and most important processes in selecting safe handling techniques to be utilized by the residents and staff. This fundamental assessment will lead to safety, best practice and falls prevention. Refer to Chapter 2 that deals with assessment for more detailed information. However, the assessment should specifically include the following:

1. medical diagnosis
2. mobility history
3. physical examination (pain, range, balance, strength)
4. mental status and cognition
5. communication
6. weight
7. other relevant features (e.g. diurnal variation, extra medical equipment - PEG feeds, urinary catheters and oxygen supplementation).

Perhaps the simplest strategies are sometimes the hardest to convey to staff. It is never superfluous to repeat the basics and to spell out some rules relating to resident handling. Some of the most important points to teach and assess in patient handling programmes are related in point format below. Educate staff to do the following:

- Refer to the mobility plan (especially if they do not know residents well or might have been away on leave and not current with resident status), get a good handover in order to be up-to-date, read any appropriate communication books/boards.
- Encourage residents to assist themselves as much as possible (this helps carers and residents). Sometimes the less help given by staff the better, even if it does take a little longer for the task to be completed.
- Emphasize good communication (get eye contact, tell the resident what the aim is and get their concurrence if possible).
- Adjust the environment for safety (manipulate bed height, ensure brakes are on equipment, clear the pathway and surrounds as necessary).
- Refer to senior staff if a resident is on the floor or seems changed or ill.
- Utilize principles of back care and joint protection in all work practices (good posture, using their legs and abdominal muscles well).
- Plan the move, confirm it verbally with the resident and their care partner if applicable and initiate the transfer on the count of three so that all parties are ready and assisting.

Summary

- The role of the physiotherapist is to assess the physical and cognitive state of the resident to determine the presence of risk factors for a fall.
- The physiotherapist also needs to educate the resident, family and carers about the environmental, personal and age-related factors that might contribute to a fall and relate this information to manual handling and caring tasks.
- Case conferences that include a pharmacist, medical practitioner, carers, residents, family and the physiotherapist may need to be initiated by the physiotherapist. All aspects of falls prevention might then be addressed and the resident and family are incorporated in the decision-making processes so all will be happy to act on decisions regarding care. (Appendix 3 discusses case conferences in more detail.)
- Physiotherapists should provide carer education regarding safe resident handling procedures.

References

Becker C, Kron M, Lindemann U et al 2003 Effectiveness of a multifaceted intervention on falls in nursing home residents. Journal of the American Geriatrics Society 51(3):306–313

Bumin G, Uyanik M, Aki E, Kayihan H 2002 An investigation of risk factors for falls in elderly people in a Turkish rest home: A pilot study. Aging Clinical and Experimental Research 14(3):192–196

Capezuti E, Maislin G, Strumpf N, Evans L K 2002 Side rail use and bed-related fall outcomes among nursing home residents. Journal of the American Geriatrics Society 50(1):90–96

Leipzig M, Cummings R, Tinetti M 1999 Drugs and falls in older people: a systematic review and meta-analysis: 1. Psychotropic drugs. Journal of the American Geriatrics Society 47:30–39

Lord S R, Dayhew J 2001 Visual risk factors for falls in older people. Journal of the American Geriatrics Society 49(4):508–515

Lord S R, Dayhew J, Howland A 2002 Multifocal glasses impair edge-contrast sensitivity and depth perception and increase the risk of falls in older people. Journal of the American Geriatrics Society 50(11):1760–1766

Menz H B, Lord S R 1999 Foot problems, functional impairment, and falls in older people. Journal of the American Podiatric Association 89(9): 458–467

Menz H B, Lord S R, McIntosh A S 2001 Slip resistance of casual footwear: implications for falls in older adults. Gerontology 47(3):145–149

Neutel C I, Hirdes J P, Maxwell C J, Patten S B 1996 New evidence on benzodiazepine use and falls: the time factor. Age and Ageing 25:273–278

Royal College of Nursing 1996 Code of Practice for Patient Handling, London

Tinetti M E 2001 Where is the vision for fall prevention? Journal of the American Geriatrics Society 49(5):676–677

Tinetti M E, Speechley M, Ginter S F 1988 Risk factors for falls among elderly persons living in the community. New England Journal of Medicine 319: 1701–1707

Weiner D K, Hanlon J T, Studenski S A 1998 Effects of central nervous system polypharmacy on falls liability in community-dwelling elderly. Gerontology 44:217–221

Yip Y B, Cumming R G 1994 The association between medications and falls in Australian nursing-home residents. Medical Journal of Australia 160:14–18

9 A theoretical framework for the assessment and treatment of balance and mobility deficits in the elderly

Nancy Low Choy

This chapter aims to:

- review the theoretical elements that contribute to balance and mobility as a basis for assessing balance and mobility in the elderly, and presenting a tailored but multidimensional approach to assessing and retraining balance and mobility deficits in the elderly
- describe a process of assessing balance and mobility in the elderly that uses observational and problem-solving skills while analysing balance and mobility tasks, identifies and measures impairments, and monitors progress and outcomes for elders of varying functional motor ability.

Introduction

Falls and injury prevention is a topical area of research in the elderly with programmes aiming to reduce the incidence of falls and related injuries in men and women over the age of 65 years (Hinman 1998, Lord et al 1994, 1995, 1996, Speechley & Tinetti 1991, Steinberg et al 2000, Tinetti et al 1994). This focus has been the result of studies that show falls occurring in one in three people aged over 65 years in any given 12-month period (Cho & Kamen 1998, Lord et al 1993, Speechley & Tinetti 1990, Woollacott & Tang 1997). One of the contributing elements to the rise in prevalence of falls in elders is the decline that may occur in the multiple mechanisms involved in postural stability and balance. The physiotherapist is ideally equipped to manage dysfunction in the postural mechanism and can use acquired knowledge, skills and experiences to address the needs of the frail aged in residential aged care along with older people who live in supervised care or independently in the community. An understanding of the theoretical basis of 'balance' provides the physiotherapist with the knowledge base from which an informed assessment can be developed. A thorough assessment of the elements contributing to balance and safe mobility identifies those aspects of balance, along with underlying impairments, that need to be addressed for each resident. The use of tools that monitor progress and outcomes and the ability to implement targeted intervention programmes on an individualized basis or effectively in a group provide the physiotherapist with the specialized skills required to meet the variable needs of older people.

Theoretical basis for assessment and interventions

The presenting balance and mobility of an individual (resident or community ambulant elder) is dependent on the integrity of the sensorimotor systems, the given task and the environment in which the individual is functioning. This triad has been given prominence by the works of Shumway-Cooke & Woollacott (2001). For the ageing adult, this means understanding the individual with varying impairments (abilities and deficits), while performing a range of tasks that require stability and demand mobility in a functioning environment such as found within an RACF, an individual's home and local community (Table 9.1). A grasp of this concept ensures that a comprehensive and multidimensional approach to both assessment and intervention for optimal management of the elderly client is offered and clearly underpins the functional and multidimensional approach to retraining balance and mobility.

A large body of research informs us of the elements that an individual requires for efficient balance and mobility. These include the role and quality of sensory input, central processing and integration of sensory cues, reaction time to stimulus response and cognitive (attention) demands during the execution of tasks. There is also the need for flexibility in the musculoskeletal system, selective activation and timing of motor units for task execution as well as strength and endurance of recruited skeletal muscle fibres. Deficits in any of these elements could contribute to decreased stability, mobility, endurance and efficiency of movement. Thus each of these changes within the individual needs to be considered as a basis for developing the practical implications for retraining balance and mobility.

Table 9.1 *The contextual framework for assessment and intervention*

The client group
Frail aged with multiple impairments who is dependent
Elder requiring supervised care
Elder who is independent
Balance and mobility tasks
Sitting balance
Capacity to stand up, balance and walk
Capacity to transfer and be wheelchair ambulant
The settings
Residential aged care facility
Supervised care within a hostel/home
Living independently at home within the community

Sensory system decline

The visual, somatosensory and vestibular systems are important components of postural control. These systems are used to monitor the relationship between the position and movement of the body in space and the forces acting upon the body that may cause displacement (Shumway-Cooke & Woollacott 2001). Older people frequently have impaired vision, vestibular function, and somatic sensation in the legs and feet. A decline in the sensory systems may cause decreased perception, integration, reaction time and feedback during tasks under varying environmental conditions. Such impairments reduce postural stability, particularly when there is concomitant impairment of central processing within the nervous system.

Decreased visual acuity adversely affects balance ability. It is recognized that a loss of visual acuity can result from cataracts, macular degeneration, and loss of peripheral vision due to ischaemic retinal or brain disease (Lord et al 2001, Shumway-Cook & Woollacott 2001). Distance acuity of less than 20/50 will have a significant effect on postural stability. Because of multiple changes within the structure of the eye itself, less light is transmitted to the retina. With a decrease in contrast sensitivity, this causes loss of visual contour and depth perception. Understanding of the type of changes in the visual system that cause decreased postural stability has been advanced by the work of Tanaka et al (1995), Wade & Jones (1997) and Lord & Menz (2000). Studies by Tanaka et al (1995) have shown that the combined effects of age, insufficiency of muscle control, and reduced vision and tactile sensitivity are associated with postural instability. The work of Lord and colleagues has demonstrated the importance of considering contrast sensitivity and depth perception, as a decline in these functions with ageing has been linked to an increased risk of slips, trips and falls (Lord & Menz 2000). Further, the issue of the type of corrective lenses has been raised, with multifocal lenses attributed with a higher incidence of falls than bifocal or distance only lenses (Lord et al 2001, 2002).

These issues are important as elders are considered to be more reliant on vision for balance than younger persons. This reliance has been demonstrated in healthy elders (Alhanti et al 1997, Manchester et al 1989, Newton 1995, Tanaka et al 1995, Teasdale et al 1991) and fallers aged over 65 years (Anacker & Di Fabio 1992, Cho & Kamen 1998, Lord et al 1991, 1992, Maki et al 1994, Tobis et al 1985, Whitney et al 2000). The somatosensory and vestibular system changes that have been documented with ageing may be important contributors to this reliance on vision.

Somatosensory changes with ageing have been extensively researched in recent decades with a number of parameters requiring consideration. Hurley et al (1998) give emphasis to the combined effect of age, strength and joint position sense on postural steadiness and function, while others have demonstrated decreased tactile sensitivity and dynamic joint positioning ability with ageing (Manchester et al 1989, Tanaka et al 1995). The work of Anacker & Di Fabio (1992) demonstrated the importance of the quality of orienting input from the ankle receptors to postural stability when balancing on firm and compliant surfaces, while Ring et al (1989) showed the relationship of foot position awareness, age and stability. Earlier researchers (Whanger & Wang 1974) had demonstrated that cutaneous vibratory sensation could best be detected at the knee in elders as reduced ankle sensation had occurred with ageing. In general, the reduced function of the proprioceptive system is considered a contributor to the rising incidence of falls with elders over 65 (Anacker & Di Fabio 1992, Brocklehurst et al 1982, Horak et al 1990, Manchester et al 1989, Tanaka et al 1995). It is clear that a decline in somatosensory function could contribute to a reduced ability to balance with changes in tactile acuity, vibration sense and joint repositioning ability needing to be considered. Other researchers give emphasis to the combined effect of a decline in somatosensory function and vestibular function on postural instability in elders (Alhanti et al 1997, Horak et al 1990, Newton 1995, Peterka & Black 1990, Teasdale et al 1991, Whitney et al 2000).

In the aged, a reduction in function of the vestibular system is evidenced by a loss of vestibular hair and nerve cells by 60 years of age (Paige 1992) but the precise contribution to unsteadiness and falls is difficult to measure (Lord et al 2001). Researchers have demonstrated the importance of efficient vestibular function while balancing on a compliant surface without vision and that postural stability is significantly different in young and older adults when ankle joint and visual input are distorted or absent (Baloh et al 1987, Horak et al 1989, 1990, Peterka & Black 1990, Teasdale et al 1991, Woollacott et al 1986). This means that older people are more prone to falls when visual conflict or poor vision presents in conjunction with a change to the ground or support surface or when deficits are present in either the proprioceptive or vestibular systems when vision is occluded.

Thus the vestibular system is an important source of information for stability during movements in 'busy' environs or when tasks are executed on stable or more challenging, unstable surfaces. It provides the individual with the capacity to know when the environment is stable or moving, thus resolving any conflict for the visual system. In a similar way the vestibular system assists the somatosensory systems to maintain balance during tasks that are faster paced, when tasks require the individual to balance over a narrower base or while working at height, and when tasks are executed on an unstable base (e.g. grass) or if lighting is poor (e.g. shaded conditions or twilight), when vision is less able to be used or not available (e.g. night-time/darkness).

Other researchers have drawn attention to the contribution of dizziness and gaze instability to unsteadiness and falls. With ageing, the otolith may become hardened, fragment and detach, setting up abnormal signal patterns in the hair cells (Baloh et al 1987). An imbalance of signals from one vestibular apparatus may contribute to the increased incidence of dizziness with unsteadiness reported in the elderly. The most common cause of dizziness with unsteadiness in the elderly is benign paroxysmal positional vertigo (BPPV) where hardened otoconia dislodge and float in one of the semicircular canals, usually the posterior canal (Baloh et al 1987, Baloh & Halmagyi 1996, Herdman 2000). A bilateral loss of vestibular cells is less likely to cause an imbalance of signals, such that unsteadiness may present without accompanying dizziness, although complaints of a shifting visual field (oscillopsia) remain common (Hillman et al 1999). Gaze stability is controlled through the vestibular ocular reflex (VOR) which provides a coordinated action between eye and head movement during motor tasks so that objects in the visual field remain clear during movement. With a decline in peripheral vestibular receptor function with ageing, the capacity of the VOR to maintain gaze stability may be reduced and the visual field appears to 'shift' or 'blur' with head movement (Hillman et al 1999). In addition to such degenerative changes within the vestibular apparatus, dizziness may be caused by medication and a number of pathologies implicating the vestibular system (Baloh & Halmagyi 1996, Herdman 2000). As dizziness may contribute to instability, unsteadiness and imbalance during gait and negatively affect functional mobility, it is important to identify the cause of dizziness. If the vestibular system is implicated it may be amenable to physiotherapy intervention. This means that an assessment of balance ability in the elderly needs to consider the status of the vestibular system and determine if gaze instability and/or dizziness are contributing to the balance difficulties experienced as well as assessing balance under environmental conditions (removal of vision and a change in the support base) that challenge vestibular function.

In summary, there is some redundancy in each of the sensory systems when the systems are efficiently functioning. This means that balance should be able to be maintained without vision, on unstable surfaces, or in sensory conflict situations. However, if more than one system is deficient, balance control is challenged and falls may result (Horak et al 1990). This may occur with pathology (Baloh & Halmagyi 1996, Herdman 2000), but in the elderly a general decline in multiple systems has been demonstrated and these changes summate in the aged to cause balance difficulties in a number of situations (Herdman 2000, Lord et al 1991, 1993, Woollacott 2000). For the elderly, situations of sensory conflict (e.g. a busy visual environment or a change in the support surface being negotiated) may tax an already impaired sensorimotor system and contribute to a loss of balance. Although it is important to assess the integrity of the sensory systems, the decline in balance is recognized in part as a problem of central processing of sensory information as much as a primary change in sensory system function.

Changes in central nervous system function associated with a decline in balance

Multiple aspects of central nervous system (CNS) function are susceptible to changes with ageing. Consideration needs to be given to: the reduced ability to process and re-weight sensory information; slower reaction times and delayed anticipatory postural responses in preparation for voluntary movement; and the decreased capacity to allocate sufficient attention to postural control during the performance of dual or multiple tasks.

Processing and organization of sensory information

Slower processing and organization of sensory information may occur with ageing and contribute to postural dyscontrol. Even if accurate sensory input is available, the CNS is less able to use accurate information in determinations of position and movement (Horak et al 1989). Elders find situations with reduced or conflicting somatosensory and visual inputs particularly challenging and when they are asked to balance in these demanding situations increased postural sway or loss of balance may occur (Alhanti et al 1997, Horak et al 1990, Newton 1995, Peterka & Black 1990, Teasdale et al 1991, Whitney et al 2000). In addition, many elders who have had a fall have impaired visuospatial perception. This change in ability to correctly perceive the vertical and other orientations may be particularly important in the anticipatory formulation of postural adjustments for a specific environmental hazard (Tobis et al 1985, Wade & Jones 1997).

Anticipatory postural responses and strategy selection

Slowed reaction time is a frequent deficit produced by ageing (McIlroy & Maki 1996), with an increased time interval between application of a stimulus and initiation of movement. In addition pre-motor time (time interval between application of a stimulus and initiation of electromyographic (EMG) activity), and motor time (time interval between onset of EMG activity and initiation of movement) is lengthened with normal ageing (Studenski et al 1991). Thus both anticipatory postural responses and those adjustments required during movement may need to be considered with ageing.

In certain dynamic situations the body uses anticipatory (proactive) postural responses to stabilize the body both during and before initiating voluntary movement. Some research has studied the age-related changes associated with these anticipatory responses in order to better understand these issues for balance. Older adults have been shown to have slowed muscle response latencies compared to younger individuals for both postural and prime-mover muscle groups in a simple single-leg flexion task. The same research found a decreased correlation between the two muscle groups and a decrease in time period between onset of the two groups when the task was increased in speed. A loss of balance was associated with prime-movers and postural muscles being activated at the same time in the very old group, which may be a factor in decreasing postural control in the elderly (Studenski et al 1991, Woollacott 2000). Subsequent research has identified slower voluntary reaction times and postural muscle reaction times, disruption in the organization of muscle synergists, increased variability in muscle response latencies and activation, and an increased incidence of co-contraction of muscles in elders. These changes serve to decrease the efficiency of the anticipatory postural response system, which clearly may cause instability and lead to falls in the elderly (Frank et al 1987, Inglin & Woollacott 1988, Stelmach & Worringham 1985).

Age-related changes in automatic postural response synergies were studied by Woollacott et al (1986). These researchers examined the muscle response synergies and strategies of older adults (61–78 years) in order to make a comparison with young adults (19–38 years). Fundamentally the older group recorded similar response organization patterns to the younger group (muscle synergies began in the ankle and moved proximally), yet differences were evident in some response characteristics. A significantly slower onset latency in ankle dorsiflexors was shown for ankle strategies in a backward sway perturbation. In some older adults the muscle response organization was upset, with response activation occurring proximally first and radiating downwards, a direct reversal of the normal pattern shown in earlier research. Co-activation in the antagonist muscles along with the agonists tended to occur more often in the older group than in the younger group, resulting in a general stiffening of joints in response to perturbation. This impaired response amongst synergistic muscles activated in response to instability is an important finding in relation to age-related changes in the elderly and balance control.

The elderly have been shown to use a hip movement strategy more often than younger controls. This may be due to related pathology such as ankle muscle weakness or stiffness, or peripheral sensory system decline. This increased usage of the hip strategy may alter movements made within the new internally mapped limits of stability and generally limit the boundaries for the use of discrete movement strategies (Horak et al 1989, Manchester et al 1989). These researchers suggested that the preferred use of the hip strategy predominantly in older adults may be implicated in falls in certain situations, for example when ambulating on difficult narrower surfaces where the shear forces generated by the feet cannot be resisted adequately to prevent falling. These findings amongst elderly subjects show that there is limited ability to adapt movements for balance in response to changing tasks and environmental demands.

More recent research (Brauer et al 2000) demonstrated a delay in gluteus medius activation during a stepping task with increasing age which was predictive of prospective fallers. Impaired control of lateral stepping reactions in older adults has also been demonstrated (Maki et al 2000). Other research has also demonstrated delayed responses and reduced ability to step maximally and rapidly, with displacement in all directions in elders compared to younger adults, and this was also significantly more impaired in those elders who had had a fall (Medell & Alexander 2000). This decline in ability to activate muscles efficiently during tasks and to control stepping responses when displaced is critical given the increased reliance of elders on the hip strategy as a mechanism for balancing when displaced. Together these findings demonstrate the vulnerability of elders when required to balance in challenging or unstable situations.

Attention demands and balance

A growing area of research relates to the cognitive aspect of postural control, i.e. the allocation of attention to balance during the performance of additional tasks. Changes to postural steadiness while standing on varying surfaces and executing a second task have been demonstrated in elderly fallers compared to young and older people who have not had a fall (Brauer et al 1999a, 1999b, Shumway-Cook & Woollacott 2000, Shumway-Cook et al 1997). Other research has shown the influence of a second task while walking (Brauer et al 2000, Lundin-Olsson et al 1997, 1998, Shumway-Cook et al 2000). Rankin et al (2000) have shown that a decline in muscle activity occurs when performing a secondary (dual) task while Shumway-Cook & Woollacott (2000) give emphasis to the increasing attention demands for postural control with ageing, with elders unable to allocate sufficient attention to postural control during the performance of multiple tasks.

Cognitive control may strongly impact on the ability of the elderly to balance. Dual-task situations, decreased confidence and a fear of falling are important aspects to examine in the elderly and more research is needed in this area. Fear of falling or apprehension about movement is a likely result of difficulty in maintaining balance. This may result in the voluntary decrease in movement often seen in the aged. Often it is not an inability to move that is witnessed but a fear of moving. A pattern of disuse may result with a negative cycle of events leading to further disability. Some research has been directed at the impact of fear of falling on postural control and falls risk (Maki et al 1991) but further work is warranted.

Musculoskeletal system decline

An understanding of how the decline in joint range of movement, muscle strength and endurance contributes to the deterioration of balance and postural stability is important in directing the management of aged clients.

Strength changes with age

Age-related deterioration in sensorimotor function of muscle has been established (Aniansson et al 1980, Hyatt et al 1990, Lexell 1993, Murray et al 1985, Vandervoort & McComas 1986). Decreased strength is the result of several factors that may contribute to decreased muscle hypertrophy and subsequent decline in function with ageing. These include a loss of alpha motor neurons, atrophy of type I and II myofibres, diminished oxidative capacity of exercising muscle, and a subsequent reduction in ability to produce torque (Grimby & Saltin 1983, Murray et al 1985, Rutherford & Jones 1992). Such changes in muscle morphology, together with a decrease in the daily level of muscle loading, leads to a decline in strength (Lexell 1993). Lower extremity muscle strength can be reduced by as much as 40% between the ages of 30 and 80 years with weakness even more severe in older nursing home residents with a history of falls (Whipple et al 1987). This research found a marked reduction in measures of mean ankle and knee strength in fallers compared to non-fallers.

Skeletal muscle strength has been shown to be very important for function, with Buchner & de Lateur (1991) demonstrating that over 20% of the variance in functional status is explained by relative strength in the lower limb muscles. Other studies support this view and have shown that age is correlated negatively with strength, postural stability and mobility tasks (Hurley et al 1998, Lord & Castell 1994). Quadriceps strength has been emphasized in most of the research linking lower limb strength, postural stability and mobility tasks (Hurley et al 1998, Lord et al 1991, 1994). Limited research has been carried out on the strength of the hip muscles. Further work associated with hip muscle strength, particularly the hip abductor muscles, and balance performance with ageing is required, given the work of Brauer et al (2000) that demonstrated the delay in gluteus medius activation in prospective fallers. In addition, very little attention has been paid to eccentric muscle strength and age-related changes although this type of contraction is important in maintaining postural stability and while performing tasks such as sitting down from standing.

Soft tissue compliance and ageing

The compliance of tissues with ageing has received some attention from researchers. Increased tightness of muscle and stiffness of joints is particularly evident toward the end range of motion and may influence the overall skill in coordinated movement (Studenski et al 1991). Loss of flexibility has been linked to degenerative changes in collagen fibres, dietary deficiencies, general paucity of movement, and arthritic joint changes (Lewis & Phillippi 1993).

Diminished strength and flexibility have been considered precursors to poor postural alignment, and the importance of joint range of movement, muscle strength and endurance for postural stability has been documented (Hurley et al 1998, Skelton et al 1994). Decreased range of motion and loss of spinal flexibility may lead to a characteristic flexed or stooped posture. Faulty posture is further influenced by inactivity and prolonged sitting. Of particular importance is the potential loss, owing to stiffness, of ability to efficiently accomplish preparatory postural adjustments prior to execution of a movement.

In summary, unsteadiness and the increased potential for a fall may be a consequence of the multiple changes that could occur with ageing. Challenging surface and visual environments, dual-task situations, inefficient responses when tasks or situations impose speed demands along with reduced strength and flexibility may collectively contribute to poor balance and decreased confidence with fear of falling emerging in certain situations (Tinetti et al 1990).

Multiple problems may underlie decreased balance ability with ageing, which clearly reflects the complexity and multisystem control of postural stability and balance. A growing body of evidence guides our understanding of these changes and supports a holistic and comprehensive approach to assessment which links the individual deficits with specific tasks and environmental situations. In this way the physiotherapist can confidently demonstrate the problems as they relate to each individual resident or community ambulant elder, identify which tasks are problematic or ably executed and in which environmental conditions the task can be performed safely and independently, or when supervision or assistance is required for safety.

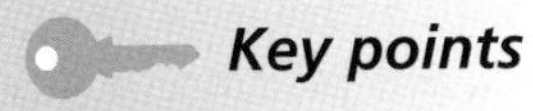

Key points

Multiple elements need to be assessed in an examination of balance to determine those aspects that require attention during intervention. Factors relating to the individual include:

capacity to move from positions with larger base of support to those with smaller base of support (e.g. sitting ability; standing up; standing balance; weight shift and step)
quality of alignment and ability to hold a position with a decreasing base of support (e.g. standing with standard base of support; feet together; stride stand; tandem stand)
ability to hold varying positions under a variety of conditions involving visual/proprioceptive conflict (e.g. eyes open/closed; firm/soft surface)
ability to control internally generated displacement (e.g. weight shift; reach and step) and determine limits of stability
ability to control responses to external forces: quality of responses (ankle; hip and stepping strategies) and response time to displacement (efficient; delayed; absent)
capacity to manage dual/multi-tasks
contribution of specific sensory and motor systems to balance: sensory system function (visual, somatosensory and vestibular system function) and visuospatial perception; functional strength and flexibility; musculoskeletal/cardiovascular-respiratory endurance.

The assessment process used by physiotherapists considers these multiple elements during the performance of motor tasks in a variety of environments. In turn, interventions can provide an opportunity to integrate all aspects to improve balance and safe mobility in relevant environments for each individual resident. This would also include a need to identify those tasks and environmental conditions that require supervision or assistance from care staff for safe execution.

Assessment of balance and mobility

The resident who has a fall or who is at risk of a fall requires a comprehensive evaluation to determine the causal factors and identify those aspects amenable to physiotherapy intervention. Multiple factors have been shown to increase the risk of a fall and associated injuries in elders over 65 years. These factors include environmental challenges, postural hypotension, multiple pathologies, four or more medications, depression, declining sensorimotor function as well as the difficulty elders have with dual tasks and the external environment (Brauer et al 1999a, 1999b, Hinman 1998, Shumway-Cooke et al 1997, 2000, Speechley & Tinetti 1991, Tinetti et al 1988, Woollacott & Tang 1997).

A medical review provides the physiotherapist with a profile of general health, medical and surgical history, co-morbidities and pharmacological management as a basis for interpreting the presenting balance and functional mobility. From a physiotherapy assessment the contribution of sensory/perceptual, cognitive (attention to dual task) and motor dysfunction to the performance of balance/mobility tasks within the functioning environment can be determined. The environmental considerations include ability to walk over a variety of floor surfaces; ability to manage from a variety of seating and negotiate chair/table access; indoor and outdoor surface challenges; management of stairs, slopes, uneven surfaces; and capacity to manage under conditions of variable lighting (sunlight and shadows) or poorly lit conditions. The clinical reasoning skills of the physiotherapist enable the identified problems to be interpreted and prioritized into a management plan that addresses the reduced postural control evident during balance and mobility tasks in a variety of environmental and lighting demands.

Understanding the conditions in which the balance performance is compromised provides the basis for intervention and, as required, for modifying the environment to minimize 'falls risk'. Essentially the physiotherapist seeks the reasons for poor balance and increased falls risk and identifies the tasks and environmental conditions required for safe execution of tasks in positions such as sitting, standing or walking. Reliable and valid clinical measures can be used to identify the underlying impairments contributing to reduced stability and mobility and to objectively monitor the performance of the different aspects of balance and mobility. Such steps provide us with the information required for a future review of the resident and enable us to determine if interventions have been effective as well as the need for assistance during activities of daily living.

Analysis of balance and mobility tasks: use of observational skills

As physiotherapists we frequently commence the evaluation of balance and mobility tasks using our observational skills while analysing movement. Subsequently we document the quality of the movement control during the performance of the selected motor task. An examination of sitting and standing balance as well as walking is critical but it may also be necessary to consider bed mobility tasks for the resident functioning at a lower level. During the analysis of tasks, clinical reasoning skills will be used to consider the likely problems that could be disturbing balance and mobility. The impairments are confirmed by applying specific tests, and a summary of suitable measures is provided. An objective measure of performance of the task completes the review of the resident.

1. Balanced sitting: consider the effect of the type of chair/bed surface on sitting ability

(i) Observe, describe and palpate sitting posture and alignment

- Are the feet supported on the floor or dangling? Does support change all further observations?
- Is weight evenly distributed; adequate anterior pelvic tilt; adequate trunk and neck extension; head balanced on level shoulders?

- If resident leans or falls – why? Which direction?
- Is he/she aware of falling? Sensory loss? Spatial neglect? Verticality problems?
- Is he/she afraid?
- Is the resident visually dependent?
- Is dizziness a problem – reason?

(ii) Observe resident-initiated displacements in sitting

Internal displacement These include movement of head and trunk, reaching forward, to side, back, overhead and to the floor. Note the cues/assistance required and the ability of the resident to move outside the base and return, to determine if the resident can be safely left unsupervised in sitting.

- Head/trunk movements while moving in a position.
- Postural adjustments during reaching tasks forward/side/back directions and return to a stable position.
- Forward reach towards floor and return; the ability to pick an object up from the floor.
- Ability to reach sideways towards floor and return to upright or need to sit in chair with arms.
- Ability to balance in sitting while lifting up right/left legs alternately; ability to put on shoes.

(iii) Observe responses to external displacements

- Note the quality of trunk and limb responses to external displacement applied in anterior-posterior and lateral directions. Are the reactions reliable? Delayed/slow? Or efficiently used to enable the client to safely undertake tasks in sitting?
- For more able residents the ability of clients to balance, move and respond to displacement while sitting on a softer surface (e.g. over the side of a bed) could be made. Is the resident able to control this seated position with feet on/off the floor?

(iv) Clinical measures of sitting ability

- Timed sitting for 30 seconds (eyes open/eyes closed).
- Seated reach: measure the distance reached forward/sideways in unsupported sitting.
- Use the relevant component of a functional motor scale, e.g. Motor Assessment Scale (MAS) (Carr et al 1985), Clinical Outcomes Variable Scale (COVS) (Seaby & Torrance 1989) or Physical Mobility Scale (PMS) (Nitz & Brown, in preparation).

In summary, the analysis of sitting ability will determine if the resident is safe and independently able to sit unsupervised and their capacity to carry out tasks in sitting with or without supervision; the assessment needs to consider the type of seating required and the instructions required for individual carers and other staff.

2. Standing up and sitting down: consider the effect of the type/height of chair/bed on standing and sitting ability

If the resident is independent, observe the task of sit to stand and return to sitting, or provide the close supervision/assistance needed to complete these tasks. Analyse the tasks and identify the likely causes of instability or inability associated with the performance of these tasks. If assistance is required, consider why it is necessary so that appropriate recommendations for care staff to provide assistance will ensure safety for residents and the carers.

(i) Consider the following during standing up from a chair/bed (varying heights) as a sole task and then while carrying out a second task

- Is the foot placement appropriate with feet positioned under/behind knees?
- Is the calf/ankle flexible to enable heel contact with the floor when feet are correctly positioned?
- Is the base (foot position) too wide, too narrow or appropriate?
- Is forward inclination of the trunk controlled with appropriate anterior pelvic tilt?
- Is anterior translation of knees, with passive dorsiflexion of the ankle present to prepare for weight acceptance over the base (feet) prior to buttock off?
- Is force generation in the plantarflexors (foot stability)/quadriceps sufficient for buttock off?
- Is extension of hips and knees over the base (feet) appropriate for the upright position to be attained?

(ii) Observe sitting down and consider the control/problems while performing this task alone and then while completing a second task, e.g. holding an object

- Forward trunk inclination with sufficient anterior pelvic tilt.
- Initial anterior translation of knees, with passive dorsiflexion of the ankle during controlled lowering towards new base (buttock/thigh).
- Quality of weight distribution during sitting down to prepare for weight acceptance at buttock-on.
- Posterior translation of weight from feet to buttock/thigh.
- Realignment of trunk to upright.

(iii) Clinical measures of standing up and sitting down

- Use the relevant component of the MAS, COVS or PMS.
- Use the time taken to complete a number of cycles of sit to stand to sit, e.g. five repetitions with and without holding an object.

In summary, the analysis of standing up and return to sitting will determine if the resident is safe and independent; whether supervision or assistance is required; the effect of surface on this performance; and whether the patient has the capacity for multiple stands (functional strength and endurance) and whether a second task can be executed while standing up and sitting down.

3. Balanced standing

(i) Standing alignment and weight distribution

- Can the patient stand unsupported or do they require assistance? Why? What type of assistance?
- Is base of support wide or narrow?
- Is weight evenly distributed or asymmetrical?
- If the resident is unstable, note direction and reason for losing balance.
- Is the resident afraid of falling?
- Does range or muscle length affect alignment/balance?

(ii) Internal displacement – self-generated movements in standing
Observe movements and quality of control as the resident moves in standing using a standard base; progress the more able resident to the stride position or narrow the base during the following tasks.

- Stand and turn head and body to the right and then to the left. Is dizziness a problem?
- Weight shift from right to left leg.
- Ability to stand, reach outside base of support and return to a stable position (forward/side/back/across midline and return).
- Ability to step and touch/pick up objects and shift to a new position.
- Ability to lower towards floor/pick up an object.
- Ability to reach overhead/adding toe stand during reach.
- Speed of execution of these tasks.
- Measure using appropriate objective tools.

(iii) External displacement in standing Residents who are independently ambulating are frequently challenged by surface changes, uneven surfaces as well as unexpected forces such as jostling in a crowd or while standing in a moving bus or train. For such higher level clients, the capacity of an individual to manage an external force may be assessed by the physiotherapist identifying the quality of response to displacement and then grading this response.

The physiotherapist gently displaces the resident forward/laterally and backward and records the quality of ankle, hip and stepping strategies to this displacement (Shumway-Cooke et al 2001). This level of challenge to balance is carried out if the resident is able to step and is a critical aspect to include when the resident is mobile. The responses may be absent, or a gentle force may elicit a reliable or unreliable response. Without reliable stepping responses there is limited capacity for an older person to safely walk without supervision and their reliance on assistance from a person or walking aid is apparent. Use of an objective scale to record the response to displacement helps to quantify the response.

- Pastor, Day & Marsden Scale (1993). The examiner displaces the resident backwards and grades the response. (Always have a reliable person behind the resident to prevent a fall.)
- The quality of stepping response to lateral displacement is graded (Maki et al 2000).

In summary, the analysis of standing balance will determine if the resident is safe and independent in standing; whether supervision or assistance is required; the effect of support base and surface challenge on this performance; and whether the resident has the capacity to stand and carry out dual/multiple tasks in standing. The functional strength and endurance for ongoing work in standing can be identified. Guidelines for carers can then be established.

4. Gait

During the analysis of gait, the physiotherapist determines whether the resident can walk alone, requires physical assistance and/or use of a walking aid. You will have determined the ability of the resident to step as part of your balance assessment and thus will know how best to support the resident during the initial assessment of gait. The stability at mid-stance, where momentary single limb stance is required during stepping, is of particular interest and will help you to decide on the amount of support required or the capacity of the resident to manage unaided. Our focus is on whether the resident can safely mobilize or whether there is a falls risk during walking. Stability during turning is of particular interest as people turn frequently whilst walking (Dite & Temple 2002, Thigpin et al 2000) and falling while turning is common. The level of independence and use of aids and/or orthoses needs to be recorded. As appropriate, an objective measure of gait is used.

(i) General observations Note the speed of gait (measure this objectively); cadence; rhythm/symmetry; step length; arm swing; trunk rotation. Record the type of surfaces walked on and progression to different floor surfaces (e.g. carpet), stairs, ramps and outside (pavers, road, grass, gravel).

(ii) Analyse the gait cycle to identify the specific component(s) that require attention

Stance phase Observation of the movements and muscle control at heel-strike, foot flat, mid-stance, heel rise and toe-off provides the clinician with a strategy to analyse gait and observe:

- anterior-posterior trunk/pelvic/hip/knee control
- mediolateral trunk/pelvic/hip/ankle control
- knee control at heel strike, mid-stance and heel rise to toe off
  controlled knee flexion from heel strike to mid stance
  knee extension in mid-stance, then controlled flexion to toe off
- control of the foot during:
  heel strike and while lowering foot to floor
  rollover with development of leverage for push-off during heel rise
  push off.

Swing phase Observations of propulsion for toe off and control of the trunk, pelvis, hip, knee and foot during mid-swing and late swing determines the quality of:

- hip, knee flexion and dorsiflexion to enable adequate ground clearance in early to mid swing

- rotation of pelvis during swing
- knee extension with dorsiflexion of the ankle during late swing as the foot reaches towards the floor.

Turning during walking An inherent aspect of walking is the need to turn. Impaired turning ability has been linked to falls. Preliminary research demonstrates that dependent elderly are unable to pivot safely, take more steps to turn, stagger on turning and frequently pause or hesitate during turning (Thigpin et al 2000). Dite & Temple (2002) recommend assessing four aspects of turning:

- steadiness throughout the turn
- fluency of movement between the turn and walk when exiting the turn - no hesitancy
- the number of steps taken to turn
- the time taken to turn.

(iii) Clinical measures of balance and walking in an indoor environment For those residents who are able to ambulate with the assistance of a walking aid or independently, additional tools and specific measures are available:

- the Timed 'Up and Go' test (TUG) (Podsiadlo & Richardson 1991)
- the TUG(manual) and TUG(cognitive) (Shumway-Cooke et al 2000)
- timed 10 metre walk (Wade et al 1987)
- the 10 metre walk with head rotation (Herdman 2000) (the time to walk 10 metres is recorded and the ability to keep within a 25 cm wide walkway when the head is actively rotated every three to four steps is noted).

(iv) Higher level activities/mobility disability An analysis of tasks in which the more independent resident may be participating is important to ensure safe execution within the RACF or general community. A review of tasks at this level enables the mobility disability to be determined. The research of Patla & Shumway-Cooke (1999) has increased the awareness of the level of disability associated with community ambulation. These researchers define mobility disability as a product of the interaction between the individual and critical environment factors that impact on the individual's ability to safely and independently manage mobility tasks critical to that individual. At this level the environment (extrinsic factors) is increasingly contributing to the challenge of walking.

Tasks within a residential environment

- Can the elder walk indoors and safely change from a firm to a softer surface?
- Can the elder walk throughout the residential environment, accessing bathroom/toilet; dining table/chair etc.?
- Can the elder change speed safely, slowing for obstacles or hurrying to meet a time constraint, i.e. efficiently respond to environmental constraints or task demands?

- Can the elder walk over a thick mat?
- Can the elder walk up stairs? Use of rail/s? Use of a walking aid?
- Can the elder walk on firm outdoor surfaces?
- Can the elder change from daylight to shade safely while walking outdoors?
- Can the elder manage a ramp/incline?
- Can the elder walk outside over uneven surfaces.
- Can the elder open a door (both pushing the door away and pulling it towards them)?
- Can the elder turn 360 degrees to left/right? Is dizziness provoked?
- Can the elder safely walk in poor/dim/light? Is a night-light required?
- Can the elder safely walk while carrying an object or while talking?
- Can the elder run safely for short periods in response to a task demand?

Tasks outside the RACF

- Can the elder walk on firm outdoor surfaces?
- Can the elder change from daylight to shade safely?
- Can the elder manage a ramp or incline?
- Can the elder walk outside on uneven surfaces?
- Can the elder manage time constraints for traffic crossings?
- Can the elder manage shopping environments?
- Can the elder manage crowds?
- Can the elder manage the effect of traffic?

In summary, the analysis of walking will determine if the resident is safe and independent or whether supervision or assistance is required; the effect of a variety of surfaces and walking tasks on this performance; the role of lighting and visual conditions; and whether the resident has the capacity to carry out a sole or dual task. Guidelines for carers can then be developed.

Identify impairments that may contribute to balance and mobility problems

There are a number of impairments that may compromise the performance of functional motor tasks and in particular the ability to balance and ambulate. Research findings may provide a basis for prioritizing the testing of some impairments, particularly when the predictive capacity of the impairment can be demonstrated. To date variable results have been demonstrated with strength of lower limb muscles as a predictor of gait outcome (Nadeau et al 1997, Perry et al 1995). While the strength of the plantarflexors and knee extensors correlates with some gait parameters, the quality of sensory function has been shown to correlate more consistently with gait parameters in elders and after stroke (Lord et al 1996, Nadeau et al 1997, Perry et al 1995). Recent research associates changes in visual acuity, contrast sensitivity and depth perception with slips, trips and falls (Lord & Menz 2000, Lord et al 2001). In the absence of vestibular pathology, the link between gaze instability and falls is less clear (Hillman et al 1999, Lord et al 2001, Whitney et al 2000).

Measures of motor and sensory function provide the clinician with objective baseline data of the cause(s) of the balance/mobility problem. These findings are generally used by the clinician to target interventions. The clinician frequently grades muscle strength and records sensory function as intact, impaired or absent. New clinical measurement tools are increasingly available at moderate cost to provide the clinician with the capacity to objectively measure impairments and monitor changes with intervention. An outline of the available objective clinical measures of impairments is provided with the reliability of the measures identified.

1. Measures of muscle strength

(i) A spring gauge or a handheld dynamometer This could be used to record the strength of the lower limb muscles as an option instead of the use of manual muscle tests. The average of three maximal contractions is determined by setting the spring gauge or handheld dynamometer at right angles to particular muscle groups such as the hip abductors and extensors, the quadriceps and foot dorsiflexors/plantarflexors. Both tools provide repeatable and reliable measures of strength.

(ii) Functional strength

- The wall squat test: the time is recorded before fatigue of quadriceps is apparent (only 60% of this time is used during training).
- The number of sit to stands that could be carried out in 10 or 30 seconds could also be used as a functional strength measure.

2. Measures of lower limb flexibility/ROM

Length of all muscles can be checked but an emphasis is placed on calf flexibility in relation to balance.

(i) An inclinometer measure of ankle range This is made by positioning an inclinometer on the shin about 15 cm below the tibial tuberosity.

- Clients who are unable to participate in a standing measure could have the ankle flexibility measured in sitting. The heel is positioned at 90 degrees under the knee (inclinometer at zero) and then the heel is moved back while maintaining heel contact with the floor (inclinometer measures the available range).
- More able clients can perform a lunge/squat test (while supporting themselves on a rail or table) where the heel of the posterior limb is kept flat on the floor (Bennell et al 1998).

(ii) Distance of the big toe from a wall Another method of measuring the calf is the distance of the big toe from a wall with the knee flexed to touch the wall and the heel flat on the floor (Collins et al 2003).

3. Measures of visual function

Elders are heavily reliant on their vision for balance and mobility and thus it is important to understand the quality of available vision. The use of corrected lenses should be noted and any optometry/ophthalmology reports should be reviewed. Several tests are available and two important tests that allow the quality of visual acuity and contrast sensitivity to be measured have been developed (Lord et al 1996). These aspects need to be considered as one of the impairments that may contribute to reduced ability to interact with the functioning environment, e.g. cracks in footpaths or edges of curbs/gutters. Tests for visual field loss are more likely to be carried out when CNS dysfunction is being considered or has been diagnosed.

(i) Visual acuity

- **High and low contrast sensitivity tests.** This test is undertaken with or without corrected lenses depending on normality of vision. The line of greatest clarity is recorded while reading from a Snellen chart which has high and low contrast sensitivity sections (Lord & Clark 1996). Elders with poor visual acuity have more than two lines difference between the high/low contrast sensitivity tests. These older people have an increased falls risk as the subtle differences in floor surfaces may not be detected (Lord & Menz 2000).
- **Contrast sensitivity.** Normal vision or use of corrected lenses is used during the Melbourne Edge Test, which assesses contrast sensitivity and depth perception (Lord et al 1996). A score of 20 to 24 is normal but scores progressively less than 20 correlate with an increased risk of a fall from hesitating/tripping at surface changes or curbs/gutters where a height change occurs. Fallers typically score less than 16 on this test (Lord & Menz 2000, Lord et al 2001).

(ii) Tests of ocular control – observational tests

- **Smooth pursuit.** Note the control of eye movements in all directions (side to side and up/down in periphery). The quality of smooth pursuit is observed and any nystagmus crossing the midline or with a change of direction suggesting CNS dysfunction.
- **Saccadic movements.** Ask the resident to look repeatedly between two objects in the visual field and note the ability to do the task with one corrective saccadic eye movement - additional beats to fixate on the object suggest vestibular dysfunction.
- **The optokinetic response.** Observe the ocular response when a striped fabric is moved across the visual field. The observed nystagmus demonstrates the re-fixing ability of the oculomotor system, which may be reduced in elders and could contribute to reduced stability of elders while walking in a dynamic visual field, e.g. when people or traffic are moving past the elder who is walking.
- **Observe end-point nystagmus.** This is a normal fatigue response to the eyes being held at the end of ocular range.

(iii) Visual field Testing for visual field loss determines the functioning visual field in which the elder can interact - definitive field losses are associated with specific sites of CNS lesions, although elders often have reduced peripheral vision.

(iv) Perception of upright When balance loss is associated with poor orientation, fear of movement towards the midline or loss of balance, then difficulties with perception of the upright may need to be considered. Vestibular hypo-function is prevalent with advanced age and could contribute to this perceptual problem. In addition, the effect of reclined seating may also need to be considered as frequent resting in this position may increase the fear of moving towards the upright/midline. If a central lesion interferes with the relay of vestibular data, possibly as a consequence of lacunar infarcts and as part of a pattern of early dementia, or when the lesion interferes with interpretation of sensory cues in the parietal cortex more severe ipsi-propulsion/'pushing' may present (Davies 1990).

- Normal perception of upright < error range 5–7 degrees.
- Perception of upright with vestibular dysfunction > 7 degrees.

4. Measures of somatosensory function

A range of portable and clinical tests have been developed to measure vibration sensitivity, joint repositioning ability and tactile sensitivity (Lord & Clark 1996).

(i) Measurement of lower limb joint repositioning ability Physiotherapists can use standing methods of measuring joint position sense and passive movement appreciation or make use of the repositioning unit developed by Lord & Clark (1996). This test measures the ability of the resident to match the lower limb position either side of a large acrylic protractor while the eyes are closed or when blindfolded. The person is seated in front of a 60 cm by 60 cm acrylic sheet inscribed with a protractor which stands perpendicular to the floor. The person is required to position and reposition the knee by flexing and extending the knees and opposing the big toes in the same position either side of the acrylic sheet. Two practice trials are followed by five experimental trials while the eyes are closed. The score is the mean error in knee position by comparing the position of the big toes in degrees.

(ii) Tactile sensitivity Light touch can be assessed using touch localization with the client rating the intensity from 1 to 10. Lord & Clark (1996) have developed a pressure aesthesiometry testing kit where the size of the monofilament is recorded once the tactile pressure is perceived. Filaments can be applied to the medial and lateral malleoli; the centre of the heel; the plantar aspect of the big and little toe; and under the head of the first and fifth metatarsal heads. The client indicates when and where the stimulus is felt and the size of the filament is recorded. The protocol was established by Holewski et al (1988) and quantified by Kumar et al (1995). Assessment usually commences with the 5.7 monofilament, which is the level at which protective sensation has been established, and then monofilaments on either side of this level (e.g. 4.17 and 6.10 monofilaments etc.) are progressively used to document the precise level of tactile sensitivity (Kelly 2000).

(iii) Measurement of lower limb vibration sensitivity A tuning fork can be used to determine the integrity of vibration sense. Alternatively, vibration perception can be detected using an electronic device that generates a 120 Hz vibration of varying amplitude (Lord & Clark 1996). The vibration is applied to the tibial tuberosity and is measured in microns of motion. Subjects are asked to indicate when they first feel the vibration and then it is turned down to the threshold level and the amplitude recorded.

5. Tests of vestibular function

In addition to balance tests that implicate the vestibular system, dizziness and gaze stability need to be assessed. A range of clinical tests of gaze stability can be used to test the integrity of the vestibular ocular reflex (VOR). Observable nystagmus at rest or during head movements suggests a peripheral vestibular disorder or CNS dysfunction.

A more objective measure of gaze stability can be made by using the Dynamic Visual Acuity (DVA) test (Herdman 2000).

(i) Tests of gaze stability establish the integrity of vestibular ocular reflex (VOR) Testing for gaze instability is usually carried out if the client complains of difficulty reading or of a shifting visual field despite having corrected lenses and intact eye movement control (Hirvonen et al 1997). It is possible that instability of the VOR could cause the words to shift on the page while reading, or labels to move on cans/objects while elders are shopping. These experiences can cause postural instability and add to the falls risk while ambulating.

- **Gaze stability during slow side to side and vertical head movements.** Observe the ability to maintain gaze on the examiner's nose during slow, passive head rotations and vertical movements. Difficulties with fixation (positive response) while moving the head slowly may occur in chronic vestibular disorders (e.g. bilateral hypofunction with ageing) but the ability to fixate is usually retained during slow movements with unilateral loss of vestibular function.
- **Halmagyi impulse test.** Observe VOR instability in response to a single rapid head thrust from about 30 degrees cervical rotation towards the midline (Baloh & Halmagyi 1996). This test is a test of dynamic VOR stability and is usually positive with peripheral vestibular disorders when a single catch-up saccades follows the single head thrust to the midline. The status of the VOR in elders may be normal or compromised depending on the degree of unilateral/bilateral degeneration of receptor function.
- **The Dynamic Visual Acuity (DVA) test** is a more objective clinical measure of gaze stability. In this test the resident reads from the top of a Snellen chart until the smallest correct line is determined. The head is kept still while reading initially and then the reading task is repeated while the head is gently but passively rotated, at a rate of about 2 Hz/second – a metronome can be used to standardize speed (Herdman 2000). A normal response causes a drop of one to two lines while a greater drop is evidence of VOR instability. Uncompensated unilateral

vestibular loss typically causes three to four lines of visual acuity degradation during passive head movements.

Protocols to improve gaze stability need to be implemented when deficits are observed (Herdman 2000, Krebs et al 1993).

(ii) Nystagmus With peripheral lesions the direction of nystagmus is away from the side of unilateral lesion, i.e. a right-sided lesion causes nystagmus to beat to the left (>2 beats is abnormal).

- Gaze evoked: nystagmus with eye movement at about 30 degrees occurs with peripheral lesions – an increase in nystagmus occurs when looking in the direction of nystagmus; a decrease occurs when looking away from nystagmus (i.e. towards the lesion).
- Skew deviation of eyes (tonic/static response) suggests an acute unilateral loss.
- Spontaneous nystagmus suggests an acute peripheral lesions or CNS problem.
- Direction changing; periodic alternating or down beating nystagmus suggests CNS dysfunction.

Nystagmus induced with head shaking Observe the ocular response following rapid head shaking while the eyes are closed.

- Normal – no nystagmus, immediate suppression and ocular stability.
- Bilateral lesion – no response.
- Unilateral lesion – beats away from side of decreased function.
- The oculomotor examination outlined above can be carried out with Frenzel lenses to reduce the ability to visually fixate during testing and enable clearer observation of the ocular response during eye/head movements.

(iii) Dizziness As dizziness may be prevalent with ageing as well as with specific vestibular pathology, it is necessary to determine the cause of the dizziness (e.g. benign paroxysmal positioning vertigo – BPPV; peripheral vestibular pathology; motion sensitivity, CNS dysfunction, medication etc.). Accurate history-taking is critical to link the dizziness with either specific patterns of movement (e.g. BPPV) or general sensitivity to motion (CNS may be implicated). Both are amenable to physiotherapy intervention but different treatment protocols are required.

- BPPV. A positioning response to the Hall-Pike Dix test confirms BPPV involving the posterior canal (Herdman 2000) where otoconia are thought to be floating as particles in the canal and causing intermittent dizziness. The onset of nystagmus will be delayed (3–5 seconds) and continue for a variable period before ceasing by around 30 seconds. This problem can be managed using an Epley manoeuvre (Blatt et al 2000, Epley 1992, Lynn 1995) or a series of exercises developed by Brandt & Daroff (1979). When nystagmus continues for more than

30 seconds and up to several minutes, particles may be more adherent to the cupula and a Semont Libatory manoeuvre may be more appropriate treatment (Herdman 2000).

- General sensitivity to motion will present with less specificity and a number of functional motor activities can be disturbed. The intensity and duration of dizziness is recorded against each motor task to determine which movements should be targeted to foster habituation and an improved tolerance to motion (Herdman 2000). An habituation programme is the protocol of choice in order to desensitize the response to motion. The tasks that are least problematic are addressed initially and as the tolerance to motion improves then the more problematic movements are targeted.

The impact of dizziness on postural stability as well as on the quality of life can be determined by using either the Dizziness Handicap Inventory (Jacobson & Newman 1990) or the short form of this tool (Tesio et al 1999).

In summary, identification of the underlying impairments enables the physiotherapist to understand the causes contributing to the balance and movement disorder and to include these aspects in a management programme. The perceived needs of each resident along with the physiotherapist's problem-solving skills are used to develop priorities for management. Objective recordings of appropriate balance and mobility tasks are made to provide a baseline from which progress can be monitored.

Objective measures of functional motor tasks

A large range of tools are available to monitor physical mobility, with the physiotherapist responsible for selecting the tool(s) that monitor the physical ability/difficulty of the client group. The selected tool is used to provide a baseline measure, assist with goal setting, and monitor progress and outcome after treatment intervention.

Measures of postural stability and dynamic balance and functional mobility

1. Clinical measures of sitting ability

For the client who cannot stand, timed measures of sitting ability can be used.

(i) Timed sitting Note the quality of alignment while holding the seated position for 30 seconds.

(ii) Seated reach Measures of the distance reached can be made in sitting when the client is unable to stand unsupported.

(iii) MAS, COVS or PMS The relevant component of the Motor Assessment Scale (MAS) (Carr et al 1985), the Clinical Outcomes Variable Scale (COVS) (Seaby & Torrance 1989) or Physical Mobility Scale (PMS) (Nitz & Brown, in preparation) may be used.

2. Clinical measures of standing ability (postural stability)

A number of tests are available to monitor the ability to stand on firm and soft surfaces (postural stability) as well as measure dynamic balance and functional mobility. The tests will be applicable for the resident who can stand unsupported, and progressively available for those able to take at least one step alone, or able to mobilize with or without a walking aid. The information provided by the test conditions will be summarized to develop the implications for intervention programmes.

(i) Timed standing on a firm surface For the resident who can stand unsupported it is appropriate to introduce a timed stand with feet apart as an objective measure (Bohannon et al 1984, Newton 1989). For those residents who are able to stand for 30 seconds and take at least one step, standing ability can be challenged by either changing the base of support (feet together or stride) or by closing the eyes. Some clients may be able to be challenged by introducing the single limb stance test. The time the resident can hold the position without support is recorded. Normative data for age is available (Bohannon et al 1984, Newton 1989) to determine if the balance ability of the individual resident is typical for age or if they are less able and requiring attention to ensure added stability in standing. These tests require both anteroposterior control and considerable mediolateral stability at both the hip and ankle. During preliminary observations of stance you will note the control of hip and knee muscles, in addition to the ankle musculature, to allow you to judge when it is safe to introduce these tests.

(ii) Responses to changing sensory cues during timed standing Shumway-Cooke & Horak (1986) developed the Clinical Test for the Sensory Integration of Balance (CTSIB) to monitor the capacity of the individual to process and use the information from the somatosensory and vestibular systems during standing. The test involves standing on a firm, then a high density foam surface. For those residents who are able to manage standing on a firm floor for 30 seconds, particularly if the test can be managed with eyes closed, then it is appropriate to introduce the complete CTSIB and apply the six conditions (eyes open, eyes closed and use of a conflict dome on a firm, then foam surface). The introduction of the foam surface will challenge the somatosensory receptors even with eyes open and will help you to predict the capacity of the resident to change surfaces safely. A further progression to managing with the eyes closed will determine those able/unable to rely on their vestibular function under dark conditions when a softer surface is underfoot (e.g. carpet). A fall frequently presents with elders when testing on foam, particularly with the eyes closed, and should only be undertaken if additional stand-by support is available.

Implications of test findings for management There are a number of implications for residents who cannot manage these test conditions. Standing in dim/dark conditions may compromise balance ability and thus it is important to stand, transfer and mobilize these elders on firm surfaces in well-lit environs. For the mobile resident, advice regarding standing when showering (e.g. eyes closed while washing hair), while walking on carpeted surfaces and the need for a light for safe mobility at night could be outcomes of this test. For residents who are more independent interventions may need to consider challenging the individual and introducing a variety of surfaces to balance on and/or negotiate while walking during treatment sessions. Dynamic visual environs could also be gradually introduced (e.g. engaging with a balloon floating through the air; interacting with multiple obstacles; walking past/around a number of people who are also moving; pass/bounce/throw/catch a light ball). For these residents, the physiotherapist is aiming to prevent the decline in the sensory systems that are typically associated with advancing age.

3. Clinical measures of internal displacement

Initially a self-initiated weight shift can be observed with the selected strategy (ankle/hip strategy) noted during the weight shift. A well-controlled ankle strategy is appropriate during weight shift while those clients with trunk/pelvic instability are more likely to demonstrate a combined ankle/hip movement during weight shift (Herdman 2000). The following tests are appropriate for the resident who can stand unsupported and initiate reaching outside the base of support or is able to take a step without support.

(i) Functional reach The capacity to reach forward outside the base of support can be measured using the protocol established by Duncan et al (1990) while the ability to reach sideways outside the base of support can be measured using the guidelines set down by Brauer et al (1999c). Both tests have established normative data which can be used to predict the risk of a fall (Duncan et al 1992, Brauer et al 2000). For those clients whose ability to reach is compromised (forward <25 cm; laterally <18 cm), there is an increased risk of a fall. For forward reach a significant difference between fallers and non-fallers has been demonstrated, with healthy elderly able to reach more than 25 cm while frequent fallers reach less than 15 cm.

Implications for intervention

- When compromised forward and lateral reach is identified, initially in the treatment objects should be located so that the distance to be reached is reduced for safe performance of tasks.
- Interventions will aim to introduce tasks that gradually and safely challenge these limits and restore the capacity to reach outside the support base.
- Underlying impairments should also be identified and addressed.

(ii) The Step Test (Hill et al 1996) This test requires the resident to repeatedly place the whole foot up on to a 7.5 cm block and then back to the floor as many times as possible in 15 seconds. The number of times the stepping leg is placed on to the block in 15 seconds is recorded. The resident should not be supported but requires close supervision to ensure safety. The test challenges mediolateral stability and requires efficient strength in the stance leg, particularly the hip abductors. Normative data is available that shows that healthy elders (>60) take about 16–18 steps in 15 seconds (Hill et al 1996), although Isles et al (2004) provide a differential stepping ability for elders (>60 years: right = 15.6, left = 15.9; >70 years: right = 13.7, left = 14.1).

Implications of test findings Performances under these norms for age suggest that mediolateral stability may require attention, with interventions targeting strength/flexibility and endurance of the musculature about the trunk/pelvic/hip/knee regions to improve the performance of this test.

4. A measure of reaction time: the rapid step test

A recent addition to the available battery of tests has emerged with the development of the rapid step test: the time to complete 24 random steps forward, backward and to the side in response to a verbal command is measured (Medell & Alexander 2000). This test determines the maximum step distance for an individual, then uses 80% of this distance to set target points to which the individual steps during the execution of the test. The test is considered to be a measure of the protective elements of balance, with increased time recorded for elders compared to young adults to initiate (react to a command)/prepare to step and execute repeated steps. The test also discriminates between healthy elders and impaired elders. The test is repeatable and reliable and performance correlates with single limb stance ability as well as strength of the quadriceps and calf muscles.

5. Response to external displacement

Clients who are independently ambulating are frequently challenged by surface changes, uneven surfaces as well as unexpected forces such as jostling in a crowd or while standing in a moving bus/train. For such higher level clients, the capacity of an individual to manage an external force may be gained by applying the following tests.

(i) Pastor, Day and Marsden Scale (Harburn et al 1995, Pastor et al 1993) The examiner stands behind the person and gives a brief tug backwards at the shoulders. The patient has eyes open and is told what to expect and is instructed to resist the pull in order to prevent backward movement. The response is rated according to a scale (0–4). Inter-rater reliability is low and the force applied by the tester may be problematic. This means that several repeated tests are recommended to rate the response to displacement to improve the reliability (Harburn et al 1995).

(ii) Stepping response to lateral displacement (Maki et al 2000) The lateral stepping response to displacement is graded according to the control of the stepping response and the pattern of stepping response – a crossover response is typical of a young adult while multiple steps and increased use of arms is frequently associated with the response in elders (Maki et al 2000).

(iii) Quality of ankle/hip/stepping responses (Shumway-Cook & Woollacott 2001) These also encourage the clinician to note the ankle, hip, combination ankle/hip, stepping strategy or the inability to activate a response resulting in a fall without support during the displacement. In addition, the relationship of force applied to the chest/thorax to the quality/type of response yielded should be noted. For example, does a mild force yield an ankle strategy to maintain balance or does the resident step or over-balance, which is more typically associated with a moderate force? With the application of a moderate/vigorous force the resident would be expected to use a hip/stepping response but may be unable to respond and may fall.

6. Measures of balance, gait and endurance

(a) Tools that monitor balance and mobility within an indoor environment For those residents who are able to ambulate with or without a walking aid, additional tools are available to evaluate and measure performance.

(i) Berg Balance Scale (Berg et al 1989) This is used to monitor balance with elderly clients.

(ii) TUG (Podsiadlo & Richardson 1991) The test may be carried out using a walking aid, which makes it more suited to those residents who need to use an aid. The resident walks at a safe speed to complete the set task.

Normative data for the TUG:

- healthy elders (75 years): 8.5 seconds
- fallers: >20 seconds.

Shumway-Cooke et al (1997) recommend that the test be carried out as fast as the person can safely walk to improve the discrimination between fallers and non-fallers.

(iii) TUG(manual) and TUG(cognitive) (Shumway-Cooke et al 2000) For more able residents, the dual-task Timed 'Up and Go' test allows the effect of a second task (manual or cognitive) to be monitored during the test. An increase in time by 2 seconds is considered significant.

(iv) Timed 10 metre walk (Bohannon 1997, Wade et al 1987, Wolfson et al 1990) The test is usually performed without an aid but could be adapted to the functional level of the resident. A study by Dean et al (2001) demonstrated that walking speed over 10 metres overestimates locomotor capacity after stroke.

A further modification of the test could be the time to wheel 10 meters in a manual wheelchair. This has been used to monitor the speed of wheeling a wheelchair for ageing clients with cerebral palsy (Low Choy et al 2003) and could be applied to any client who is independently mobile in a wheelchair.

(v) 10 metre walk with head rotation (Herdman 2000) For those residents who can ambulate without an aid this test challenges the vestibular function. The time to walk 10 metres is recorded and the ability to keep

within a 25 cm wide walkway when the head is actively rotated every three to four steps is noted.

(vi) The Modified Elderly Mobility Scale (Prosser & Canby 1997, Smith 1994) This scale is used with older people with balance and mobility problems.

(vii) The gait items of the MAS (Carr et al 1985) *and COVS* (Seaby & Torrance 1989) These items can be selected and used independently of the total scales.

Implications of findings for management A number of elements are associated with these tests and require consideration in balance programmes. Functional strength is required to stand and during walking, with mediolateral control particularly challenged during the turning components of this task. Linear motion and particularly rotational motion is experienced during turning, which adds a vestibular challenge to the task. In addition, as the test is performed as fast as the client can safely manage, reaction time, the capacity to remain stable during attempted increased speed and the added functional strength and control required with added speed need to be considered. As appropriate, these elements can be progressively introduced during retraining programmes.

(b) Ambulation measures associated with challenges encountered in community environments Patla & Shumway-Cook (1999) give emphasis to the importance of tools being applied in less predictable community environs and conditions. In the absence of adverse conditions, it is recommended that the examiner interpret the performance of community ambulant clients with caution as the performance in ideal conditions may underestimate the ability of community ambulant clients.

(i) Dynamic Gait Index Eight Gait Items are scored (Shumway-Cooke et al 1997). The test has good inter-rater and test–retest reliability and can be used to predict falls among the elderly (Shumway-Cooke et al 1997):

- scores for healthy aged: 21 ± 3
- scores for aged fallers: 11 ± 4.

(ii) Fukuda Stepping Test This test was developed to monitor vestibular function in the ambulant client (Uttenberger's test). The patient takes 50 high steps on the spot with the eyes closed and the arms held forward at shoulder height. The test lacks sensitivity, with a normal response allowing rotation up to 45 degrees and travel up to 1 metre with an abnormal response being rotation >45 degrees in the direction of the peripheral vestibular problem and/or travel >1 metre (Bonanni & Newton 1998).

(iii) Singleton's test A test that challenges balance following a 360 degree turn. The elder is asked to walk 3 metres towards you, turn quickly and hold steady with eyes open, then repeat the test and hold steady with eyes closed (Herdman 2000).

(iv) Dual tasks while walking These include: time to execute an obstacle course/perform dual/multiple tasks while manipulating objects; throw/catch ball; picking up objects from floor (Herdman 2000).

(v) Duke Mobility Skills Profile This was developed to measure the gait performance of older adults. The test has good inter-rater and test-retest reliability (Duncan et al 1993).

(vi) Rivermead Mobility Index (Colleen et al 1991) Monitors a range of tasks associated with indoor/outdoor activities.

(c) Tinetti Fear of Falling Scale Fear of falling can also be monitored to determine the anxiety/perceived risk associated with a variety of home- and community-based tasks (Manning et al 1997, Tinetti et al 1990).

(d) Endurance The functional endurance of each client could be measured using the 3- or 6-minute walk test (Butland et al 1982, Schenkman et al 1997, Shumway-Cooke et al 1997). The baseline measure could be used to determine the benefits of an intervention programme (e.g. walking programme, or use of treadmill/ergometer).

Tools that monitor general physical performance and mobility

Management for the frail elderly often means a focus on bed mobility, sitting ability, transfers, wheelchair skills and/or gait training. It will thus be important to select a tool that includes this range of functional tasks for the more dependent resident. Several tools are available and include the following.

- **The Physical Mobility Scale (PMS)** currently being investigated for reliability and validity for use in residential aged care facilities (Nitz & Brown, in preparation).
- **The Physical Performance and Mobility Examination (PPME)** developed to monitor physical function and mobility in frail older adults (Winograd et al 1994).
- **The Mobility Scale for Acute Stroke Patients** (Simondson et al 1996).
- **The Motor Assessment Scale (MAS)** (Carr et al 1985) developed for use with stroke clients.
- **The Clinical Outcomes Variable Scale (COVS)** (Seaby & Torrance 1989) developed for use with ortho-geriatric and neurological clients.

Each of these scales includes measures of bed mobility; sitting ability; standing and walking ability. The MAS and COVS also include upper limb function while the COVS and PMS provide scores for transfers and wheelchair management. These latter tools also offer a greater capacity to measure the amount of assistance required within each task. This is considered an advantage for use with clients in residential aged care facilities where some clients will require assistance for all tasks. Such scales also enable the burden of care to be monitored, an important component to consider for those physiotherapists working in residential care facilities (Low Choy et al 2003).

Summary

- The information gleaned from the assessment process and the selected tests will help you to decide on the stability and safe mobility of each elder.
- There will be a need to identify the safe level of mobility for each resident/elder and for those in an RACF it will be necessary to document clearly the level of supervision or assistance required for all balance and mobility tasks.
- The information should also be used to identify situations when residents are at risk of a fall. An example might be when the resident is unable to divide attention between walking and talking while remaining stable. In this instance care plan instructions should document that the carer should not ask questions or carry out a conversation with the resident as this could compromise the safety of the resident by increasing the risk of a fall.
- The assessment process also enables targeted interventions to be offered and the education of elders about the limits to their safe mobility.
- More specific findings from the assessment will have determined the time the resident could participate in standing activities, the visual and support conditions that should form part of the set-up for task practice and the capacity of the resident to be worked in standing. This latter aspect has implications for use of tasks where residents can move and reach safely within their ability and then be challenged (under supervision) to progress towards a new limit of stability.
- This may mean working the elder while moving over a stationary base (e.g. reach and weight shift with the feet apart on a firm surface) or use of a dynamic base (e.g. working on a soft surface or stepping while reaching for an object).
- Finally, the number of steps that could be encouraged, the speed at which tasks could be safely practised, the distances that could be walked, the obstacles/surfaces that could be introduced during a walking task and the capacity to manage dual tasks could be determined from some of the more advanced tests discussed in this section.
- Thus the assessment process determines those aspects related to the elder that are amenable to intervention, the motor tasks that require attention in any given environment and the way the environment impacts on task performance. The observational analysis of balance and mobility tasks determines the quality of the performance and identifies possible impairments using problem-solving skills; the

objective examination and use of tools to measure the impairments confirms the contribution of the impairment to balance and mobility dysfunction; and objective recordings of appropriate balance and mobility tasks are made to provide a baseline from which progress can be monitored.

- The perceived needs of each elder/resident along with the assessment process using your problem-solving skills are used to develop priorities for management.

References

Alhanti B, Bruder L A, Creese W et al 1997 Balance abilities of community dwelling older adults under altered visual and support surface conditions. Physical and Occupational Therapy in Geriatrics 15:37–52

Anacker S L, Di Fabio R P 1992 Influence of sensory inputs on standing balance in community-dwelling elders with a recent history of falling. Physical Therapy 72:575–584

Aniansson A, Rundgren A, Sperling L 1980 Evaluation of functional capacity in activities of daily living in 70 year old men and women. Scandinavian Journal Rehabilitation Medicine 12:145–154

Baloh R W, Halmagyi G M 1996 Disorders of the vestibular system. Oxford University Press, New York

Baloh R W, Hornrubia V, Jacobson K 1987 Benign positional vertigo: clinical and oculographic features in 240 cases. Neurology 37:371–378

Bennell K, Talbot R, Wajswelner H, Techovanich W, Kelly D 1998 Intra-rater and inter-tester reliability of a weight-bearing lunge measure of ankle dorsiflexion. Australian Journal of Physiotherapy 44:175–180

Berg K, Wood-Dauphine S, Williams J I 1989 Measuring balance in the elderly: preliminary development of an instrument. Physiotherapy Canada 41:304–311

Blatt P J, Georgakakis G A, Herdman S J, Clendaniel R A, Tusa R J 2000 The effect of the canalith repositioning maneuver on resolving postural instability in patients with benign paroxysmal positional vertigo. American Journal of Otology 21:356–363

Bohannon R W 1997 Comfortable and maximum walking speed of adults aged 20–79 years: reference values and determinants. Age and Ageing 26:15–19

Bohannon R, Larkin P, Cook A, Gear J, Singer J 1984 Decrease in balance scores with ageing. Physical Therapy 64:1067–1070

Bonanni M, Newton R 1998 Test–retest reliability of the Fukuda Stepping Test. Physiotherapy Research International 3(1):58–68

Brandt T, Daroff R B 1980 Physical therapy for benign paroxysmal positional vertigo. Archives of Otolaryngology 106:484–485

Brauer S, Woollacott M, Shumway-Cook A 1999a Balance impaired elderly: secondary task influences EMG response to perturbation. Gait and Posture 9(1):S33

Brauer S, Woollacott M, Shumway-Cook A 1999b Balance impaired elderly change response strategy with cognitive load. Society Neuroscience Abstracts 25(1):108

Brauer S, Burns Y, Galley P 1999c Lateral reach: a new clinical measure of medio-lateral balance. Physiotherapy Research International 4(2):81–88

Brauer S, Burns Y, Galley P 2000 Postural stability measures predict falls in community-dwelling elderly. Journal of Gerontology Medical Science 55(8):M469–M476

Brocklehurst J C, Robertson D, James-Gordon P 1982 Clinical correlates of sway in old age: sensory modalities. Age and Ageing 11:1–10

Buchner D M, de Lateur B J 1991 The importance of skeletal muscle strength to physical function in older adults. Annals of Behavioral Medicine 13:91–98

Butland R J A, Pang J, Gross E R, Woodcock A A, Geddes D M 1982 Two, six and 12 minute walking tests in respiratory disease. British Medical Journal 284:1607–1608

Carr J, Shepherd R, Nordholm L, Lynne D 1985 A Motor Assessment Scale for stroke. Physical Therapy 65:175–180

Cho C, Kamen G 1998 Detecting balance deficits in frequent fallers using clinical quantitative evaluation tools. Journal of the American Geriatrics Society 46:426-430

Colleen F M, Wade D T, Robb G F, Bradshaw C M 1991 The Rivermead Mobility Index: a further development of the Rivermead Motor Assessment. International Disabilities Study 13:50-54

Collins N, Vicenzino B, Teys P 2003 The initial effects of a Mulligan mobilisation with movement technique on dorsiflexion and pain in subacute ankle sprains. Manual Therapy (in press)

Davies P M 1990 Right in the middle. Springer, Berlin

Dean C M, Richards C L, Malouin F 2001 Walking speed over 10 metres overestimates locomotor capacity after stroke. Clinical Rehabilitation 15:415-421

Dite W, Temple V A 2002 Development of a clinical measure of turning for older adults. American Journal of Physical Medicine and Rehabilitation 81(11):857-866

Duncan P, Weiner D K, Chandler J 1990 Functional reach: a new clinical measure of balance. Journal of Gerontology 45:M192-M197

Duncan P W, Studenski S, Chandler J, Prescott B 1992 Functional reach: predictive validity in a sample of elderly male veterans. Journal of Gerontology 47:M93-M98

Duncan P W, Shumway-Cook A, Tinetti M E et al 1993 Is there one simple measure for balance? PT Magazine 1:74-81

Epley J M 1992 The canalith repositioning procedure for treatment of benign paroxysmal positional vertigo. Otolaryngology Head Neck Surgery 107: 399-404

Frank J S, Patla A E, Brown J E 1987 Characteristics of postural control accompanying voluntary arm movement in the elderly. Society for Neuroscience Abstracts 13:335

Grimby G, Saltin B 1983 The ageing muscle. Clinical Physiology 3:209-218

Harburn K, Hill K, Kramer J et al 1995 Clinical applicability and test-retest reliability of an external perturbation test of balance in stroke subjects. Archives of Physical Medicine and Rehabilitation 76(4):317-323

Herdman S J 2000 Vestibular rehabilitation. F A Davis, New York

Hill K, Bernhardt J, McGann A, Maltese D, Berkovits D 1996 A new test of dynamic standing balance for stroke patients: reliability, validity and comparison with healthy elderly. Physiotherapy Canada 48: 257-262

Hillman E J, Bloomberg J J, McDonald V P, Cohen H S 1999 Dynamic visual acuity while walking in normals and labyrinthine deficit patients: a measure of oscillopsia. Journal of Vestibular Research 9(1):49-57

Hinman M R 1998 Causal attributions of falls in older adults. Physical and Occupational Therapy in Geriatrics 15:71-84

Hirvonen T P, Aalto H, Pykko I, Juhola M, Jantil P 1997 Changes in VOR of elderly people. Acta Otolaryngology (Stockholm) Supplementary 529:108-110

Holewski J, Stress R, Graf P et al 1988 Aesthesiometry: quantification of cutaneous pressure sensation in diabetic peripheral neuropathy. Journal of Rehabilitation Research and Development 25:1-10

Horak F, Schupert C, Mirka A 1989 Components of postural dyscontrol in the elderly: a review. Neurobiology and Aging 10:727-745

Horak F, Nashner L M, Diener H C 1990 Postural strategies associated with somatosensory and vestibular loss. Experimental Brain Research 82: 167-177

Hurley M, Rees J, Newham D 1998 Quadriceps function, proprioceptive acuity and functional performance in healthy young, middle-aged and elderly subjects. Age and Ageing 27:55-67

Hyatt R, Whitelaw M, Bhat A, Scott S, Maxwell J 1990 Association of muscle strength and functional status in elderly people. Age and Ageing 19:330-336

Inglin B, Woollacott M H 1988 Age-related changes in anticipatory postural adjustments associated with arm movements. Journal of Gerontology 43: M105-M113

Isles R C, Nitz J C, Low Choy N L 2004 Normative data for clinical balance measures in women aged 20 to 80. Journal of the American Geriatrics Society (in press)

Jacobson G P, Newman C W 1990 The development of the dizziness handicap inventory. Archives of Otolaryngology Head and Neck Surgery 116:424-427

Kelly C B 2000 Conservative management of vulnerable feet. In: Lusardi M M, Nielsen C (eds) Orthotics and prosthetics in rehabilitation. Butterworth Heinemann, Boston

Krebs D E, Gill-Body K M, Riley P O, Shumway-Cook A 1993 Double-blind, placebo-controlled trial of rehabilitation for bilateral vestibular hypo-function: preliminary report. Otolaryngology Head and Neck Surgery 109:735-741

Kumar S, Fernando D, Veves A et al 1995 Semmes-Weinstein monofilaments: a simple, effective and inexpensive screening device for identifying diabetic patients at risk for foot ulceration. Diabetes Research Clinic Practitioner 13:63–68

Lewis C, Phillippi L 1993 Postural changes with age and soft tissue treatment. Physical Therapy Forum 9:4–6

Lexell J 1993 Ageing and human skeletal muscle: observations from Sweden. Canadian Journal of Applied Physiology 18:2–9

Lord S, Castell S 1994 Physical activity programme for older persons: effect on balance, strength, neuromuscular control and balance reaction time. Archives of Physical Medicine and Rehabilitation 75:648–652

Lord S R, Clark R D 1996 Simple physiological and clinical tests for the accurate prediction of falling in older people. Gerontology 42:199–203

Lord S R, Menz H B 2000 Visual contributions to postural stability in older adults. Gerontology 46: 306–310

Lord S R, Webster I W 1990 Visual field dependence in elderly fallers and non-fallers. International Journal of Ageing and Human Development 31:267–277

Lord S R, Clark R D, Webster I W 1991 Physiological factors associated with falls in an elderly population. Journal of the American Geriatrics Society 39:1194–1200

Lord S R, McLean D, Strathers G 1992 Physiological factors associated with injurious falls in older people living in the community. Gerontology 38:338–346

Lord S R, Caplan G A, Ward J A 1993 Balance, reaction time and muscle strength in exercising and non-exercising older women: a pilot study. Archives of Physical Medicine and Rehabilitation 74:837–839

Lord S R, Sambrook P N, Gilbert C 1994 Postural stability, falls and fractures in the elderly: results from the Dubbo osteoporosis epidemiology study. Medical Journal of Australia 160:684–691

Lord S R, Ward J A, Williams P, Strudwick M 1995 The effect of a 12 month exercise trial on balance, strength and falls in older women. Journal of the American Geriatrics Society 43:1198–1206

Lord S R, Ward J A, Williams P 1996 Exercise effect on dynamic stability in older women: a randomised controlled trial. Archives of Physical Medicine and Rehabilitation 77:232–236

Lord S R, Sherrington C, Menz H 2001 Falls in older people: risk factors and strategies for prevention. Cambridge University Press, Cambridge

Lord S R, Dayhew J, Howland A 2002 Multifocal glasses impair edge-contrast sensitivity and depth perception and increase the risk of falls in older people. Journal of the American Geriatrics Society 50(11):1760–1766

Lundin-Olsson L, Nyberg L, Gustafson Y 1997 'Stops walking when talking' as a predictor of falls in elderly people. Lancet 349:617

Lundin-Olsson L, Nyberg L, Gustafson Y 1998 Attention, frailty and falls: the effect of a manual task on basic mobility. Journal of the American Geriatrics Society 46:758–761

Lynn S, Pool A, Rose D, Brey R, Suman V 1995 Randomised trial of the canalith repositioning procedure. Otolaryngology Head Neck Surgery 113: 712–720

McIlroy W E, Maki B E 1996 Age-related changes in compensatory stepping in response to unpredictable perturbations. Journal of Geriatrics 51: M289–M296

Maki B E, Holliday P J, Topper A K 1991 Fear of falling and postural performance in the elderly. Journal of Gerontology Medical Science 46:M123–M131

Maki B E, Holliday P J, Topper A K 1994 A prospective study of postural balance and risk of falling in an ambulatory and independent elderly population. Journal of Gerontology Medical Science 49: M72–M84

Maki B E, Edmonstone M A, McIlroy W E 2000 Age-related differences in laterally directed compensatory stepping behaviour. Journal of Gerontology Medical Science 55A:M270–M277

Manchester D, Woollacott M, Zederbauer-Hylton N, Marin O 1989 Visual, vestibular and somatosensory contributions to balance control in the older adult. Journal of Gerontology Medical Science 44: M118–M127

Manning J, Neistadt M, Parker S 1997 The relationship between fear of falling and balance and gait abilities in elderly adults in a subacute rehabilitation facility. Physical and Occupational Therapy and Geriatrics 15(2):33–47

Medell J L, Alexander N B 2000 A clinical measure of maximal and rapid stepping in older women. Journal of Gerontology Medical Science 55A: M429–M433

Murray M P, Duthie E H, Gambert S R, Sepic S B, Mollinger L A 1985 Age-related differences in knee muscle strength in normal women. Journal of Gerontology 40:275–280

Nadeau S, Gravel D, Arsenalt A, Bourbonnais D, Goyette M 1997 Dynamometric assessment of the plantarflexors in hemiparetic subjects: relations between muscular, gait and clinical parameters. Scandinavian Journal of Rehabilitation Medicine 29:137–146

Newton R 1989 Review of tests of standing balance abilities. Brain Injury 3:335–336

Newton R A 1995 Standing balance abilities of elderly subjects under altered visual and support conditions. Physiotherapy Canada 47:25–29

Nitz J C, Brown A The physical mobility scale to show dependency in frail elderly people: a reliability and validity study (in preparation)

Paige G D 1992 Senescence of human visual-vestibular interactions with ageing. Journal of Vestibular Research 2:133–151

Pastor M A, Day B L, Marsden C D 1993 Vestibular induced postural responses in Parkinson's Disease. Brain 116:11–17

Patla A E, Shumway-Cook A 1999 Dimensions of mobility: defining the complexity and difficulty associated with community mobility. Journal of Aging and Physical Activity 7:7–19

Perry J, Garrett M, Gronley J K, Mulroy S J 1995 Classification of walking handicap in the stroke population. Stroke 26:982–989

Peterka R, Black F 1990 Age related changes in human posture control: sensory organisation tests. Journal of Vestibular Research 1:73–85

Podsiadlo D, Richardson S 1991 The timed 'Up and Go': a test of basic functional mobility for frail persons. Journal of the American Geriatrics Society 39(2):142–148

Prosser L, Canby A 1997 Further validation of the Elderly Mobility Scale for measurement of mobility of hospitalised elderly people. Clinical Rehabilitation 11:338–343

Rankin J K, Woollacott M H, Shumway-Cook A, Brown L A 2000 Cognitive influence on postural stability: a neuromuscular analysis in young and older adults. Journal of Gerontology Medical Science 55A:M112–M119

Ring C, Nayak U S L, Isaacs B 1989 The effect of visual deprivation and proprioceptive change on postural sway in healthy elders. Journal of the American Geriatrics Society 37:745–749

Rutherford O M, Jones D A 1992 The relationship between muscle and bone loss and activity levels with age in women. Age and Ageing 21:286–293

Schenkman M, Cutson T M, Kuchibhatla M, Chandler J, Pieper C 1997 Reliability of impairment and physical performance measures for persons with Parkinson's disease. Physical Therapy 70:19–27

Seaby L, Torrance G 1989 Reliability of a physiotherapy functional assessment in a rehabilitation setting. Physiotherapy Canada 41(5):264–271

Shumway-Cook A, Horak F 1986 Assessing the influence of sensory interaction on balance: suggestion from the field. Physical Therapy 66:1548–1550

Shumway-Cook A, Woollacott M 2000 Attentional demands and postural control: The effects of sensory context. Journal of Gerontology Medical Science 55A:M10–M16

Shumway-Cook A, Woollacott M 2001 Motor control: theory and practical applications. Williams & Wilkins, Baltimore

Shumway-Cook A, Woollacott M, Kerns K A, Baldwin M 1997 The effects of two types of cognitive tasks on postural stability in older adults with and without a history of falls. Journal of Gerontology Medical Science 52A:M232–M240

Shumway-Cook A, Brauer S, Woollacott M 2000 Predicting the probability for falls in the community-dwelling adults using the Timed Up & Go Test. Physical Therapy 80(9):896–903

Simondson J, Goldie P, Brock K, Nosworthy J 1996 The Mobility Scale for acute stroke patients: intrarater and inter-rater reliability. Clinical Rehabilitation 10:295–300

Skelton D, Greig C, Davies J, Young A 1994 Strength, power and related functional ability of healthy aged 65–89 years. Age and Ageing 23:371–377

Smith R 1994 Validation and reliability of the Elderly Mobility Scale. Physiotherapy 80(11):744–747

Speechley M, Tinetti M 1991 Falls and injuries in frail and vigorous community elderly persons. Journal of the American Geriatrics Society 39:46–52

Steinberg M, Cartwright C, Peel N, Williams G 2000 A sustainable programme to prevent falls and near falls in community dwelling older people: results of a randomised trial. Journal of Epidemiology and Community Health 54:227–232

Stelmach G E, Worringham C 1985 Sensorimotor deficits related to postural stability: implications for falling in the elderly. Clinical Geriatric Medicine 1:679–694

Studenski S, Duncan P W, Chandler J 1991 Postural responses and effector factors in persons with unexplained falls: results and methodological issues. Journal of the American Geriatrics Society 39:229–234

Tanaka T, Hashimoto N, Noriyasu S et al 1995 Ageing and postural stability: changes in sensorimotor function. Physical and Occupational Therapy in Geriatrics 13:1–16

Teasdale N, Stelmach G, Breunig A 1991 Postural sway characteristics of the elderly under normal and altered visual and support surface conditions. Journal of Gerontology 46:B238–B244

Tesio L, Alpini D, Cesarani A, Perucca M 1999 Short form of the dizziness handicap inventory. American Journal of Physical Medicine and Rehabilitation 78:233–241

Thigpin M T, Light K E, Creel G L, Flynn S M 2000 Turning difficulty characteristics of adults aged 65 years and older. Physical Therapy 80(12):1174–1187

Tinetti M E, Speechley M, Ginter S E 1988 Risk factors for falls among elderly persons living in the community. New England Journal of Medicine 319: 1701–1707

Tinetti M E, Richman D, Powell L 1990 Falls efficacy as a measure of fear of falling. Journal of Gerontology Medical Science 45:239–243

Tinetti M, Baker D, McAcay 1994 A multifactorial intervention to reduce the risk of falling among elderly people living in the community. New England Journal of Medicine 331:821–827

Tobis J S, Reinsch D, Swanson J M, Byrd M, Scharf T 1985 Visual perception dominance of falls among community dwelling older adults. Journal of the American Geriatrics Society 33:330–333

Vandervoort A, McComas A J 1986 Contractile changes in opposing muscles of the human ankle joint with ageing. Journal of Applied Physiology 61:361–367

Wade M, Jones G 1997 The role of vision and spatial orientation in the maintenance of posture. Physical Therapy 77(6):619–627

Wade D, Wood V, Heller A, Maggs J, Hewer R 1987 Walking after stroke. Scandinavian Journal of Rehabilitation Medicine 19:25–30

Whanger A D, Wang H S 1974 Clinical correlates of the vibratory sense in elderly psychiatric patients. Journal of Gerontology 4:39–45

Whipple R H, Wolfson L I, Amerman P M 1987 The relationship of knee and ankle weakness to falls in nursing home residents: an isokinetic study. Journal of the American Geriatrics Society 35:13–20

Whitney S L, Hudak M T, Marchetti G F 2000 The association between observed gait instability and fall history in persons with vestibular dysfunction. Journal of Vestibular Research 10:99–105

Winograd C H, Lemsky C M, Nevitt M C 1994 Development of a physical performance and mobility examination. Journal of the American Geriatrics Society 42:743–749

Wolfson L, Whipple R, Amerman P 1990 Gait assessment in the elderly: a gait abnormality rating scale and its relation to falls. Journal of Gerontology 45:M12–M19

Woollacott M H 2000 Systems contributing to balance disorders in older adults. Editorial. Journal of Gerontology Medical Science 55A(8):M424–M428

Woollacott M, Tang P 1997 Balance control during walking in the older adult: research and implications. Physical Therapy 77:646–659

Woollacott M H, Shumway-Cook A, Nashner L 1986 Ageing and posture control: changes in sensory organization and muscular coordination. International Journal of Aging and Human Development 23:97–114

10 Retraining balance using task-focused workstations

Nancy Low Choy

This chapter aims to:

- present a task-oriented approach to retraining balance and mobility using workstations as an effective mode of delivering tailored interventions to individual or small groups of residents or community-based elders who are: frail aged; elders who ambulate with supervision within residential care facilities; or elders who are independently ambulant in the community
- provide an outline of workstations that illustrate varying levels of challenge but address the multiple aspects of balance and mobility that need to be considered while retraining balance and mobility in elders.

Introduction

Management of balance dysfunction in the older person requires an holistic approach to which physiotherapy makes an important contribution through falls prevention programmes as well as effective remedial intervention when falls and injuries occur. An assessment by a physiotherapist identifies those causal factors amenable to intervention and identifies and provides strategies to minimize future falls risk. It has been argued that the management of balance dysfunction in older people requires multiple systems to be considered and that addressing the impairments inherent in each individual in conjunction with varied task practice and environments enables elders to maintain and regain the ability to mobilize safely. Where the ability to mobilize safely is compromised it is critical that the limitations to balance and the need for supervision or assistance for safe mobility are identified.

Task-oriented approach to retraining balance and mobility

A task-oriented approach to retraining balance and mobility has emerged as an effective model of intervention over the last decade with a range of basic sciences used to provide the theoretical foundation for this model. Carr & Shepherd (1987, 1998, 2000, 2003) and Shumway-Cook & Woollacott (2001) are strong advocates of the need to consider a broad science basis for practice and believe that functional task training offers an efficient mode of regaining motor control by integrating the capacity of the brain to reorganize after injury (Johansson 2000, Nudo & Friel 1999, Nudo et al 2001, Shepherd 2001) as well as through application of principles of skill acquisition (Gentile 2000, Magill 2001). Such a model fosters specificity of task training, with muscle actions practised in the context of function, repeated task practice using different forms of feedback that can gradually be withdrawn, and varied task practice to enable transfer of learning to meet the functional demands of different environments. The challenge for the physiotherapist has been to know when to provide more direct assistance for the practice of motor tasks, when to operate more as a 'coach or trainer' and when to effectively incorporate part practice or 'sub-tasks' (Carr & Shepherd 2003).

Task-oriented training is promoted by Carr & Shepherd (2003) and Shumway-Cook & Woollacott (2001) and the efficacy of such training has been evaluated in a number of studies. The efficacy of task-related training has been established after stroke (Dean et al 2000, Dean & Shepherd 1997, Richards et al 1993), when retraining balance and mobility in fallers (Nitz & Low Choy 2004, Shumway-Cook et al 1997b) and for retraining functional motor tasks in cerebral palsy clients who are ageing (Low Choy et al 2003). The triad of addressing individual needs during varied task practice and in different environments is integrated within each of these programmes. Consideration of this triad is recommended when delivering balance and mobility programmes to other clients with neurological disorders and to those elders requiring intervention within residential care facilities and other community-based environments.

A review of intervention programmes that have been delivered to improve balance and mobility and decrease the falls risk of elders living in the community reveals that while an appropriate emphasis has been placed on strength, flexibility and resistance training (Buchner et al 1997, Chandler et al 1998, Lord & Castell 1994, Lord et al 1993, 1995, 1996, Rooks et al 1997, Sauvage et al 1992, Skelton et al 1995) few programmes have addressed the sensory processing and challenges that the environment (visual and surface challenges) places on balance systems or the cognitive demand inherent in many functional motor tasks requiring both balance and mobility (Brauer et al 2001, Lundin-Olssen et al 1997, 1998, Nitz & Thompson 2003, Shumway-Cook et al 1997a, 1997b, Shumway-Cook & Woollacott 2000). Most programmes include an exercise regime that can be delivered to groups of elders in community facilities although some programmes have been offered within the home (Campbell et al 1997, Jette et al 1996, McMurdo & Johnstone 1995, Sherrington & Lord 1997) with variable levels of supervision and support for the participants in the programmes. Less prevalent in the literature are programmes that provide a comprehensive, multidimensional, task-oriented approach to upgrading balance and mobility in elderly fallers. Such programmes have been successfully delivered to individual clients (Shumway-Cook et al 1997a) and to groups of elders (Nitz & Low Choy

2004) who had a falls history. In the latter study, workstations were used to provide a comprehensive programme that addressed all aspects of balance and mobility. A significant reduction in falls was achieved for the intervention group. It is possible that the added attention to balance strategy training, progressively increasing sensory challenges to tasks in varying environs and the added demand of dual tasks while practising motor tasks could have provided additional capacity for these elders to manage in community environs without recurrent falls. The delivery of such programmes within a residential care facility is advocated and considered cost-effective given the prevalence of falls in such facilities (Lipsitz et al 1991, Liu et al 1995, Lord et al 1991, Rubenstein et al 1988) and the high cost of care associated with falls and subsequent injury. With the prevalence of falls persisting in the general community despite the attempts to increase participation rates in activity programmes (Hill et al 2002), it is important to invest in strategies that might reduce the recurrence of falls.

Using workstations as a mode to deliver balance and mobility programmes

Workstations are considered the optimal mode for delivering multi-dimensional task-focused programmes that are specific to the client's need. Proponents of the workstation mode of intervention (Carr & Shepherd 2003, Dean & Shepherd 1997, Dean et al 2000, Low Choy et al 2003, Nitz & Low Choy 2004) recognize that task training can be delivered in an integrated and holistic programme, that the intensity and duration of rehabilitation programmes can be increased without adding to the cost of delivering a physiotherapy programme, and that the group dynamics generated may enhance motivation and compliance to training (Ada et al 1999). While this form of intervention is also considered to reduce the dependency on physiotherapists, the functional ability of individual clients will need to be considered, particularly in the context of frail older people living in residential care facilities.

The challenge for physiotherapists working in residential or community-based aged care is to deliver interventions that integrate the multiple elements of balance, target the needs of individual clients yet ensure a cost-effective mode of delivery. Clinicians could work with individual residents at their functional level and work capacity or overlap residents who could feasibly be managed in a small group. An appropriate assessment would provide the clinician with the necessary information to decide on the feasibility of overlapping residents or the need to work on an individualized basis. Once the focus of a workstation has been determined it is feasible to adapt the station to the activities of daily living encountered by a resident so that the individual can practise the functional task during care activities under the supervision of the carer. In addition, other more ambulant residents or community-dwelling elders could reasonably be worked in a small group under supervision, with respective workstations adjusted to safely challenge these clients. The need to include training for carers who work with frail aged or other highly dependent residents to ensure effective carryover of functional gains made with training was supported by the findings of a study with cerebral palsy residents who are ageing with a disability (Low Choy et al 2003).

Workstations set up in the form of a circuit would appear to provide an effective option for the physiotherapist to deliver variable task experiences while addressing the elements of balance under different environmental conditions. The multiple aspects of balance that may need to be addressed when delivering such a balance and mobility programme to an individual within a residential care facility or community environment were discussed in the preceding chapter. Interventions may need to:

- improve functional strength and flexibility
- ensure specificity of practice to meet task and environmental demands
- increase control at the limits of stability in all planes with particular attention to mediolateral stability for safe mobility during walking and particularly turning
- decrease reaction times by increasing speed of response to stimuli while balancing and walking
- develop reliable postural responses and varied strategies according to direction/force of displacement
- activate, foster integration and use sensory information/challenges for improved balance during task execution and/or conditions involving altered visual/proprioceptive input or conflict
- increase ability to manage dual/multiple tasks or recognize the inability of residents to safely manage multiple tasks
- improve endurance by increasing musculoskeletal and cardiovascular-respiratory capacity.

There are four practical steps to apply when planning a workstation mode of intervention for an individual resident or for a number of older people who could participate in a small group intervention:

- assess each resident to determine the aspects of balance and mobility that require attention and use tools that can objectively measure the impairments and functional motor abilities/limitations of the resident prior to the programme being implemented
- set up workstations that ensure all elements of balance and mobility are addressed and can be tailored to meet the specific problems of the individual
- plan how to make each station easier or more difficult to cater for the individual abilities that could present in the group through use of variable tasks which can be practised under different environmental conditions at each station
- reassess residents at the end of the programme or at intervals that are determined by their changing medical status to determine improvement and further areas for intervention.

In developing a workstations programme, a number of key principles need to be considered. The programme is driven by the individual needs of each participant and their active participation rather than being dependent on the physiotherapist being available for active practice of functional tasks. It is important therefore that each participant is provided with sufficient knowledge so that they are able to maximally benefit from their own programme. This is just as applicable for more independent/able residents as for those with a high level of functional dependence. Each participant therefore needs to be able to understand the purpose of each individual station and the relevant aim and goal for themselves. The relevance of the activity to specific functional tasks needs to be clear, as do the means of varying the activity. This should include not only making the task easier or harder (i.e. progressions or regressions) but also task variations so as to assist with transference of learning and promote interest during the repeated practice critical to a successful outcome.

By providing the resident with such knowledge and skills, the likelihood of carryover beyond the therapy setting is increased. This is further enhanced by the functional context of activities which are similar to work in real life and thus addressing the issue of specificity of training.

Each workstation should have a clear, easily understood instruction sheet. Key words, photos or diagrams may be used to name and give purpose to the workstation (e.g. sit-to-stand station, reaching station). The activity is best placed into a relevant functional context (e.g. to make it easier to reach into the bedside cupboard). The purpose needs to be clearly explained. The means of varying the task, making it easier or harder need to be clearly illustrated with words or pictures.

A second important principle is that the therapist acts as a 'coach' or 'trainer'. The supervising therapist is responsible for the initial detailed assessment and subsequent reassessment. This is vital so as to allow a targeted, individualized approach. Based upon the assessment findings the therapist is then responsible for developing workstation tasks to address specific identified issues. The therapist is responsible for training each participant in the task to be practised and for providing strategies for solving everyday functional problems and so place the training activity into a functional context which increases the likelihood of carryover. Safety remains a primary issue and all tasks need to be designed so that each individual is challenged but is able to perform the activities safely. This will often provide challenges to the therapist when designing the programme.

Residents at different functional levels may have different goals from individual workstations. More independent residents are able to take responsibility for learning the tasks and are able to work their way independently through the stations. Such individuals may gradually be able to independently adapt, modify and progress each task so as to optimally challenge themselves. Residents at a lower functional level will be more reliant upon the physiotherapist to set up each task to suit individual needs. They may be more reliant on equipment and/or the physiotherapist/carer to ensure safety. This is clearly the case for those residents with impaired cognitive function, perceptual deficits, behavioural problems or poor sitting or standing balance. Tasks and activities for these residents will need to be carefully evaluated and participation in challenging aspects of a workstation programme will require individualized attention. For example, residents with very poor sitting balance may perform preparatory tasks in lying, actively move and reach while sitting in a chair but practise sitting tasks without such supportive seating when the physiotherapist is available. Use of a tilt table with modified support to enable the upper body to actively participate in reaching activities, or standing with body weight support (if available), may allow such residents to be challenged in a safe and supported environment.

Thus workstations can be used to deliver comprehensive, multidimensional and targeted interventions to improve balance and mobility in elderly residents, with the content and level of delivery adjusted to meet the functional level of each individual. This means that the more dependent resident, those who can be worked under supervision and those who can be progressively extended and challenged are able to benefit from the same workstation. Thus the frail elderly living in residential care are as able to participate in such programmes as are those living in supervised care or those living independently in the community. The challenge is for physiotherapists to apply their acquired knowledge and skills in a flexible and effective programme to meet the needs of participating elders.

Specific workstation foci

With the aim of these interventions being an improved ability to balance and mobilize the workstations need to address:

- flexibility of the trunk and limbs with specific attention to the lower limbs
- functional strength training using tasks that involve the lower limbs (sit to stand; stepping activities and walking tasks)
- internal perturbations through reaching tasks that require variable weight shift, in lying at the lowest level or load/de-load of the lower limbs in both sitting and standing, and stepping if working in standing
- challenges at the limits of stability with particular attention to mediolateral stability during walking and turning
- introduction of dual tasks that increase the motor and cognitive demands
- preparing for external perturbations by retraining the ankle, hip, suspension and stepping strategies
- introducing external perturbations (changing surfaces, visual conflict, external forces)

- improving balance under different sensory (visual, tactile/proprioceptive and vestibular) demands, e.g. walking on varying surfaces, interacting with objects in the environment such as different height blocks and chairs, and managing to interact with objects moving in the visual field (e.g. catch/throw a ball)
- decreasing reaction times for internally and externally paced activities, and
- improving endurance by increasing musculoskeletal and cardiovascular-respiratory capacity.

Thus the following workstations have been developed to include these varied demands on balance and mobility, and the ways to adjust each workstation to increase the challenge are illustrated. Availability of other equipment such as a treadmill, overhead harness system to enable body weight to be supported or a bicycle or arm ergometer would allow additional tasks to be included.

Workstations

Seated reach (Fig. 10.1)

Purpose

To promote weight shift and control at the limits of stability while encouraging lower limb loading and weight acceptance.

Starting position

Sitting in the middle of a plinth with feet on floor.
Table in front and on one side with block at shoulder height; stool at other side.
Multiple objects on table to be shifted from lower stool or to top of stool on other side.

Tasks

Practise moving to limits of stability in all planes.
Practise controlled weight shift in different directions.
Ensure lower limb load during weight shift.
Improve range of movement and trunk flexibility.

Variations

Move objects further away.
Alter the direction of reaching, e.g. high to low, behind to in front.
Reach with both hands.

Sit to stand (Fig. 10.2)

Purpose

To practise standing up and sitting down from a standard seat.
To improve functional strength in lower limb muscles.
To improve ability to stand up/sit down on a different surface.
To improve work capacity, exercise tolerance and fitness.
To encourage dual task ability.

Set-up

Sitting in the middle of a plinth with feet on floor.
Table in front or side for use or to provide a safer work set-up.

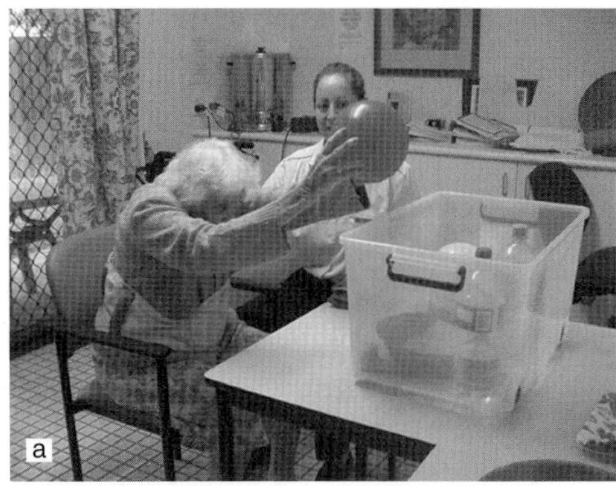

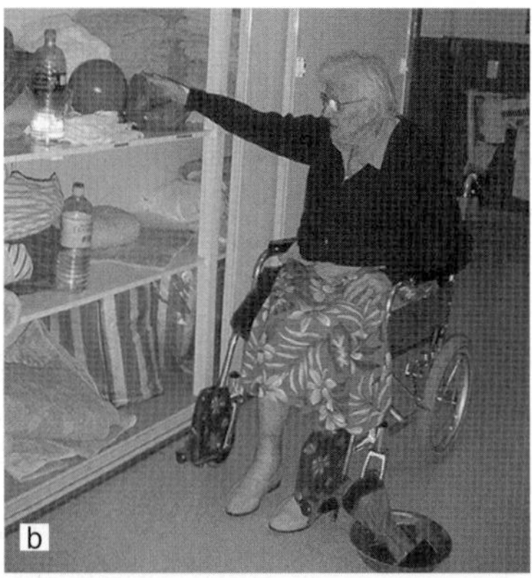

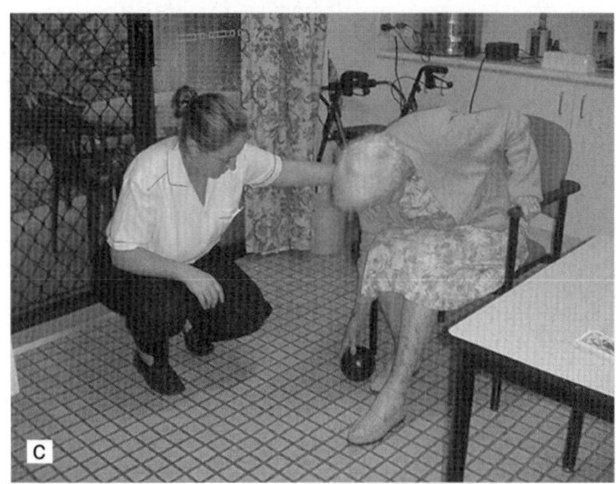

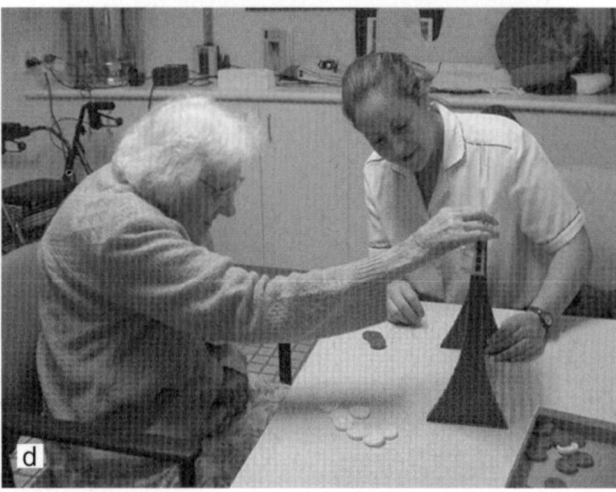

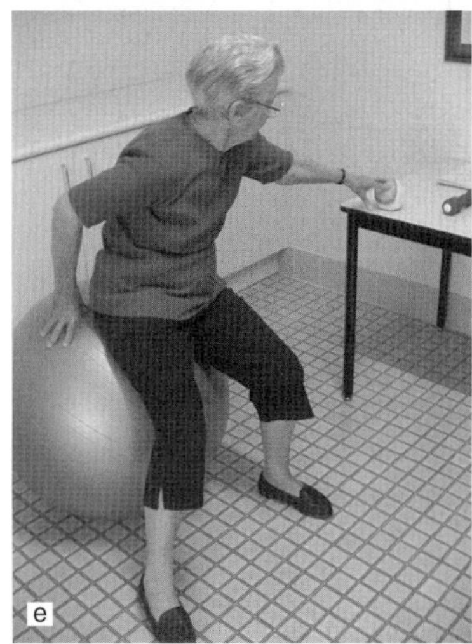

Figure 10.1a–e

Examples of the progression of exercises that may be utilized in a seated reach workstation. (a) Forward reach using both arms to gain trunk extension. (b) Lateral reach to encourage weight shift and trunk mobility. (c) Reach to floor for trunk control and flexibility. (d) Reach and participate in problem-solving task. (e) Use of less stable base to challenge balance control during reach.

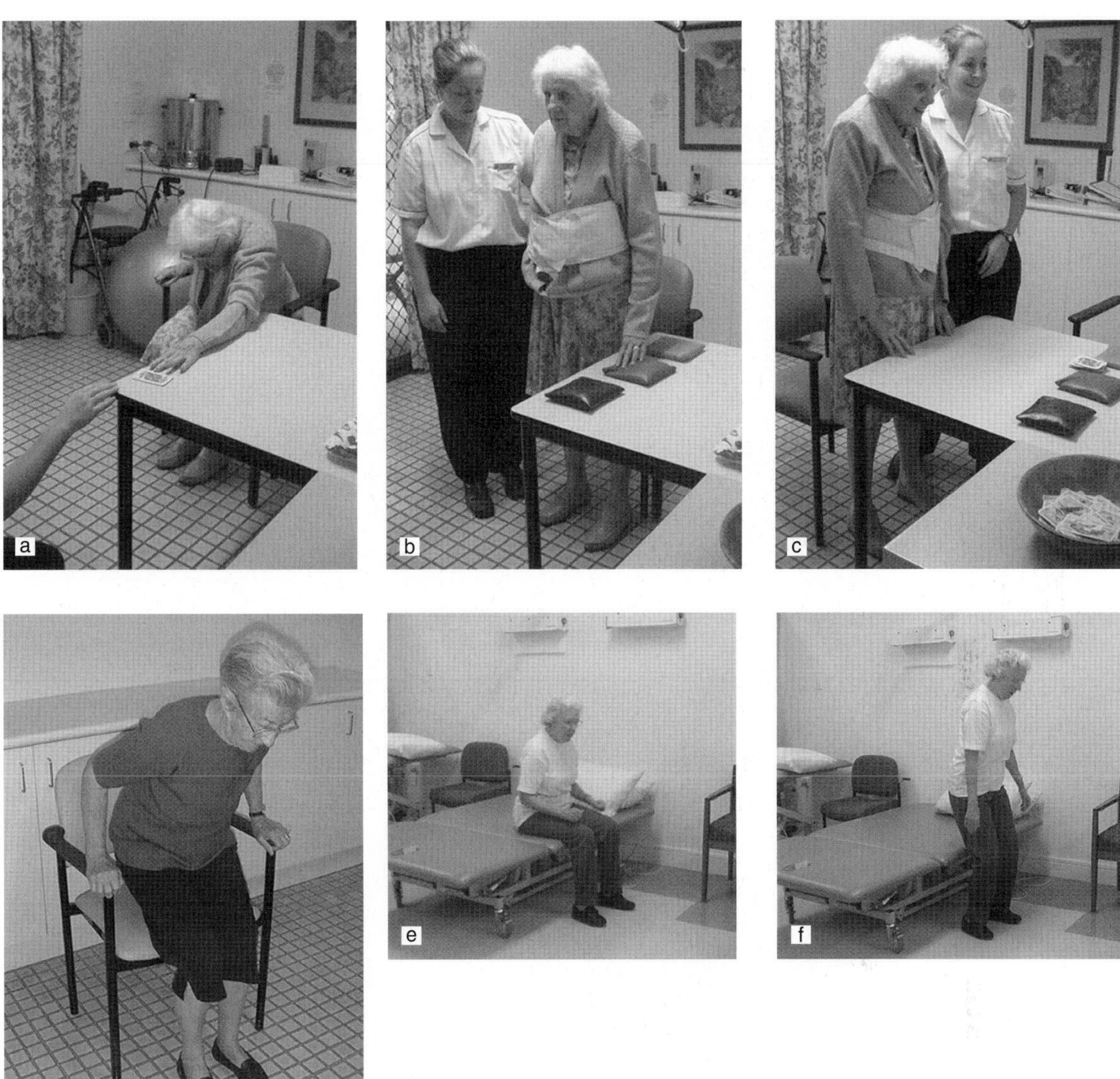

Figure 10.2a–f
Examples of the progression of exercises that may be utilized in a sit-to-stand workstation.

Variations Change the height of the bed/chair (lower to make it harder).
Stand/sit without using hands for support.
Stand/sit while holding objects, e.g. cup of water on a tray; objects of varying size/weights to add the demand of a second task.
Stand/sit with softer surface (e.g. mat) under feet.
Stand from a chair/table arrangement.
Stand/sit with one leg in front of the other.
Stand/step towards object on one side.

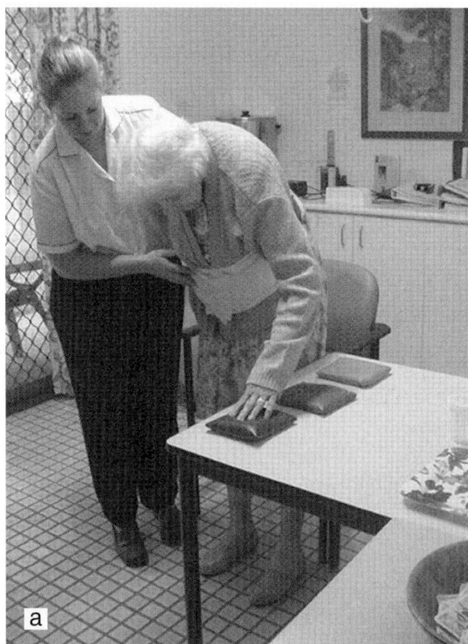

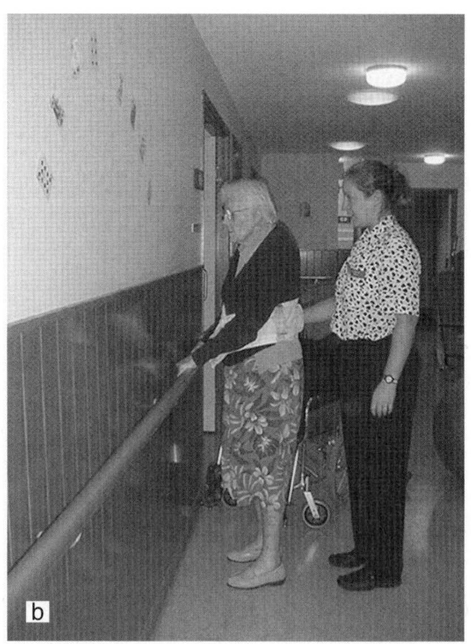

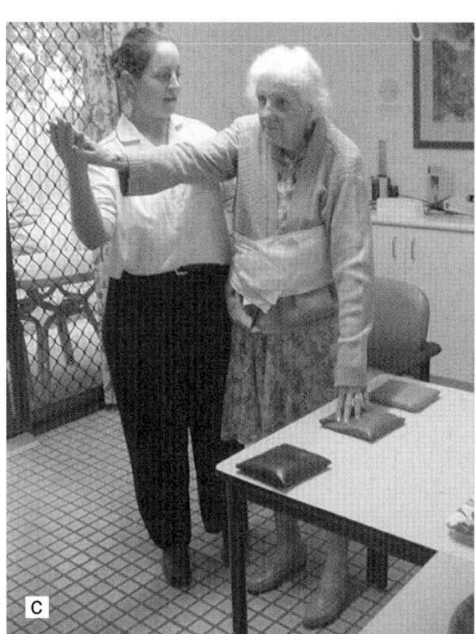

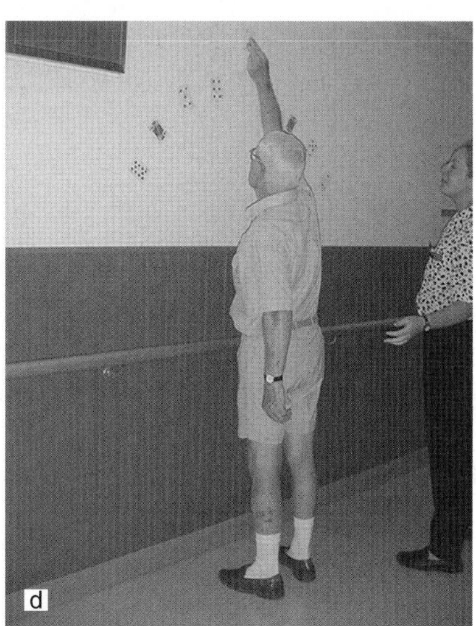

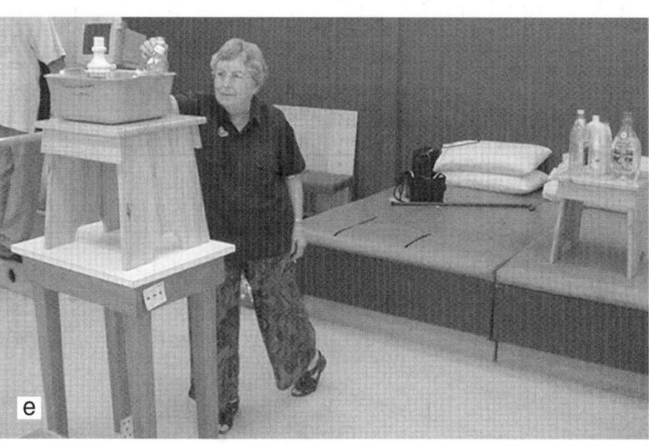

Figure 10.3a–e *Examples of the progression of exercises that may be utilized in a reach/step and reach workstation.*

Reach/step and reach in standing (Fig. 10.3)

Purpose

To improve the ability to reach and shift objects in standing and while stepping and reaching.

To promote weight shift in all planes and towards the limit of stability.

To promote mediolateral stability.

To improve functional strength (eccentric/concentric control) of the lower limbs.

To improve ability to manage multiple tasks.

Set-up

Standing at a table/bench with a lower plinth behind for safety.

Trolley with shelving to one side, table/stool 1–2 metres away on other side.

Firm/mat as floor surface related to ability level.

Variations

Move objects further away, higher, lower.

Alter the direction of reaching, e.g. high to low, behind to in front.

Reach with both hands.

Shift light/heavy objects.

Add a softer surface.

Block work (Fig. 10.4)

Purpose

To increase functional strength, concentric and eccentric control of the lower limb extensors, abductors and adductors.

To improve mediolateral stability by stepping up and over blocks of varying heights and walking sideways over the blocks.

To improve ability to carry out a dual task.

Set-up

Two small blocks between parallel bars.

Variations

Walk forward, sideways and backwards with care.

Introduce a variety of blocks with added height challenges.

Add a soft foam square between the blocks.

Carry an object while walking forward/sideways and backwards.

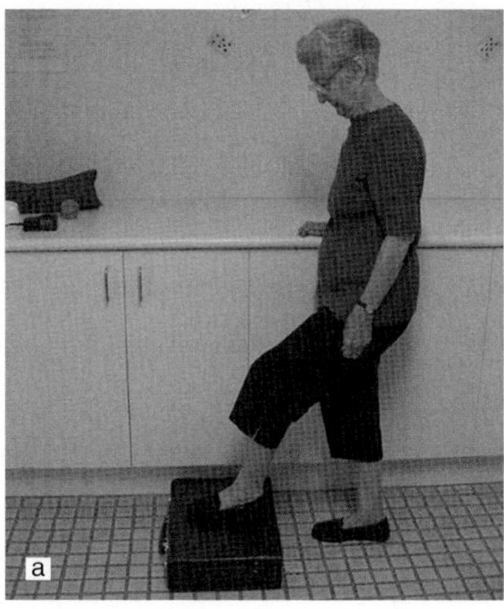

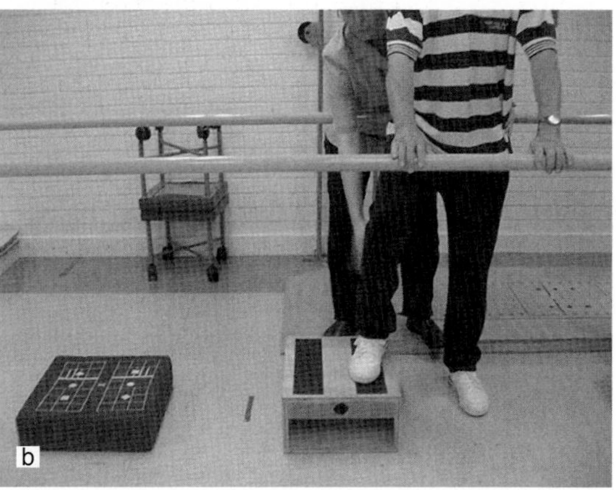

Figure 10.4a–d

Examples of the progression of exercises that may be utilized in a block work workstation.

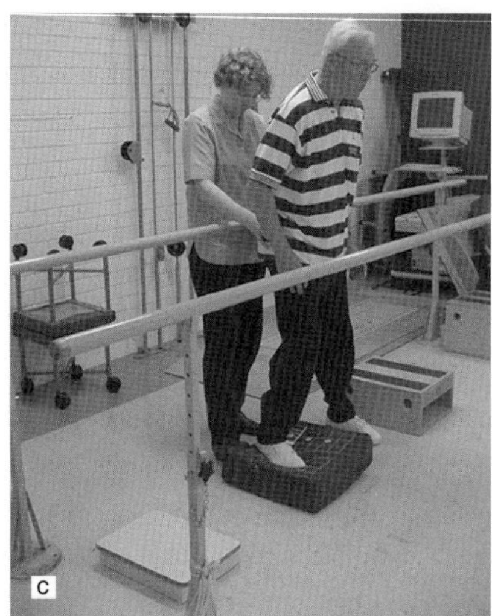

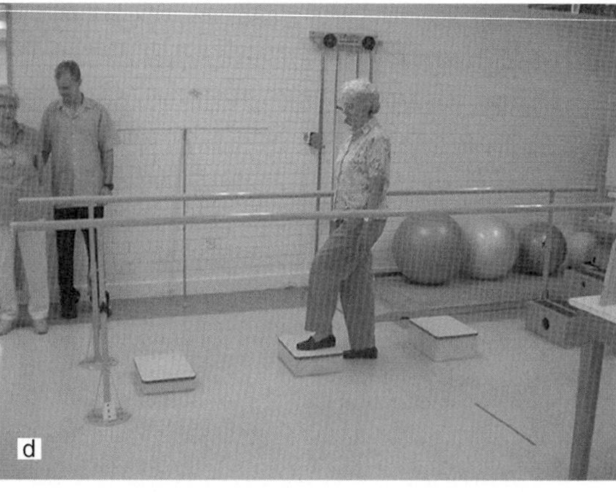

Figure 10.4a–d
Continued.

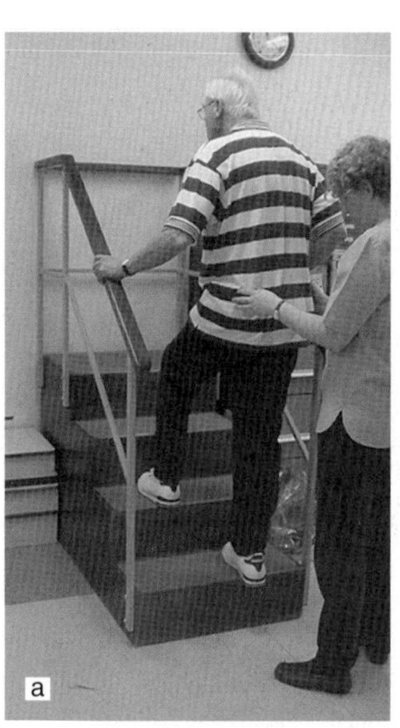

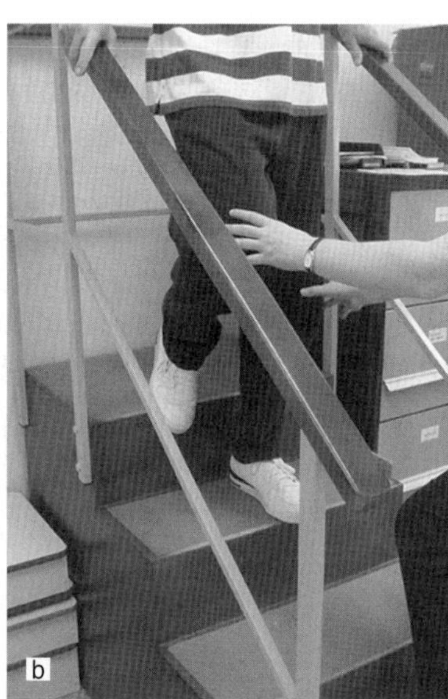

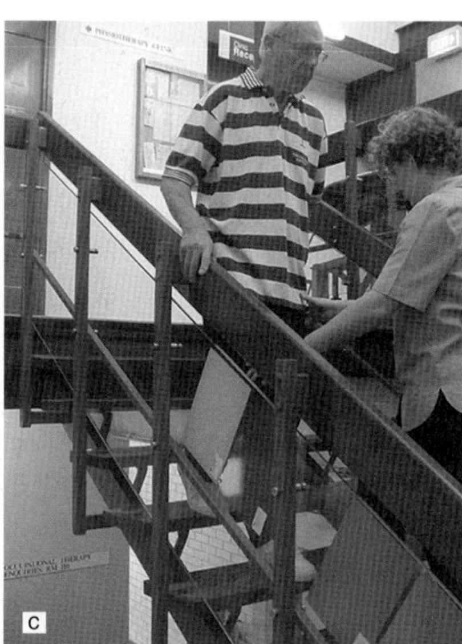

Figure 10.5a–c
Examples of the progression of exercises that may be utilized in a stairs workstation.

Stairs (Fig. 10.5)

Purpose

To improve functional strength, added flexibility and controlled force generation of the plantarflexors by lowering heels over stair edge, then carrying out a controlled toe-stand.

To promote concentric/eccentric control of the lower limb extensors with reciprocal stair walking.

Set-up

Small set of stairs with rails.

Variations

Number of times the stairs are practised with use of rails.
Number of heel drops/toe-stands.
Walking slowly up and down stairs without use of rails.
Walking at a comfortable speed up and down stairs without use of rails.

Stepping out of the square (Fig. 10.6)

Purpose

Stepping out of the square to promote weight shift and an efficient stepping response.
To promote the ability to efficiently plan a step.

Set-up

Square marked on floor with tape.
Markers set around the square at about 60% of the client's maximum ability to step.

Variations

Stepping to targets within a set time.
Use of targets with random number sequence to introduce a second component to this task.

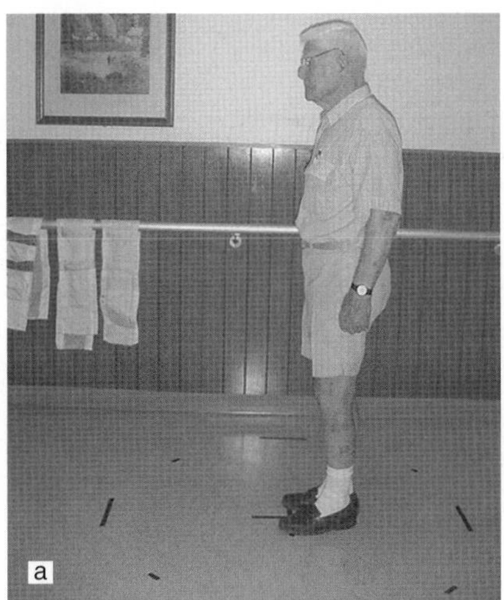

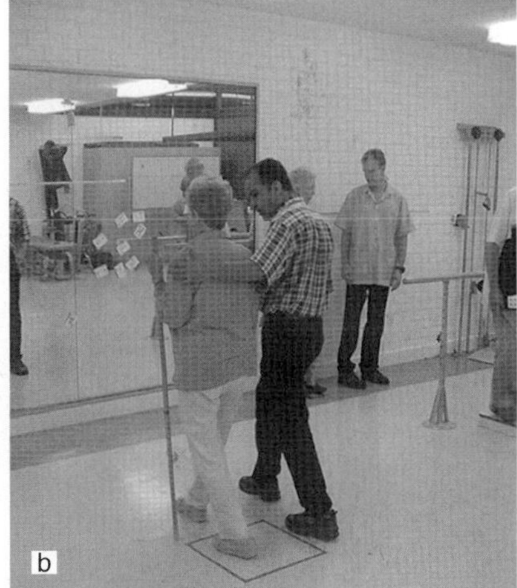

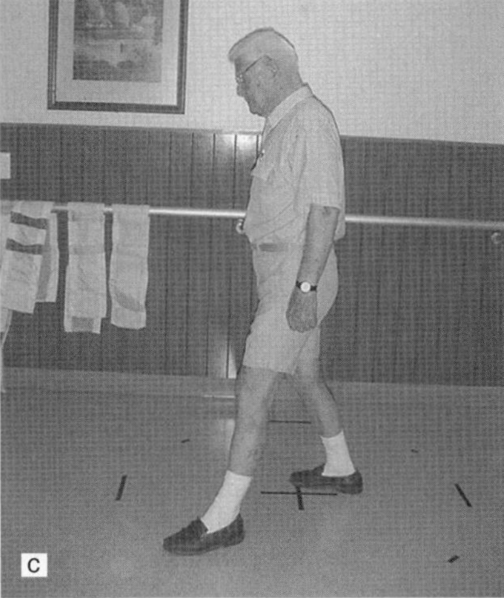

Figure 10.6a–c *Examples of the progression of exercises that may be utilized in a stepping out of the square workstation.*

Ankle/hip strategy training (Fig. 10.7)

Purpose

To promote efficient use of ankle and hip strategies in response to displacement backwards.

Set-up

Use of a blank wall to lean on when moving backwards.
Feet set out from wall.
Table in front of patient.

Variations

Leaning on wall, reach to table and stand up without pulling on the table.
Stand out from the wall and move hips backwards to touch the wall, then reach forwards/pick up toes and stand up.
Start out from wall and lower hips towards wall but pull up toes and stand up again without touching wall.

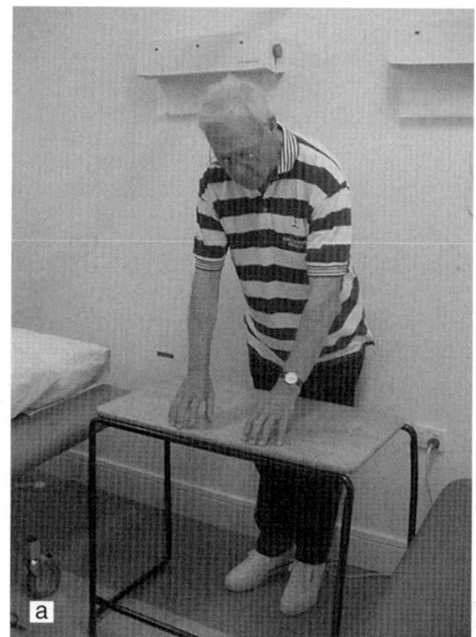

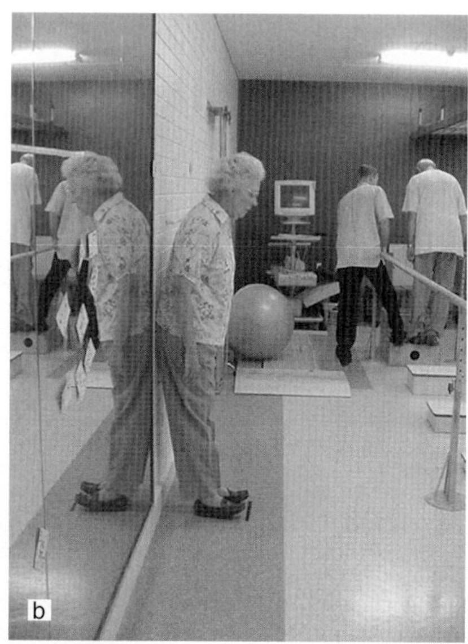

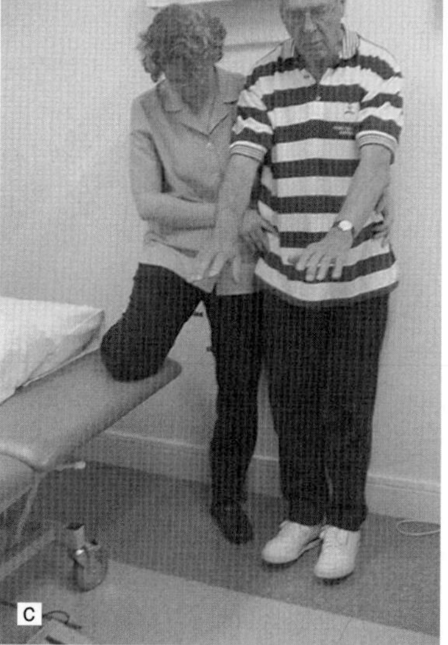

Figure 10.7a–c *Examples of the progression of exercises that may be utilized in an ankle and hip strategy workstation.*

Walking (Fig. 10.8)

Purpose

To promote efficient walking over a variety of surfaces and environmental demands.

Set-up

Set out blocks, rubber mat/foam square, within parallel bars for lower level client.

Set out blocks, rubber mat/foam square, small tilt board within parallel bars for more able client.

Set up equipment in open space for higher level client.

Variations

Walk over different surfaces (stable/unstable).

Turning around an obstacle.

Search for a series of objects, e.g. find a card series in sequence while executing a walking circuit, Walk and tap a balloon/while catching/ throwing a ball.

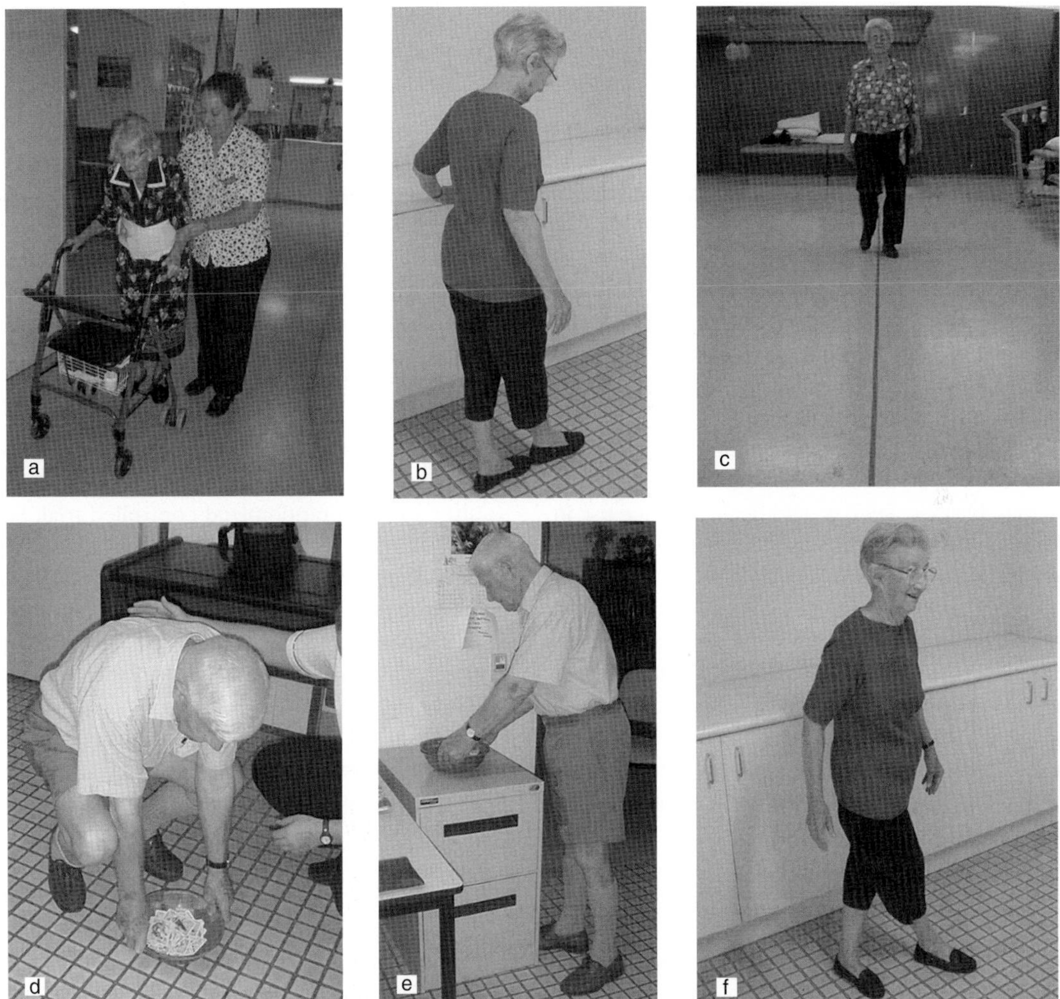

Figure 10.8a–f

Examples of the progression of exercises that may be utilized in a walking workstation.

Summary

- Physiotherapists play an important role in the field of balance, mobility and falls prevention.
- An effective assessment identifies causal factors leading to impaired mobility and balance and identifies factors which may be amenable to treatment.
- There are multiple systems which may be involved in balance dysfunction. By addressing impairments in varied environments and task-oriented activities we may enable elders to maintain or regain the ability to safely mobilize.
- Workstations are an efficacious mode of delivering multidimensional task-focused programmes. These can be delivered through individual or small group situations.

References

Ada L, Mackay F, Heard R, Adams R 1999 Stroke rehabilitation: does the therapy area provide a physical challenge? Australian Journal of Physiotherapy 45:33–38

Brauer S, Woollacott M, Shumway-Cook A 2001 The interacting effect of cognitive demand and recovery of postural stability in balance impaired elderly. Journal of Gerontology Medical Science 56(8):M489–M496

Buchner D M, Cress M E, de Lateur B J et al 1997 The effect of strength and endurance training on gait, balance, fall risk, and health service use in community-living older adults. Journal of Gerontology Medical Science 52(4):M218–M224

Campbell A J, Robertson M C, Gardner M M et al 1997 Randomised controlled trial of a general practice programme of home based exercise to prevent falls in elderly women. British Medical Journal 315:1065–1069

Carr J H, Shepherd R B 1987 A motor relearning programme for stroke, 2nd edn. Butterworth-Heinemann, Oxford

Carr J H, Shepherd R B 1998 Neurological rehabilitation: optimizing motor performance. Butterworth-Heinemann, Oxford

Carr J H, Shepherd R B 2000 A motor learning model for rehabilitation. In: Carr J H, Shepherd R B (eds) Movement science foundations for physical therapy in rehabilitation. PPO-ED, Austin, TX, p 33–110

Carr J H, Shepherd R B 2003 Stroke rehabilitation: guidelines for exercise and training to optimize motor skill. Butterworth-Heinemann, Oxford

Chandler J M, Duncan P W, Kochersberger G, Studenski S 1998 Is lower extremity strength gain associated with improvement in physical performance and disability in frail, community-dwelling elders? Archives of Physical Medicine and Rehabilitation 79:24–30

Dean C, Shepherd R 1997 Task-related training improves performance of seated reaching tasks after stroke: a randomized controlled trial. Stroke 28:722–728

Dean C M, Richards C L, Malouin F 2000 Task-related training improves performance of locomotor tasks in chronic stroke: a randomised controlled pilot trail. Journal of the American Geriatrics Society 81(4):409–417

Gentile A M 2000 Skill acquisition: action, movement and neuromotor processes. In: Carr J H, Shepherd R B (eds) Movement science foundations for physical therapy in rehabilitation. PPO-ED, Austin, TX, p 111–187

Hill K, Kerse N, Lentini F et al 2002 Falls: a comparison of trends in community, hospital and mortality data in older Australians. Aging 14:18–27

Jette A M, Harris B A, Sleeper L 1996 A home-based exercise programme for non-disabled older adults. Journal of the American Geriatrics Society 44:644–649

Johansson B B 2000 Brain plasticity and stroke rehabilitation. The Willis lecture. Stroke 31(1):223–230

Lipsitz L A, Jonsson P V, Kelley M M, Koestner J S 1991 Causes and correlates of recurrent falls in ambulatory frail elderly. Journal of Gerontology 46:114–122

Liu B A, Topper A K, Reeves R A, Gryfe C, Maki B E 1995 Falls among older people – relationship to medication use and orthostatic hypotension. Journal of the American Geriatrics Society 43(10):1141–1145

Lord S, Castell S 1994 Physical activity program for older persons: effect on balance, strength, neuromuscular control and balance reaction time. Archives of Physical Medicine and Rehabilitation 75:648–652

Lord S R, Clark R D, Webster I W 1991 Physiological factors associated with falls in an elderly population. Journal of the American Geriatrics Society 39:1194–1200

Lord S R, Caplan G A, Ward J A 1993 Balance, reaction time and muscle strength in exercising and non-exercising older women: a pilot study. Archives of Physical Medicine and Rehabilitation 74: 837–839

Lord S R, Ward J A, Williams P, Strudwick M 1995 The effect of a 12-month exercise trial on balance, strength and falls in older women. Journal of the American Geriatrics Society 43:1198–1206

Lord S R, Ward J A, Williams P 1996 Exercise effect on dynamic stability in older women: a randomised controlled trial. Archives of Physical Medicine and Rehabilitation 77:232–236

Low Choy N, Isles R, Barker R, Nitz J 2003 The efficacy of a work-station intervention program to improve functional ability and flexibility in ageing clients with cerebral palsy. Journal of Disability and Rehabilitation 25:1201–1207

Lundin-Olsson L, Nyberg L, Gustafson Y 1997 'Stops walking when talking' as a predictor of falls in elderly people. Lancet 349:617

Lundin-Olsson L, Nyberg L, Gustafson Y 1998 Attention, frailty and falls: The effect of a manual task on basic mobility. Journal of the American Geriatrics Society 46:758–761

Magill R A 2001 Motor learning concepts and applications, 6th edn. McGraw-Hill, New York

McMurdo M E, Johnstone R 1995 A randomized controlled trial of a home exercise programme for elderly people with poor mobility. Age and Ageing 24:425–438

Nitz J C, Low Choy N L 2004 The efficacy of a specific balance-strategy training programme for preventing falls among older people: a pilot randomised controlled trial. Age and Ageing 33:52–58

Nitz J C, Thompson K 2003 'Stops walking to talk': A simple measure of predicting falls in the frail elderly. Australasian Journal on Ageing 22(2):97–99

Nudo R J, Friel K M 1999 Cortical plasticity after stroke: implications for rehabilitation. Review Neurology 9:713–717

Nudo R J, Plautz E J, Frost S B 2001 Role of adaptive plasticity in recovery of function after damage to motor cortex. Muscle and Nerve 8:1000–1019

Richards C L, Malouin F, Wood-Dauphine S 1993 Task-specific physical therapy for optimization of gait recovery in acute stroke patients. Archives of Physical Medicine and Rehabilitation 74:612–620

Rooks D S, Kiel D P, Parsons C, Hayes W C 1997 Self-paced resistance training and walking exercise in community-dwelling older adults: effects on neuromotor performance. Journal of Gerontology Medical Science 52:M161–M168

Rubenstein L Z, Robbins A S, Schulman B L et al 1988 Falls and instability in the elderly. Journal of the American Geriatrics Society 44:273–278

Sauvage L R, Myklebust B M, Crow-Pan J 1992 A clinical trial of strengthening and aerobic exercise to improve gait and balance in elderly male nursing home residents. American Journal of Physical Medicine and Rehabilitation 71:333–342

Shepherd R 2001 Exercise and training to optimize functional motor performance in stroke: driving neural reorganization? Neural Plasticity 8:121–129

Sherrington C, Lord S R 1997 Home exercise to improve strength and walking velocity after hip fracture: a randomized controlled trial. Archives of Physical Medicine and Rehabilitation 78:208–212

Shumway-Cook A, Woollacott M 2000 Attentional demands and postural control: the effects of sensory context. Journal of Gerontology Medical Science 55A:M10–M16

Shumway-Cook A, Woollacott M 2001 Motor control: theory and practical applications. Williams & Wilkins, Baltimore

Shumway-Cook A, Gruber W, Baldwin M, Liao S 1997a The effect of multi-dimensional exercises on balance, mobility and fall risk in community-dwelling older adults. Physical Therapy 77(1):46–57

Shumway-Cook A, Woollacott M, Kerns K A, Baldwin M 1997b The effects of two types of cognitive tasks on postural stability in older adults with and without a history of falls. Journal of Gerontology Medical Science 52A:M232–M240

Skelton D A, Young A, Grieg C A, Malbut K E 1995 Effects of resistance training on strength, power and selected functional abilities of women aged 75 and older. Journal of the American Geriatrics Society 43:1081–1087

Tinetti M E, Speechley M, Ginter S F 1988 Risk factors for falls among elderly persons living in the community. New England Journal of Medicine 319:1701–1707

11 Exercise prescription in residential aged care facilities

Susan R. Hourigan

This chapter aims to:

- outline the benefits of exercise in the residential aged care population
- reiterate the importance of good clinical reasoning by means of thorough and appropriate assessment, treatment, exercise prescription and re-evaluation
- overview exercise prescription and how it applies to physiotherapists working with residents living in RACFs
- show how exercise programming and exercise protocols may be integrated into the nursing and activities systems of facilities
- suggest issues that will apply to both mobile and immobile residents (although the chapter is aimed more specifically towards those residents who are mobile and have a higher level of physical functioning than the extremely frail or fully dependent RACF resident)
- relate principles of exercise prescription to the older population, various issues encountered in RACFs, theoretical background and treatment ideas for this special group.

Introduction

One of the main roles of the physiotherapist working in residential aged care is to prescribe exercise to residents. The physiotherapist individually assesses the need for therapy amongst the residents and through clinical reasoning develops personalized therapy plans. Other staff such as physiotherapy, nursing or activities assistants, who are under the physiotherapist's direction, often implement the exercise programmes. The ongoing role of the physiotherapist, in regard to exercise programming, includes regular re-evaluation to determine the effectiveness of the given regimen. It is important that objective measurements are used so that outcome measures can be recorded for accountability and documentation requirements.

With employees other than physiotherapists carrying out the prescribed exercise programmes to varying degrees of effectiveness this system is clearly less than ideal, yet it does enable a broader access to limited physiotherapy assessment and treatment than would otherwise be available.

In Australia at least, the lack of physiotherapy services stems from government funding constraints within the aged care sector, the appropriation of available funding to other services by management and a genuine workforce shortage of physiotherapists.

Physiotherapists working in aged care need to have a solid understanding of exercise physiology, exercise prescription and clinical reasoning in order to make judgements regarding best practice in relation to exercise programming. Physiotherapists understand the risks and benefits of various modalities and doses of exercise in relation to specific pathology and health-related goals. They are the best equipped professionals to incorporate exercise into the health care of residents within RACFs.

The value of exercise in geriatric health care has been extensively questioned. Some reviews have positively hailed exercise as a means of preventing and treating diseases associated with old age whilst others have questioned whether there are any benefits to exercise in late-life and whether exercise prescription has been over-sold (Fiatarone Singh 2002). It seems critical to point out that there are numerous studies which represent benefits associated with activity and health status in older adults. It is equally as important to highlight that as there are many different people, diseases and health issues; there are as many different modalities of exercise, methods of programming, doses of activity and lengths of programmes. The literature is scattered with both positive and negative research results pertaining to the usefulness of different exercise regimens.

Advancing age is associated with a decline in both functional abilities and fitness component measures. Changes to the cardiovascular system, respiratory system, musculoskeletal system, central and peripheral nervous systems, posture and gait in the elderly population have been well documented and were summarized in Chapter 1 of this text (McArdle et al 1996, Shephard 1997, Shumway-Cook & Woollacott 1995, Trew & Everett 1997). The ability to exercise and efficiency of movement inevitably decreases with the passage of years. Effects on lifestyle and quality of life of this reduction in movement capabilities and functional activities may be catastrophic. The maintenance of physical function and mobility in the elderly is of great importance. Perhaps the most important issue related to quality of life is that of independent function and ambulation – it is the key factor which enables residents to make their own decisions and to go where they please. This self-determination enables them to bring themselves to activities of choice or remove themselves from unwanted places, people or situations. It is often the key to maintaining dignity, privacy and happiness.

It is clear that a number of age-induced changes can be prevented, slowed down or even reversed with appropriate activity (Trew & Everett 1997). Some research has suggested that half of the loss of functional decline associated with ageing is a result of disuse, which is easily modifiable with regular exercise (Pardini 1984). It is generally accepted that regular exercise enhances physical adaptability, mobility and coordination, all of which contribute to an enriched life in old age (Rissel 1987).

Evidence does exist which supports the notion that exercise can be used as therapy to:

- minimize the physiological changes associated with ageing
- contribute to psychological health and wellbeing
- increase longevity and decrease the risks of many common chronic diseases, e.g. diabetes and cardiac disease
- primarily treat, or adjunctively assist certain chronic diseases (especially in regard to 'disuse' syndromes)
- counteract specific side effects of standard medical care (iatrogenic complications)
- prevent and treat disability (Fiatarone Singh 2002, Pardini 1984, Rissel 1987, Trew & Everett 1997).

The benefits of exercise are many, and include but are not limited to:

- improved strength
- increased range of motion
- improved flexibility
- improved functional mobility
- improved cardiac status
- improved respiratory status
- better sleep
- improved gastrointestinal function
- increased self-esteem
- improved tone management
- improved postural control
- improved social interaction
- decreased falls risk
- increased fun and laughter
- stress release/endorphin release
- improved immunity
- improved skin integrity
- improved posture
- improved gait
- improved efficiency of movement
- increased exercise tolerance
- decreased fear of falling
- increased endurance
- improved quality of life
- improved dexterity.

Several other chapters in this text relate specifically to diseases or conditions experienced in the age strata residing in RACFs. We have illustrated the likely benefits of exercise throughout this text in relation to many syndromes or diseases. Exercise therapy may be utilized in the treatment of the following conditions, including but not limited to:

- frailty
- mobility impairment
- functional disability
- falls
- osteoporosis
- palliative care
- diabetes
- incontinence
- arthritis
- gout
- stroke
- cancer
- ischaemic heart disease
- cardiomyopathy
- congestive cardiac failure
- respiratory disease
- chronic renal failure
- insomnia
- hypertension
- peripheral vascular disease
- venous stasis
- obesity

- constipation
- depression
- dementia
- neurological disorders and diseases.

Changes associated with the above conditions occur in physical indices such as body weight, strength, cartilage integrity, blood pressure, anxiety, muscle and bone mass, and balance. Once problems are identified we are able to recommend exercise which assists in counteracting the given changes, for example prescribing resistance or aerobic training for sufferers of osteoarthritis, combined with balance training for those with established osteoporosis.

It is imperative to conduct a full assessment of the resident in order to decide what, if any, will be the treatment ideals and to determine their goals. Chapters 2, 8 and 9 deal in more detail with various aspects of resident assessment. A thorough assessment will allow the therapist to prescribe a relevant exercise programme in order to improve or maintain the resident's mobility, independent function and quality of life, for as long as possible.

A good understanding of different disease processes is necessary in order to modify exercise given certain considerations. Education at the undergraduate physiotherapy level provides for students to learn how to establish frames and principles in which to base further knowledge and experience. It is not within the scope of this chapter to examine conditions separately and state the given rationale for different exercises; it is expected that practising clinicians will be able to do this with prior gained knowledge or reading of other material as self-directed learning. However, the principles of exercise prescription as related to residents within RACFs will be addressed in the next section. Firstly, we examine the ability of the older person to train and benefit from exercise.

Trainability in the aged population

Traditionally, the view has been held that older individuals were not able to improve their strength and endurance capacity to the same extent as younger people. Reasons provided for this 'blunted' trainability were attributed to a decline in neuromuscular function and an age-related impairment in the cellular capability for protein synthesis and chemical regulation. However, significant research in the past two decades has enabled a modified version of the traditional view to be made.

'When a healthy person, young or old is given an appropriate training stimulus, large and rapid improvements occur in physiologic function, often at a rate and magnitude that is independent of the person's age' (McArdle et al 1997, p 643). Regardless of age, regular physical activity produces measurable physiological improvements. The magnitude of these improvements depends on many factors, including initial fitness status, medical history, age, and type and amount of training (McArdle et al 1996).

Trainability studies in the elderly concentrating on strength development reveal findings clearly indicating an impressive plasticity in physiological, structural, and performance characteristics well into the ninth decade of life (Fiatarone et al 1990). Healthy older adults show no negative metabolic or hormonal responses or any adaptive problems to regular exercise that would contraindicate participation in a standard training programme.

Exercise prescription principles in the mobile elderly

Exercise prescription is the process whereby a person's recommended regimen of physical activity is designed in a systematic and individualized manner (American College of Sports Medicine 1991). In all cases, careful consideration is given to the resident's health history, risk factor profile, behavioural characteristics, and personal goals and preferences. Specific purposes of an exercise prescription will vary according to needs, interests, health status and background. Generally the aim is to enhance physical fitness (maintain or improve functional abilities), promote health (by reducing risk factors and instilling confidence), and ensure safety during participation. Clearly these aims will vary depending on the individual and an exercise programme should reflect the specific outcomes that are sought by a particular resident and the involved physiotherapist. Importantly exercise prescription is as much an art as it is a science. The science behind exercise programming needs to be applied flexibly in order to reach the desired outcome of increasing a resident's habitual physical activity. Behaviours, likes, interests and motivation are therefore key considerations in the implementation of a successful programme.

The exercise programme designed for the mobile resident will be an integration of all of the principles we have discussed within the dimensions of not only this chapter but also Chapter 10 relating to balance training. The 'whole' (the programme) will be less than the sum of its parts such that exercises prescribed should target multidimensional factors within a simplistic task-oriented focus. For example, if a therapist wishes to train strength, balance, vestibular function, flexibility and praxis because a resident suffers from recurrent falls, osteoarthritis and has had previous neurological insult they may wisely choose a sit-to-stand exercise. This is a task-oriented approach which maximizes integration; it uses the principle of specificity to optimize independence and functional activity whilst training many different subsystems all important for the resident's outcome. Some residents will be capable of independent practice of task-focused exercise. Where possible the potential for self-management of chronic disease or prevention of the progressive effects of ageing should be identified and encouraged in residents. Independence will be rewarded by an increase in the feeling of self-worth concerning physical ability. In some instances residents might be recruited as motivators and leaders of small exercise groups. They should not be encumbered with the safety of others; this should be a staff responsibility. These residents may be able to assist, however, through organizing the attendance of other members at the exercise venue by providing reminders or by physically accompanying participants to the venue (this is particularly useful if poor vision precludes safe passage of another resident to the exercise session).

In addition to the maintenance of safety, there are five principles that are the basis of exercise prescription and must be considered when writing exercise programmes for residents.

1. Principle of specificity – the programme must be specific to achieve desired outcomes – 'it's no good doing weight training to increase one's flexibility'.
2. Principle of overload – to effect change the training stimulus must exceed the demands placed on an individual by tasks normally undertaken. There must be an additional functional demand to initiate adaptive change.
3. Principle of reversibility – once a programme is discontinued positive gains will be lost. As the body adapts to increased demands, it also adapts to decreased demands (this is the basis for the negative aspects associated with 'disuse' atrophy).
4. Principle of initial values – depending on starting levels some people with low levels of ability will have a greater capacity for percentage improvement than other residents who begin with average or above measures.
5. Principle of diminishing returns – each person has an individual biological ceiling that determines the extent of a possible training effect. As this ceiling is approached, physical gains will slow and eventually plateau. Some residents will have greater scope to improve than others.

It is useful to remember the principles of exercise prescription when writing an holistic programme which targets all systems. Perhaps the easiest method of remembering what needs to be defined within a programme is the 'FITT' principle of exercise prescription:

F: Frequency
I: Intensity
T: Type
T: Time

The frequency parameter relates to the question 'how often', i.e. how many repetitions, how many times per day or week? Intensity relates to 'how hard', i.e. what target heart rate is required, what level of perceived exertion and what speed or weight? The type points to which exercise is required, 'what type?' meaning aerobic training like walking or swimming, resistance training like hand weights or Theraband™, or flexibility work with stretching or yoga. The time of exercise relates to the question 'how long?', i.e. a 5 minute walk, 10 second stretch, 5 second hold.

Individualized programmes

Exercise programmes which are developed for residents must be based on good clinical reasoning. Once the assessment of the resident has been undertaken it is advisable to develop a problem list and comment on the aims and goals of the therapy and exercise to be completed. This is achieved by prioritizing the importance of different objectives. Finally, the physiotherapist should state which outcome measures will be utilized to objectively review the programme. See Chapters 2, 8 and 9 for information on physiotherapeutic assessment, and Appendix 2.

A balanced exercise programme in aged care may include the following:

- cardiorespiratory endurance training – aerobic conditioning
- flexibility training
- resistance training – muscle strength, power and endurance (repetition over time)
- balance and postural control training.

Cardiorespiratory training

This encompasses all activities which use large muscle groups over a sustained duration and is rhythmic and aerobic in nature (e.g. walking, swimming and cycling). The intensity generally equates to 55–90% of maximum heart rate, although this may be lower in a group such as those in RACFs due to the sedentary status and low fitness levels often found in the elderly population. The duration of activity required ranges from anywhere between 15 and 60 minutes of continuous or discontinuous aerobic activity. Again, even 5 minutes may have considerable health and functional benefits amongst residents in RACFs. Usually the activity will need to take place 3 to 5 days each week. In many cases conditioning effects, most noted over the first 6–8 weeks, will mean the exercise should be progressed by manipulating duration or intensity, or both. In the elderly, it is extremely important to individualize exercise prescription. In order to modify programmes correctly it is important to do a risk factor assessment and have knowledge of any pre-existing medical conditions.

Exercise intensity

Perhaps the most difficult part of exercise prescription is to determine and apply the appropriate intensity. This requires individualization and monitoring to ensure safety and the correct level of exertion. Usually exercise intensity is prescribed as a percentage of functional capacity and measured using heart rate (HR), rates of perceived exertion (RPE), METs, or estimated energy expenditure (VO_2). One MET is equivalent to an oxygen uptake (or VO_2) of 3.5 ml/kg/min (this represents the approximate rate of oxygen consumption of a seated individual at rest). It is conventional in clinical exercise testing to express VO_{2max} in METs. Typically healthy young adults may be prescribed exercise at a level which equates to 60–70% of their functional capacity. Within RACFs, however, where many residents have a lower functional capacity, training may be initiated at a level of about 40–60% of functional capacity.

One of the easiest ways to determine exercise intensity for the older person is through the 'talk' test. As the name implies, a person should be able to carry on light conversation whilst exercising to ensure they are not

Table 11.1 *RPE Scales (Borg 1982)*

Category RPE Scale	Category-Ratio RPE Scale
6	0 Nothing at all
7 Very, Very Light	0.5 Very, Very Weak
8	1 Very Weak
9 Very Light	2 Weak
10	3 Moderate
11 Fairly Light	4 Somewhat Strong
12	5 Strong
13 Somewhat Hard	6
14	7 Very Strong
15 Hard	8
16	9
17 Very Hard	10 Very, Very Strong Maximal
18	
19 Very, Very Hard	
20	

exercising too hard. Utilizing this easy strategy will ensure a resident is exercising at a light to moderate intensity and staying within a safe level of exertion. Additionally it may also train dual-tasking by giving a cognitive demand through conversation.

Another relatively simple method to utilize that corresponds highly to what is actually going on in the body is to measure intensity levels using Borg's Rating of Perceived Exertion Scale (RPE) (Borg 1982) (Table 11.1 – the category-ratio RPE scale (in the right hand column) is a newer adaptation of the RPE scale which equates the levels to a 0–10 scale; either scale can be used in practice but both have been included for the reader's information). By using and becoming familiar with the scale, some residents will be able to keep themselves within the desired training levels prescribed by their physiotherapist. This is a particularly useful scale as there is a strong correlation between maximal oxygen uptake percentages, heart rate reserve percentages, minute ventilation, and blood lactate levels with RPE. This may be even more important and useful with residents taking medications that restrict heart rate responses to exercise, which applies to many residents living within RACFs.

Numerous clinical studies have shown that the category RPE scale is a reproducible measure of exertion within a wide variety of individuals regardless of age, gender or cultural origin. After some training using this scale, it is possible to get residents to keep themselves around different levels of perceived exertion during exercise. The range of 10–14 (Light to Somewhat Hard) equates to a usual light to moderate training load (50–75% of heart rate range) and enables the therapist to have control over exercise intensity due to approximation of RPEs with other exercise intensity measures of cardiorespiratory and metabolic variables mentioned previously, such as METs, VO_2, heart rate and ventilation.

Another method of prescribing exercise intensity relies on heart rate measurements and target heart rate ranges as a percentage of maximal heart rate (MHR). MHR can be estimated using the following equation:

$$\text{MHR} = 220 - \text{age (in years)}$$

This relies on the linear relationship between heart rate and exercise intensity; 70–85% of maximal heart rate is equal to about 60–80% of functional capacity. As workload increases so does heart rate so that the body can pump extra oxygen around for the tissues which are in demand; this occurs to a point that is referred to as *maximal heart rate* where the heart rate cannot increase further. Therefore functional capacity levels may be estimated by percentages of MHR and exercise intensity can be prescribed as such.

Example: Mrs X (80 years old):

$$\begin{aligned} \text{MHR} &= 220 - \text{age (80)} = 140 \\ \text{70–85\% of her MHR (140)} &= \text{98–119 bpm (beats per minute)} \\ \text{98–119 bpm} &= \text{60–80\% of functional capacity} \end{aligned}$$

An indicator of 40–60% of her functional capacity would be a heart rate of approximately 60–98 bpm. As this may well be around the level of her resting heart rate value, we can see that many residents of advancing age within RACFs are already utilizing much of their functional capacity at rest. *Often exercise demands do not need to be great to allow sufficient training stimulus in the elderly population*.

The use of heart rate measurements and percentages is a more involved method of prescribing exercise intensity and may be seen as superfluous and unnecessary within RACFs. It is important to note that target heart rate range is a *guideline only* and professionals must use their decision-making skills to assess how an individual is responding to exercise with consideration to safety and comfort. Some medications alter heart rate responses to exercise, so it is important as noted previously to assess what medications a resident is on and how this will affect them physiologically.

There are many signs and symptoms physiotherapists need to monitor during exercise training to ensure safety and effectiveness. A number of measurements can also be taken to provide feedback on how a resident is coping physiologically and psychologically and whether exercise should be continued. These include, but again are not limited to:

- respiratory rate
- oxygen saturation levels
- pain
- skin colour
- claudication
- shortness of breath on exertion (SOBOE)
- angina
- gait pattern
- perceived exertion
- perceived fatigue
- movement patterns/biomechanics
- quality of movement
- safety.

Flexibility

The ability to function normally requires that all joints are able to move through an adequate range of motion. Often inflexibility will create difficulties with performance of activities of daily living in the elderly. Emphasis generally should be on flexibility training in the upper and lower trunk, neck, hip and ankle regions. Importantly, dorsiflexion range in the ankle joint is of particular importance for mobility, more specifically in the performance of a sit to stand or in ascending or descending stairs (Bohannon et al 1991, James & Parker 1989).

It is important to perform stretches slowly with a gradual progression to greater ranges of motion. A slow dynamic movement may be followed by a static stretch that is maintained for 5–10 seconds. The reader is reminded that a 20 second stretch, although sometimes prescribed in the younger population, is not advisable for older people owing to the compression of arterial blood supply that occurs when the fascial planes separating muscles and compartments are compressed during the stretch process. This compression may reduce blood supply as suggested and cause tissue injury. Thus, only hold tissues in a lengthened position for around 5 seconds at a maximum and consider the use of other techniques such as slow reciprocal movements to extremes of range. Other methods may achieve the best results in range gain. Proprioceptive neuromuscular facilitation (PNF) techniques such as hold-relax or contract-relax (Adler et al 1993) are additional active methods of increasing range of movement that are very effective for cognitively sound residents.

Programme goals

Ensure the whole programme targets the given aims and assessed problems. Think through what each exercise achieves. What systems does it use and how could it be modified to adopt a more functional task?

1. Choose low impact activities with basic movement patterns (e.g. walking).
2. Choose enjoyable and non-competitive activities (e.g. dancing or swimming).
3. Do not forget a gentle warm-up and warm-down when needed.
4. Include flexibility exercises - teach stretches - do not let residents bounce into their stretch.
5. Include resistance exercises for major muscle groups.
6. Start at low levels and progress slowly - this way the body has time to adapt. Take it easy!
7. Progress gradually by increasing time, frequency and intensity.
8. Older individuals only need light to moderate intensity exercise - do not overdo it.
9. Concentrate on breathing and postural control.
10. Encourage regular drinks of water, especially in hot weather.
11. Be careful of extremes in weather. Avoid exercising in very hot or very cold temperatures.

12. Use positive messages around the facility and get staff to encourage residents as much as possible.
13. Consider using music – it usually enhances enjoyment when exercising.

Documentation

Never has there been such an emphasis on thorough written records as now. The demand for what seems at times a copious amount of paperwork reflects several current factors. At once there is a consumer call for appropriate and excellent services, a government demand for accountability and proof of funding usages and a society becoming more litigious in nature. No doubt, record keeping is of high importance; it allows others clear access to the clinical reasoning and steps which have taken place in the minds and hands of physiotherapists when formulating programmes. It also allows for more comprehensive reviews by providing baseline data and allows for evidence-based research to be conducted in some instances. Apart from external pressures the demand illustrates the internal desire amongst physiotherapists to advance their profession and to demonstrate their autonomy and worth.

The exercise programme (or therapy care plan) itself needs to include the following information:

- resident details (name, date of birth, major diagnosis)
- date programme written and initiated
- programme aims – problem list and/or desired outcomes
- assistance required by the resident, e.g. two staff assist/daily
- importantly, details of the exercises, including:
  - frequency – (how often) how many repetitions, times per day or week
  - intensity – (how hard) target heart rate, speed, weight
  - type – (what type) resistance, flexibility, aerobic
  - time – (how long), i.e. 5 minute walk
  - date of review/s and details of such (outcome measures, changes, comments on progress)
  - appropriate pictures or diagrams which illustrate the exercises – stick figures may be useful.

This therapy care plan must be included in the total resident care plan and be reviewed regularly by the physiotherapist. The question of how frequently a care plan must be reviewed varies widely depending on the status of the resident; this should be determined by the physiotherapist. Physiotherapists should use their professional skills to determine the necessary evaluation which should take place and how often this should occur; this will depend mainly on the resident's health status and any changes to this.

Demands for review times are often placed upon physiotherapists by external bodies or persons; this may vary with different management, facilities or agencies. A brief and recent survey of Australian physiotherapists determined that generally review periods vary tremendously and are completed anywhere between every 2 and 12 months. The regularity required for reviews has been a contentious issue recently within Australia as different stakeholders lay their claims; certainly a consensus has not been definitively reached as yet. Best practice would stipulate that decisions regarding appropriate timeframes for review of exercise programmes are part of the clinical decision-making process skills needed by the physiotherapist.

Other staff involvement/ education

Staff involved in the implementation of the therapy care plan will require education and training. Guidance will be needed to ensure the safety of both residents and staff. Good handling skills must be taught and emphasized in order to ensure the effectiveness of therapy programmes. Ensure in-service education sessions are conducted where necessary. Some appropriate topics will include: how best to assist residents with exercises; active and passive movements (these are not straightforward and require a moderate amount of skill to be implemented safely); massage; positioning; patient handling/manual handling; the benefits of exercise; falls prevention; and how to run group exercise sessions.

The job descriptions of all staff that assist with therapy programmes should include the need for this to occur. Staff must be empowered to assist residents with exercise and be responsible for ensuring that it is done. Exercise sessions and resultant resident achievements can become the source of a great deal of satisfaction and enjoyment for all concerned. Exercises can assist in the development of a positive, supportive, healthy and happy environment for residents and staff. In order for this to occur there needs to be team enthusiasm, a fostering environment and the support of management in the programmes offered.

Often time will be an issue for nursing staff; usually it will be the lack thereof or the requirement for other jobs such as hygiene needs, meals or paperwork. It is important to emphasize the benefits of exercise and educate staff regarding the needs of the residents in this regard. In order to assist with the daily routine of nursing staff it may be wise to suggest when exercises should be conducted with the resident so the workload is achievable. The programme will no doubt benefit from being written into the daily work routine, i.e. state which time of day it needs to occur (between 2:00 and 2:15 pm) or specify when during the hygiene routine the exercises may be completed (e.g. 10 assisted arm lifts with underarm washing in the shower in the evening). Involving evening staff in the exercise care plan will share the load more evenly and ultimately may suit some residents better.

The use of documentation folders for the daily recording of exercises completed should be a requirement for all facilities. This enables the physiotherapist to review what is being done and allows a feedback mechanism for staff to communicate with the therapist.

It is important that staff approach exercise in a positive way. At any age, many people need some encouragement and assistance to exercise, especially those who may not have done so for many years. Importantly, above all else it is the residents' choice that matters most when deciding whether to do exercises or not. Like people of any age they can feel unmotivated when it comes to activity. With encouragement and support to participate they often feel much better for having done so. Successful outcomes in exercise programmes are often determined by the staff member's initial approach towards the older person. Good communication, a positive approach and a general willingness to assist are the key factors which gain the resident's compliance and willingness to cooperate.

Behaviour modification

Time, fatigue and pain are all reasons stated by residents for not exercising – amongst others. We shall look briefly at the myriad of excuses given for not wanting to participate in exercise and organized activities and provide some methods of counteracting the age-old avoidance strategies.

- Some residents feel they are beyond help. It may pay to write out a list of the positives and negatives of participation and compare the two; residents will then surely see that it will be worthwhile to fit daily activity into their lives.
- Lack of time? If this is the concern perhaps the person could keep a diary for a week; they will no doubt be surprised at the amount of time spent in pursuits such as waiting for meals or watching television, and revise the timetable.
- Perhaps fatigue is a worrying factor? Poor sleep habits leave people physically and mentally sluggish. If difficulty initiating or maintaining sleep is an issue then they should ensure elimination of daytime napping, go to bed at the same time each night, gradually decrease and stop caffeine intake (coffee and tea), use the bed only for sleeping (no reading or television watching), and have a light meal a few hours before retiring. See the section on sleep in Chapter 4 for further information.
- Chronic pain? This may be due to multiple medical causes such as osteoporosis, osteoarthritis or even fracture. Residents or staff should consult with the doctor and/or physiotherapist for a thorough assessment. Often aches and pains can be reduced by appropriate exercise. Physical activity specific to some complaints (such as joint or bone conditions) can contribute to improved mobility and function, and improved energy level and a sense of wellbeing (Minor & Lane 1996).
- 'Too old'! We are never too old to want to feel better and have an improved quality of life. Often the best motivation for older persons is the knowledge that there is truth in the adage 'move it or lose it'.

Examples of exercises

In order to illustrate the principles outlined in this chapter we have included examples of some exercises commonly prescribed for residents. Related information is included to highlight the systems involved and benefits to the resident. Numerous variations can be made to the basic exercises and are done so as to achieve slightly different responses or to prioritize particular aims. This list is by no means exhaustive and is only meant to illustrate some of the principles previously outlined.

1. Exercise: ***Arm raises*** (Fig. 11.1)

Variations Arm raises can be combined with deep breathing exercise in most individuals. This can be performed in lying, sitting or standing. Weights may be added.

Goal To improve upper limb strength, active range, thoracic cage expansion, trunk extension, upper limb function, upper limb strengthening.

Systems Muscle strength, power and endurance.
Flexibility and joint range training.
Balance training.

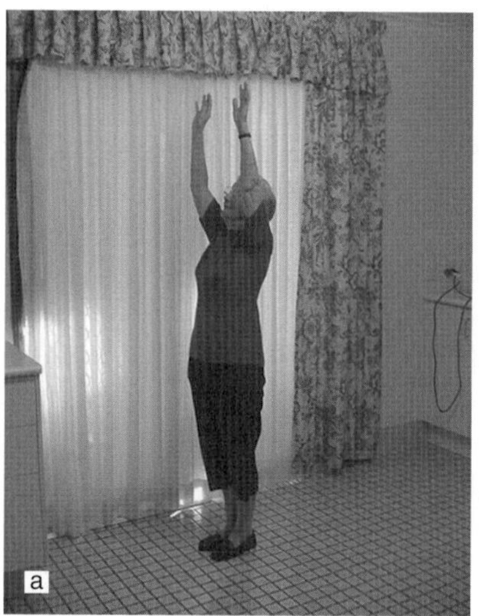

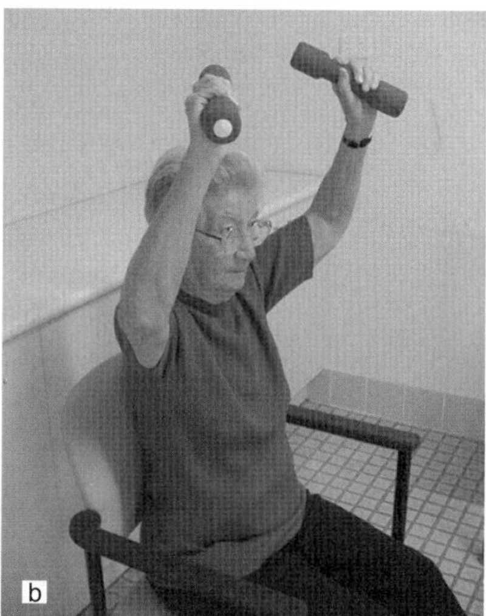

Figure 11.1a & b *Arm raises.*

2. Exercise: ***Leg extension*** (Fig. 11.2)

Variations Sitting, standing, lying, ±weights.

Goal To improve lower limb strength; assist in maintaining or improving functional mobility, balance.

Systems Muscle strength, power and endurance.
Flexibility and joint range training.

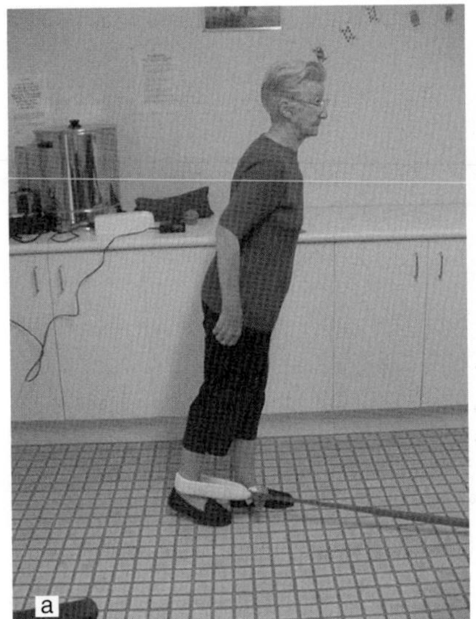

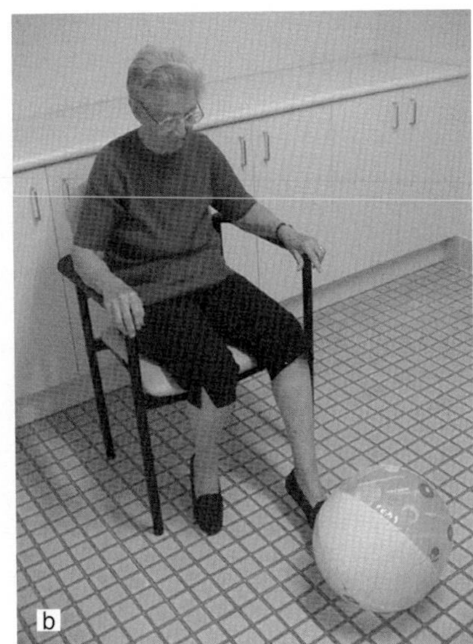

Figure 11.2a & b
Leg extension.

3. Exercise: ***Foot and ankle exercises*** (Fig. 11.3)

Variations Sitting, lying, standing, ±weights.

Goal To maintain available and necessary range in the ankle joint, improve flexibility, circulation, integrate sensory systems and responses from the feet. Maintain or improve functional mobility.

Systems Muscle strength, power and endurance.
Flexibility and joint range training.
Balance and postural control.

4. Exercise: ***Prayer position to traffic control (policeman) position*** (Fig. 11.4)

Variations This may be completed combined with deep breathing exercises, ±weights.

Goal To maintain or improve upper limb activities, scapular retraction, posture training, respiratory exercise, thoracic cage expansion, relaxation.

Systems Flexibility and joint range training.
Respiratory system training/enhancement.
Muscle strength, power and endurance.
Balance and postural control.

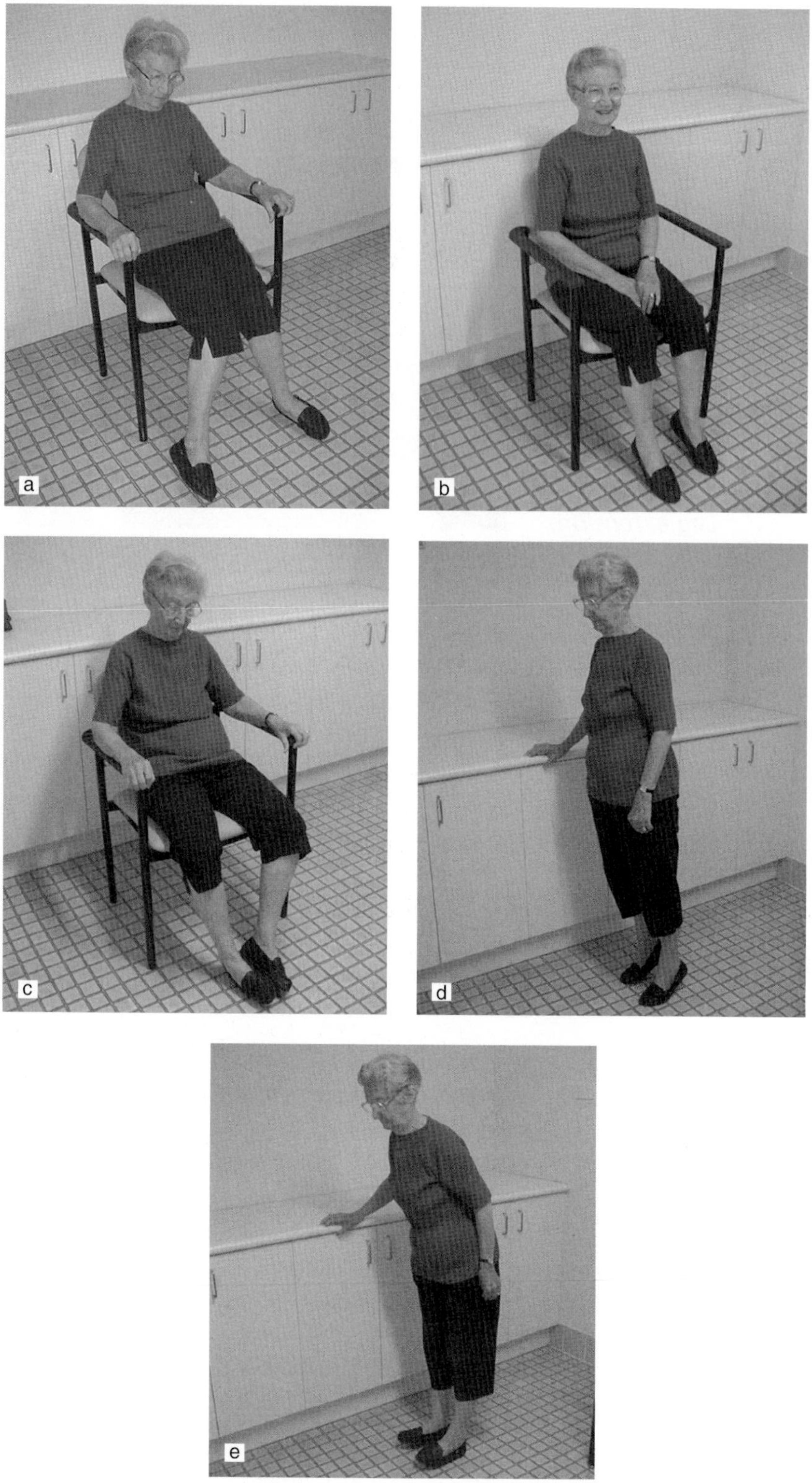

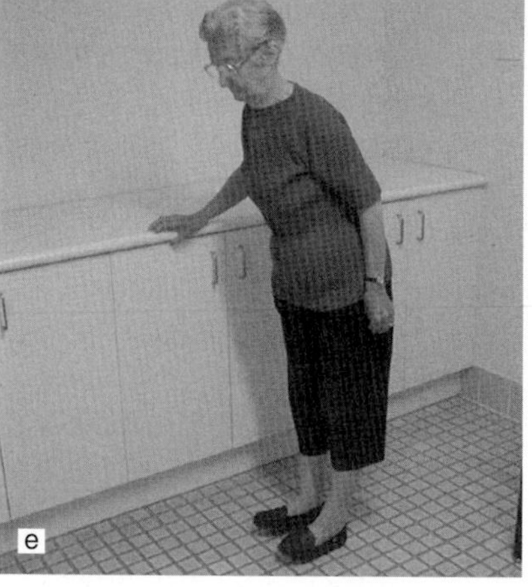

Figure 11.3a–e *Foot and ankle exercises.*

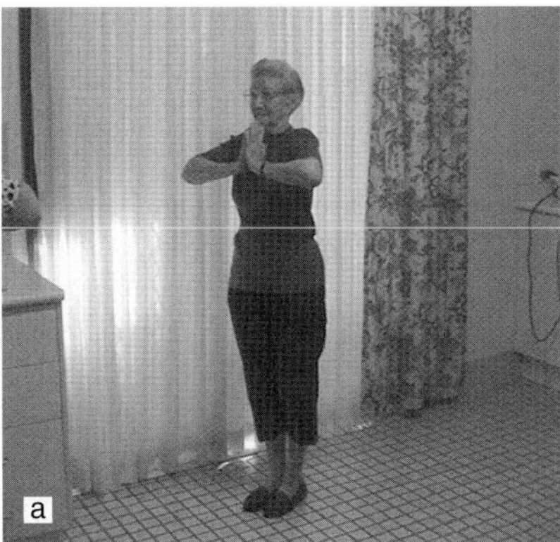
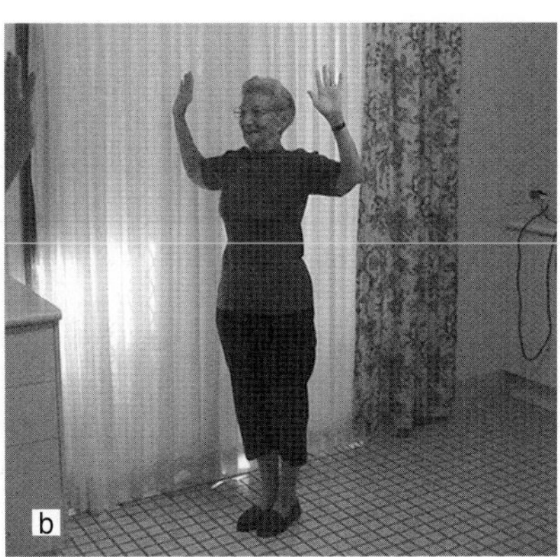

Figure 11.4a & b *Prayer position to traffic control (policeman) position.*

5. Exercise: ***Trunk rotation*** (Fig. 11.5)

Variations Sitting, standing, in water (aquatic physiotherapy). On a bed, chair, ball.

Goal To maintain flexibility within the trunk, to assist relaxation of tone, to improve gait pattern, to allow movement for activities of daily living, improve sitting balance.

Systems Flexibility and joint range training.
Postural control, balance.
Muscle strength, power and endurance.

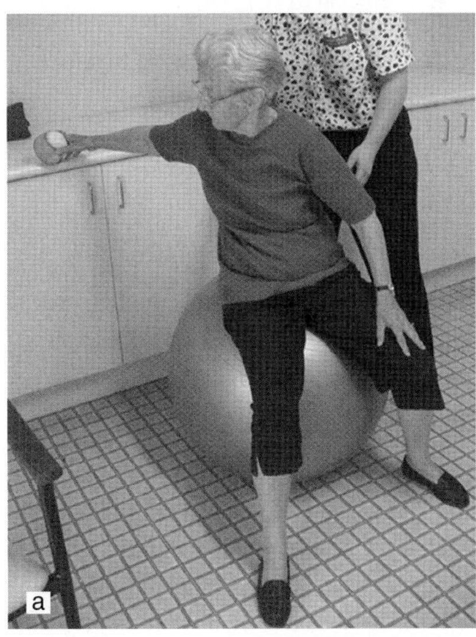
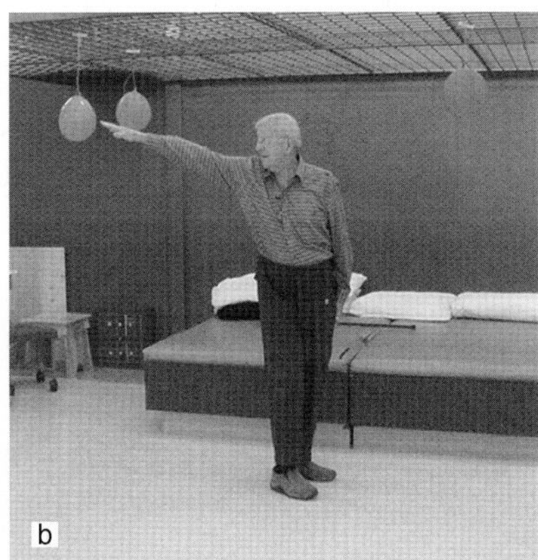

Figure 11.5a & b *Trunk rotation.*

6. Exercise: ***Passive arm and leg exercises*** (Fig. 11.6)

Variations Position (sitting, lying), in water. Often these exercises are combined with massage to good effect. One or two persons assist.

Goal To maintain joint range, flexibility, skin integrity, positioning, comfort. To facilitate requirements for hygiene assistance and other activities of daily living. To control tone and spasticity. To assist in the management of pain and neuromechanosensitivity and allow smooth movement of neural tissues within other soft tissues. Relaxation.

Systems Flexibility and joint range training.

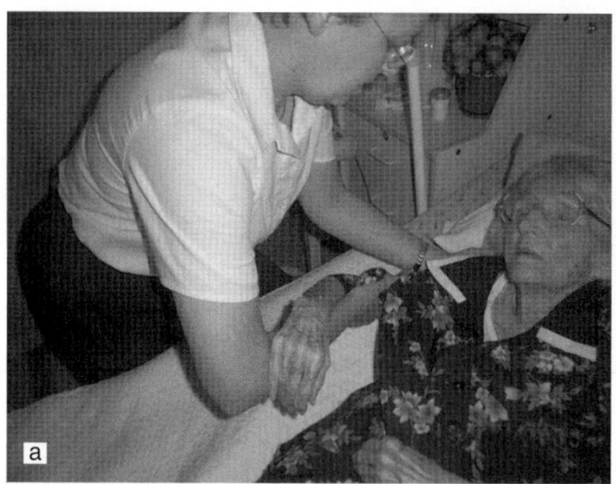

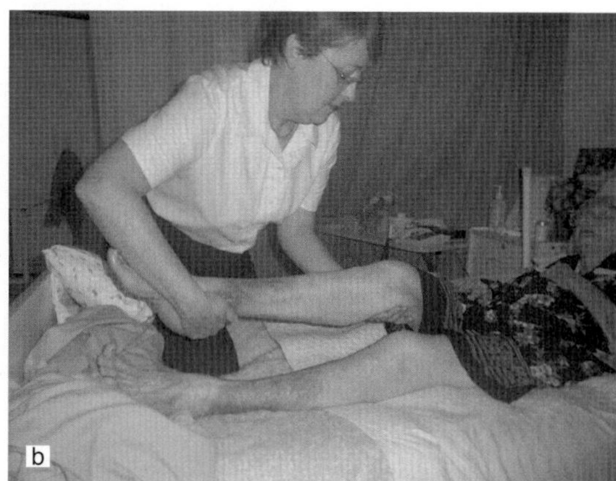

Figure 11.6a & b
Passive arm and leg exercises.

7. Exercise: ***Sit-to-stand practice*** (Fig. 11.7)

Variations At a rail, in front of a mirror, in water, from a chair, bed, or ball.

Goal To maintain or improve lower limb strength, functional mobility, motor planning, balance, sensory integration.

Systems Flexibility and joint range training.
Balance and postural control.
Muscle strength, power and endurance.
Vestibular system.
Cardiorespiratory endurance training.

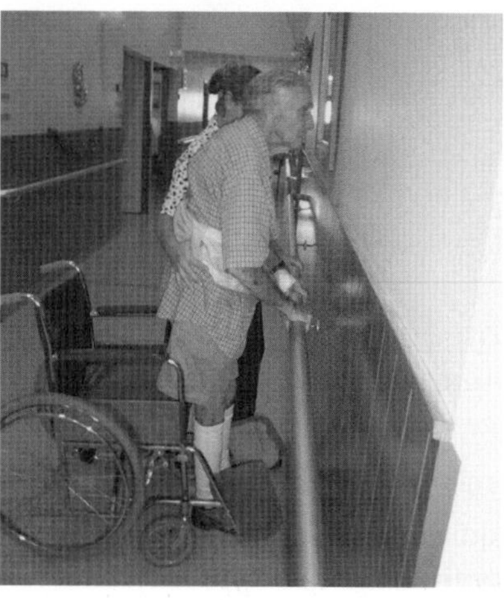

Figure 11.7
Sit-to-stand practice.

8. Exercise: ***Ball games*** (Fig. 11.8)

Variations Different sized, shaped or weighted balls (e.g. balloons, Theraballs™, beach balls, footballs). Sitting or standing. Throwing, catching, kicking. Combined with cognitive tasks. One-on-one or group exercise. Different textured or noisy balls.

Goal Stimulation, enjoyment. Upper limb function, dexterity and shoulder ranging exercise. Coordination, motor planning, and balance training. Maintain or improve functional mobility, movement.

Systems Flexibility and joint range training.
Balance and postural control.
Muscle strength, power and endurance.
Cardiorespiratory endurance training.

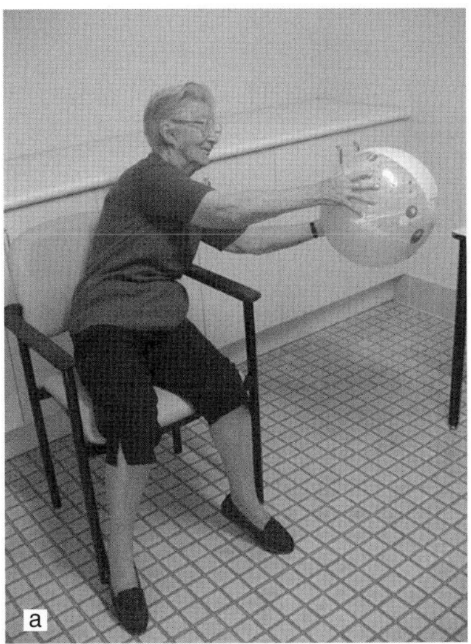

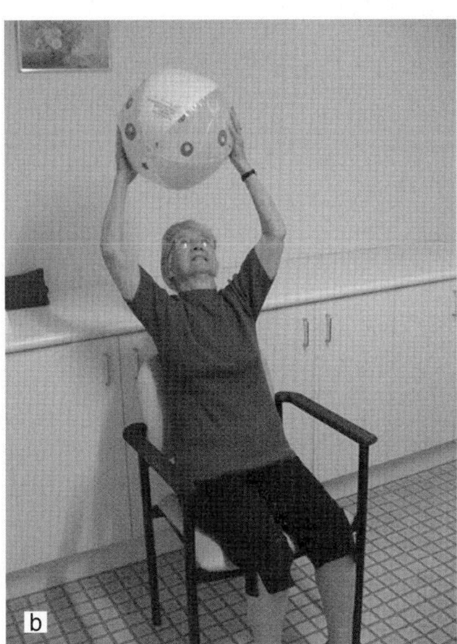

Figure 11.8a & b *Ball games.*

9. Exercise: ***Walking*** (Fig. 11.9)

Variations Indoors/outdoors, obstacle courses, different levels and surfaces. ±Weights. Individual or group training sessions.

Goal To maintain or improve fitness and functional mobility. Enjoyment. Relaxation. Rehabilitation.

Systems Cardiorespiratory endurance training.
Balance and postural control.
Muscle strength, power and endurance.

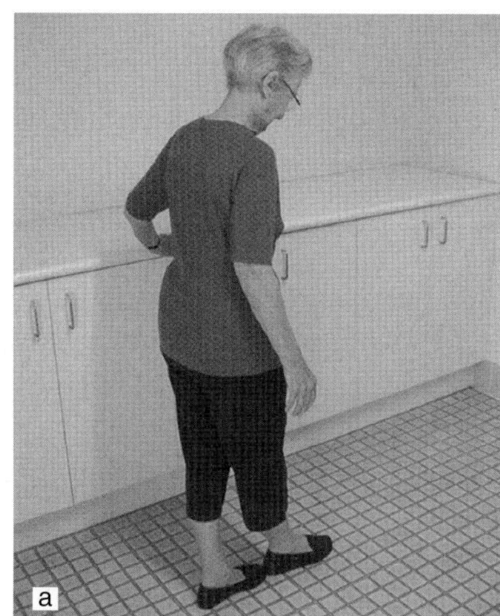

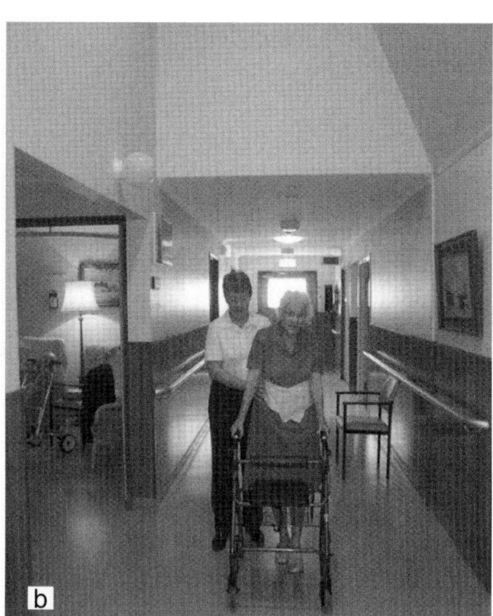

Figure 11.9a & b
Walking.

10. Exercise: ***Reaching for objects on a wall*** (Fig. 11.10)

Variations High, low and wide placements. Add sit to stand before reaching. Combine with deep breathing.

Goal To maintain or improve functional mobility. Falls prevention. Upper limb function training.

Systems Balance and postural control.
Muscle strength, power and endurance.
Flexibility and joint range training.
Coordination.
Cardiorespiratory training.

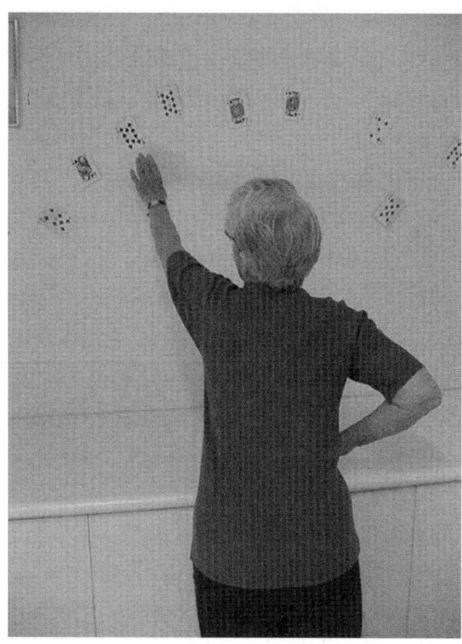

Figure 11.10
Reaching for objects on a wall.

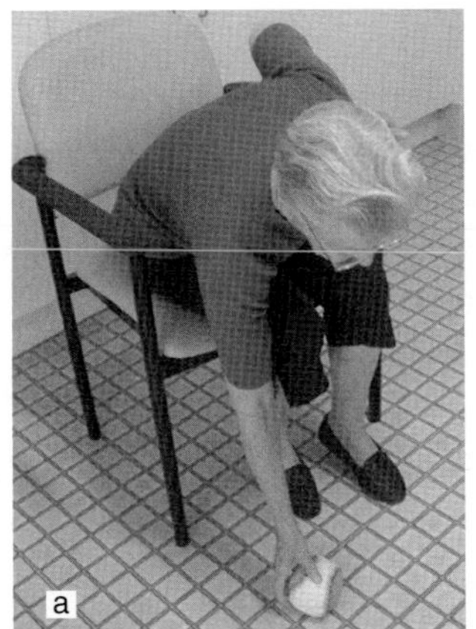

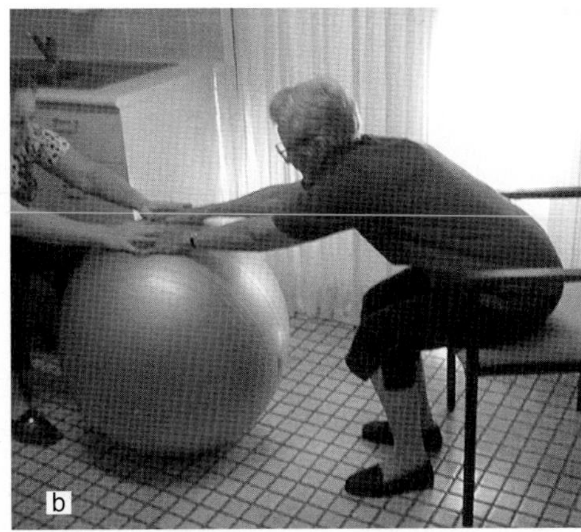

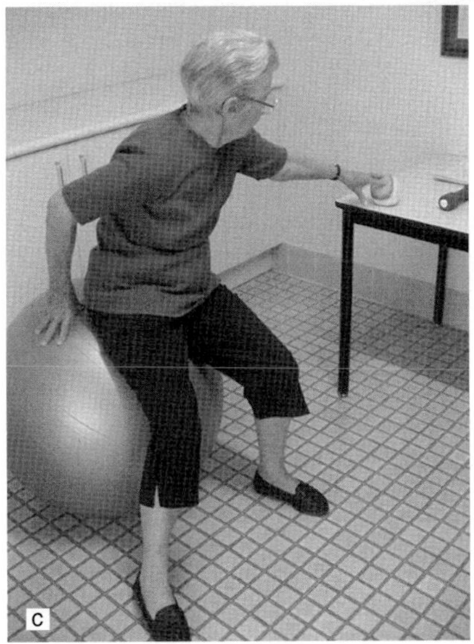

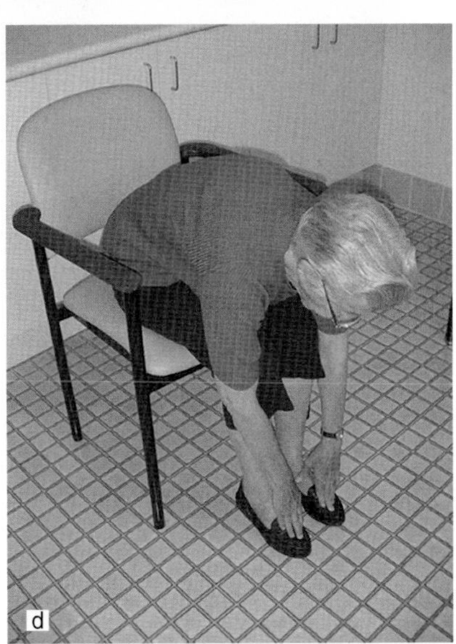

Figure 11.11a–d *Sitting balance exercises.*

11. Exercise: ***Sitting balance exercises*** (Fig. 11.11)
Forward reaching in chair – 'toe touches'/sitting bowls.

Variations From a ball, bed or chair.

Goal To maintain or improve sitting balance, flexibility, trunk movement. Sensory integration. Trunk and abdominal muscle exercise.

Systems Balance and postural control.
Muscle strength, power and endurance.
Flexibility and joint range training.
Coordination.
Cardiorespiratory training.

12. Exercise: ***Arm weights*** (Fig. 11.12)

Variations Theraband™, dumbbells, elastic tubing, cans, pulleys, sandbags. Sitting, lying, standing. Combined with walking.

Goal To improve upper limb strength and function. Bone health.

Systems Muscle strength, power and endurance.
Balance and postural control.
Flexibility and joint range training.
Coordination.
Cardiorespiratory training.

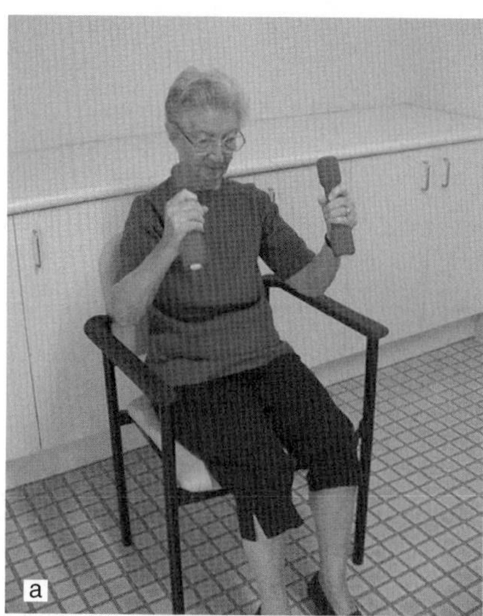

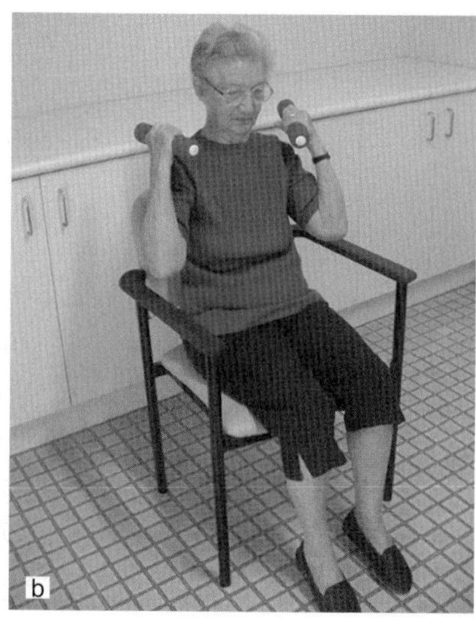

Figure 11.12a & b
Arm weights.

13. Exercise: ***Neck exercises/shoulder shrugs*** (Fig. 11.13)

Variations In water, on land. Standing, sitting or lying.

Goal To maintain or improve head and neck posture and movement; facilitate improved ergonomics and functioning; relieve postural tension, headaches. Relaxation.

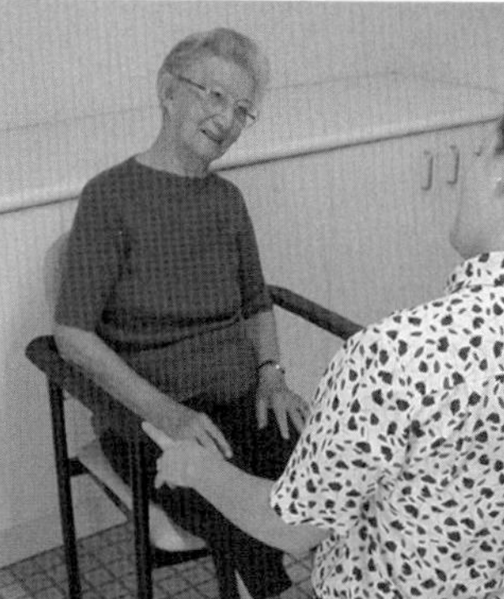

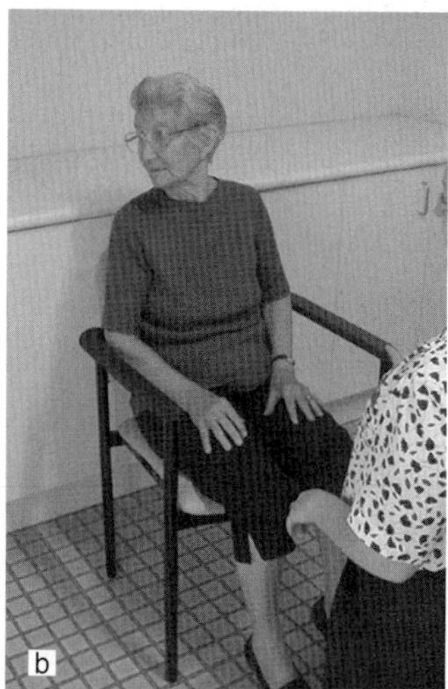

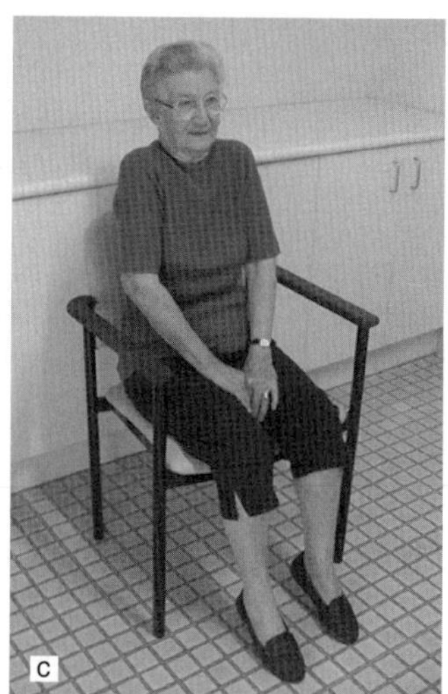

Figure 11.13a–c
Neck exercises/shoulder shrugs.

Systems Flexibility and joint range training.
Balance and postural control.
Muscle strength and endurance.
Vestibular system training.

14. Exercise: ***Hand exercises*** (Fig. 11.14)

Variations In water. Combined with wax bathing treatment.

Goal To maintain hand dexterity and function. To maintain independence with meals, crafts, writing. Coordination.

Systems Flexibility and joint range training.
Muscle strength, power and endurance.

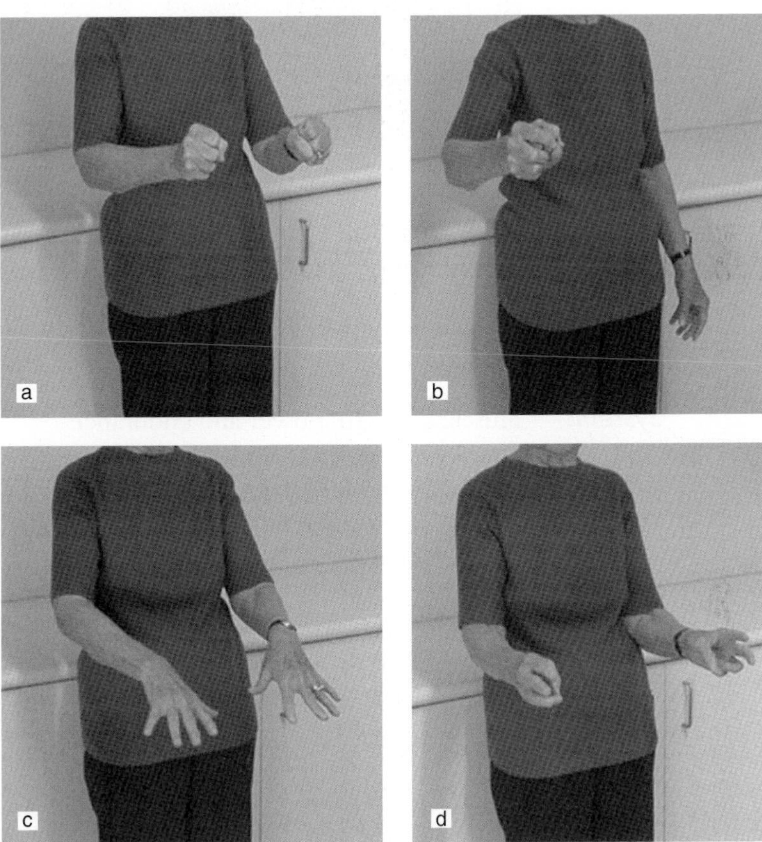

Figure 11.14a–d
Hand exercises.

15. Exercise: ***Squats/Lunges*** (Fig. 11.15)

Variations In water or on land. ±Weights. ±Hand support (rail).

Goal To maintain or improve lower limb strength and function.

Systems Muscle strength, power and endurance.
Balance and postural control.
Flexibility training.
Cardiorespiratory training.

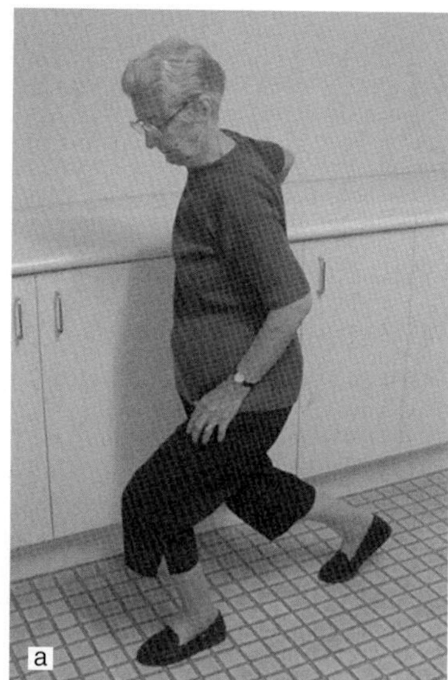

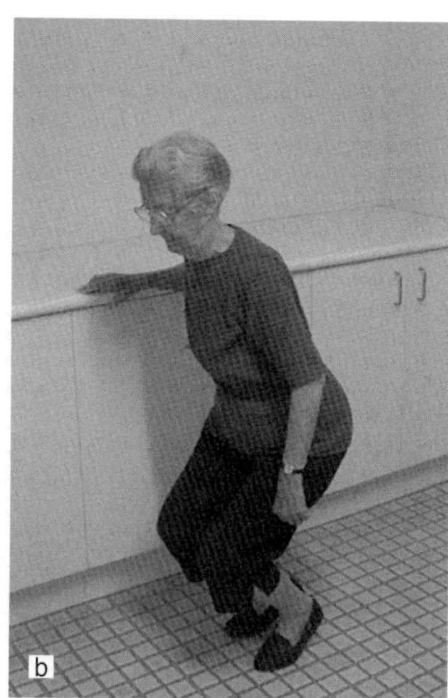

Figure 11.15a & b
Squats/Lunges.

16. Exercise: ***Step-ups*** (Fig. 11.16)

Variations In water or on land. ±Weights. Different heights. ±Hand support.

Goal To maintain lower limb strength and function. To improve or maintain functional mobility, balance and postural control.

Systems Muscle strength, power and endurance.
Balance and postural control.
Flexibility and joint range training.
Cardiorespiratory training.
Coordination.

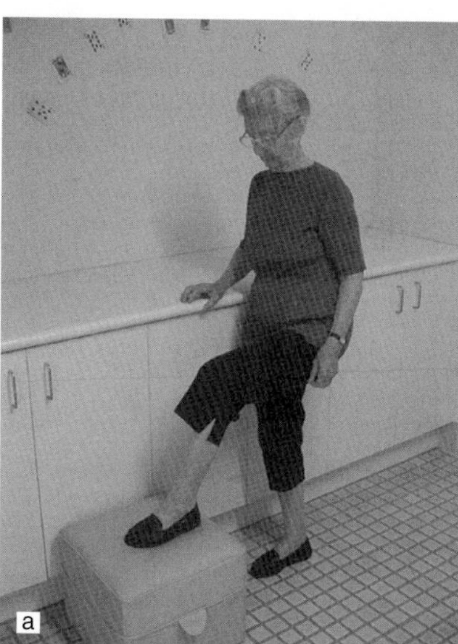

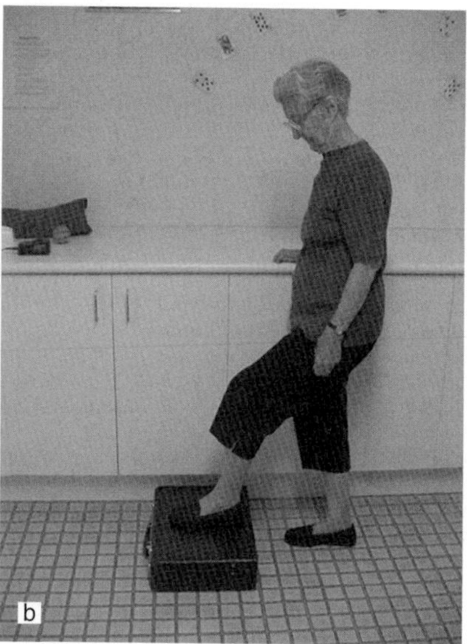

Figure 11.16a & b
Step-ups.

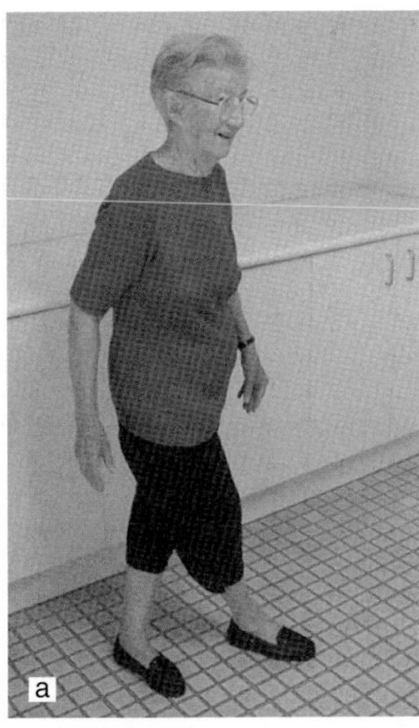

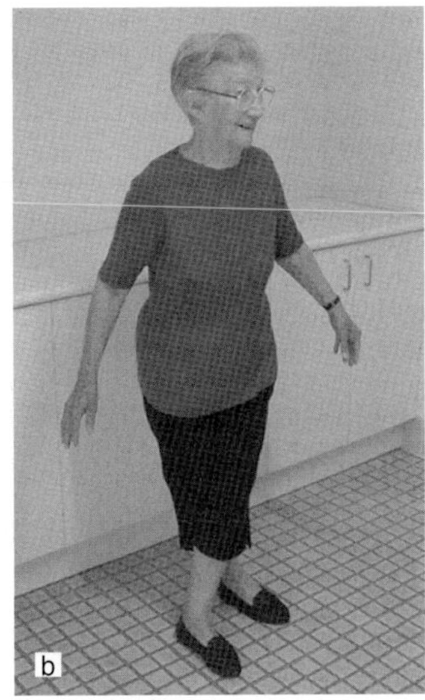

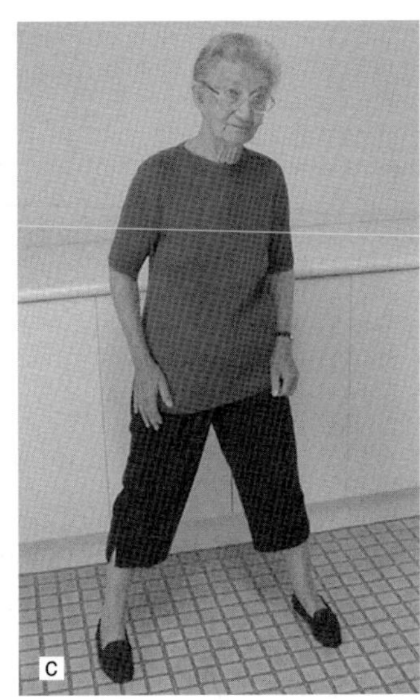

Figure 11.17a–c
Sideways walking.

17. Exercise: ***Sideways walking*** (Fig. 11.17)

Variations ±Hand support. In water or on land, feet together or crossing like a 'grapevine' step.

Goal To improve functional mobility. Falls prevention. To improve medial and lateral hip control. Gait training.

Systems Balance and postural control.
Coordination.
Muscle strength, power and endurance.
Cardiorespiratory training.

18. Exercise: ***Stirring the pot*** (Fig. 11.18)

Variations Standing, sitting. ±Weights. Can do this similarly by asking the resident to write letters of the alphabet using imagery on the floor.

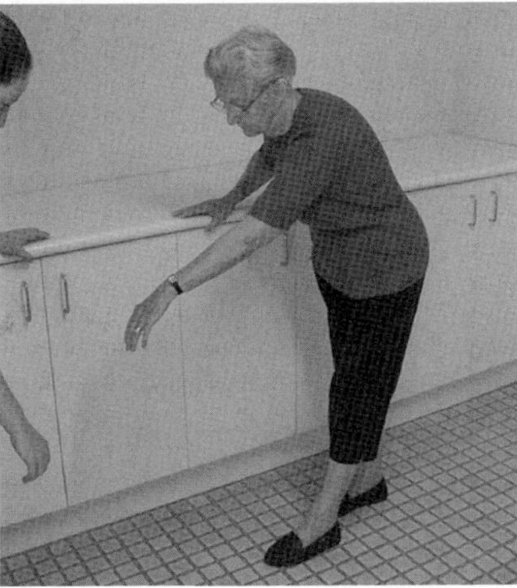

Figure 11.18
Stirring the pot.

Goal To maintain or improve upper limb function and dexterity. Useful post fractured humerus to assist in ranging of the glenohumeral joint; and also to facilitate hygiene (cleaning under the arms).

Systems Flexibility and joint range training.
Muscle strength, power and endurance.
Balance and postural control.
Coordination.

19. Exercise: ***Writing exercises – island hopping/drawing*** (Fig. 11.19)

Variations Different sized and weighted pens/pencils.

Goal Maintain or improve writing ability, coordination and motor planning and control.

Systems Fine motor control, dexterity.
Muscle strength and endurance.
Coordination.

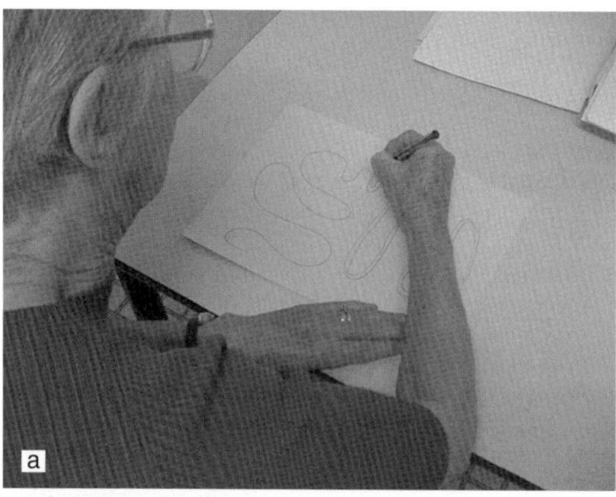

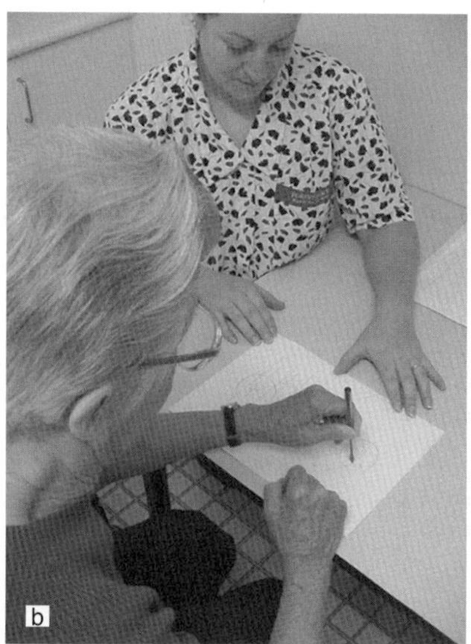

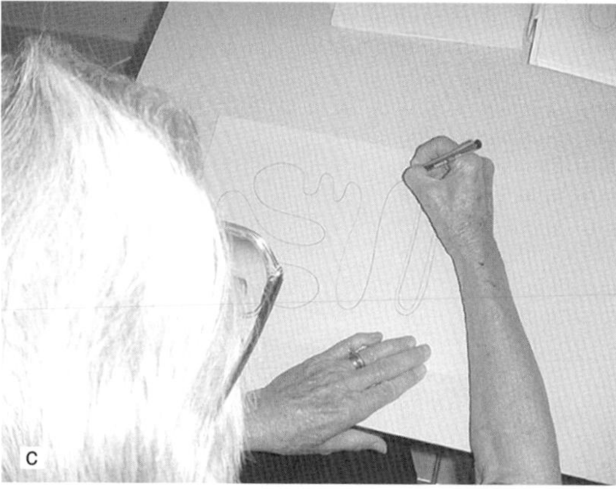

Figure 11.19a–c
Writing exercises – island hopping/drawing.

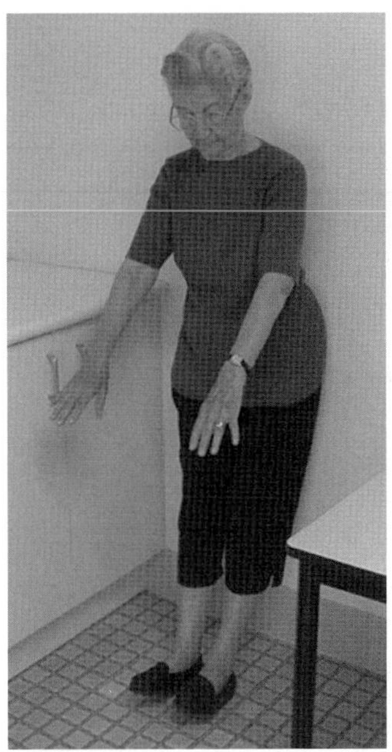

Figure 11.20 *Timber exercise (against wall).*

20. Exercise: ***Timber exercise (against wall)*** (Fig. 11.20)

Variations Vary distance from the wall, eyes open, eyes closed.

Goal To maintain or improve standing balance, mobility and function. Falls prevention. Sensory integration.

Systems Balance and postural control.
Vestibular training.
Flexibility and joint range training.
Coordination.
Muscle strength and endurance.

21. Exercise: ***Cycling*** (Fig. 11.21)

Variations Pedals as shown, stationary bike, bicycle.

Goal To maintain or improve cardiorespiratory fitness, lower limb function, mobility and postural control. Enjoyment.

Systems Cardiorespiratory training.
Muscle strength, power and endurance.
Balance and postural control.
Flexibility and joint range training.
Coordination.

Other ideas

- Parallel bar activities.
- Mini-tramp.
- Wipe on/wipe off.

The environment in which exercise is undertaken often enhances the responses. Exercise in water or on land indoors or outdoors will all have varying appeal to participants.

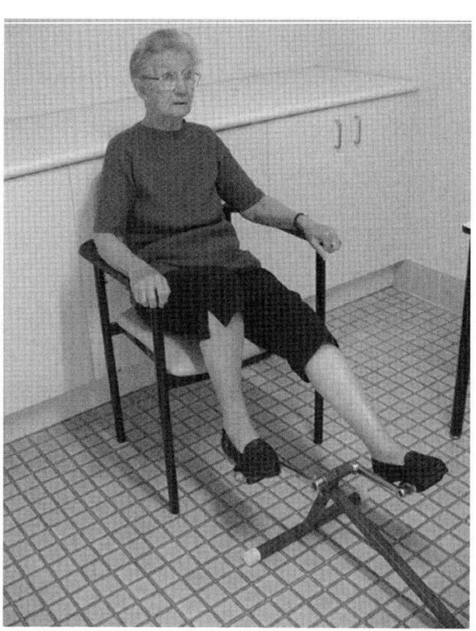

Figure 11.21
Cycling.

Aquatic physiotherapy has been shown to benefit older people living in residential aged care in improving balance and functional ability (Josephson et al 2001). Other benefits attained with aquatic therapy include increased socialization and behaviour modification. See Chapter 13 on aquatic physiotherapy for further information.

> *Speaking generally, all parts of the body which have a function, if used in moderation and exercised in labours to which each is accustomed, become thereby healthy and well developed, and age slowly; but if left unused and left idle, they become liable to disease, defective in growth, and age quickly.*
>
> Hippocrates

Summary

- Exercise can minimize the physiological changes associated with ageing in a sedentary individual.
- Exercise can contribute to psychological health and wellbeing.
- Residents in RACFs retain the ability to train and improve physically – with appropriate challenges in exercise they may have improvements in all areas of fitness similar to younger people.
- Exercise prescription must be individualized – programming is considered after careful consideration of disease processes, health status and functional goals.
- Exercise prescription must be specific; it should include modality, dose, duration of exposure and consider compliance issues and behaviour modification strategies. Following the 'FITT' principles for writing exercise programmes ensures all details are included.

- Exercise programming should be simplistic for most elderly persons; it is an art and a science. Usually the more straightforward (and therefore easy to follow) the programme is, the better. Often older persons benefit greatly from a small training demand – exercise does not need to be very hard.
- Consider all of the resident's needs (cardiorespiratory training, muscle strength, power and endurance, flexibility, balance and postural control).
- Documentation is a necessary part of good clinical practice. Notes must be timely, accurate, detailed, and easy to read.
- Ensure other staff members who may be involved in the implementation of exercise programmes are considered. They should be well trained, enthused, and compliant.
- Changing behaviours such as inactivity (especially those which may have been formed over many years) is often a difficult process. Be supportive, encouraging, persistent and understanding when assisting people with exercise programming and training.
- There are literally millions of exercises which can be performed. Do not be limited by your imagination. There are many ways to reach the same end-point in training and the more varied it is, the more interesting to both the therapist and the resident.

References

Adler S S, Beckers D, Buck M 1993 PNF in practice: an illustrated guide. Springer-Verlag, Berlin

American College of Sports Medicine 1991 Guidelines for exercise testing and prescription, 4th edn. Lea and Febiger, Philadelphia

Bohannon R W, Tiberio D, Waters G 1991 Motion measured from forefoot and hindfoot landmarks during passive ankle dorsiflexion range of motion. Journal of Orthopaedic and Sport Physical Therapy 13(1):20–22

Borg G A 1982 Psychophysical bases of perceived exertion. Medicine and Science in Sports and Exercise 14:377–387

Fiatarone Singh M A 2002 Exercise comes of age: rationale and recommendations for a geriatric exercise prescription. Journal of Gerontology 57A(5): M262–M282

Fiatarone M A, Marks E C, Ryan N D et al 1990. High-intensity strength training in nonagenarians: effects on skeletal muscle. Journal of the American Medical Association 263: 3029–3034

James B, Parker A W 1989 Active and passive mobility of lower limb joints in elderly men and women. American Journal of Physical Medicine and Rehabilitation 68(4):162–167

Josephson S R, Josephson D L, Nitz J 2001 Evaluation of a long-term water exercise program for the elderly: focusing on balance. Australasian Journal on Ageing 20(3):147–152

McArdle W D, Katch F I, Katch V L 1996 Exercise physiology – energy, nutrition, and human performance. Williams & Wilkins, Philadelphia

Minor M A, Lane N E 1996 Recreational exercise in arthritis. Musculoskeletal Medicine 2(3): 563–577

Pardini A 1984 Exercise, vitality and ageing. Ageing 344:19–29

Rissel C 1987 Water exercises for the frail elderly: a pilot programme. Australian Journal of Physiotherapy 33(4):226–232

Shephard R J 1997 Aging, physical activity and health. Human Kinetics Publishers, Champaign. IL

Shumway-Cook A, Woollacott M H 1995 Motor control: theory and practical applications. Williams & Wilkins, Baltimore

Trew M, Everett T 1997 Human movement. Churchill Livingstone, London

Further reading

Dishman R K 1994 Motivating older adults to exercise. Southern Medical Journal 87(5):79–82

Duda J L, Tappe M K 1988 Predictors of personal investment in physical activity among middle-aged and older adults. Perceptual and Motor Skills 66:543–549

Evans W, Rosenberg I H 1991 Biomarkers – The 10 keys to prolonging vitality. Simon & Schuster, New York

Gingold R 1992 Successful ageing. Oxford University Press, Melbourne

Howell R A, Howell M 1987 Foundations of health. Brooks Waterloo Publishers, Albion, Queensland

Jones J M, Jones K D 1997 Promoting physical activity in the senior years. Journal of Gerontological Nursing July:41–48

Kenton L 1985 Ageless ageing. Cox & Wyman, Reading, UK

Laura R S, Johnston B B 1997 Fit after fifty. Simon & Schuster Australia, East Roseville, NSW

Norstrom J A, Conroy W 1995 The activity pyramid and the new physical activity recommendations. The Bulletin 39:107–111

Pollock M L, Wilmore J H 1990 Exercise in health and disease – evaluation and prescription for prevention and rehabilitation. W B Saunders, Philadelphia

Pollock M L, Graves J E, Swart D L, Lowenthal D L 1994 Exercise training and prescription for the elderly. Southern Medical Journal 87(5):88–95

Siscovick D S, Weiss N S, Fletcher R H, Lasky T 1984 The incidence of primary cardiac arrest during vigorous exercise. New England Journal of Medicine 311(14):874–877

12 Osteoporosis

Susan R. Hourigan and Jennifer C. Nitz

This chapter aims to:

- define osteoporosis and identify factors likely to impact on presentation
- identify risk factors for development of osteoporosis and ways to modify risks
- consider the physiotherapy assessment aspects peculiar to osteoporosis, and
- consider exercise intervention appropriate for prevention of osteoporotic decline.

Introduction

Osteoporosis is a worldwide health issue. It is an increasing public health problem that causes loss of life and reduced quality of life in sufferers. We have dedicated a chapter to this important topic because it is so widespread amongst people living in RACFs and physiotherapists play such an important part in treatment. The prevention of fracture and injury is a paramount goal of the physiotherapist working in an RACF, as outlined in previous chapters. Osteoporosis increases a person's likelihood of injury through increased risk of fracture. It is estimated that in their lifetime, 50% of women and 33% of men will suffer a fracture related to osteoporosis.

Osteoporosis is defined as a reduction in the quantity of bone or atrophy of skeletal tissue; resulting in bone trabeculae that are scanty, thin, and without osteoclastic resorption (Stedman's Medical Dictionary, 26th edn, 1995). Harrison's Internal Medicine text defines osteoporosis as a reduction of bone mass (or density) or the presence of a fragility fracture (Braunwald et al 2002). This reduction in bone tissue is accompanied by deterioration in the architecture of the skeleton, leading to a markedly increased risk of fracture. It is a disease characterized by low bone mass and micro-architectural deterioration of bone tissue leading to enhanced bone fragility and a consequent increase in fracture risk.

Osteoporosis is defined operationally as a bone mass density that falls 2.5 standard deviations below the young adult reference mean, also referred to as a T-score of -2.5 or less.

Osteopenia is variously defined as decreased calcification or density of bone, due to inadequate osteoid synthesis. It is a descriptive term applicable to all skeletal systems in which such a condition is noted; it carries no implication about causality. The relevant T-score referred to as osteopenic is the range between −1.0 to −2.5.

Strategies to improve bone density and reduce the likelihood of falls are important in the prevention of osteoporosis. Physiotherapists have an important role to play in this condition through exercise prescription, therapeutic modalities, specific techniques and education. Appropriate treatment goals can be established following a thorough assessment of signs and symptoms, risk factors for osteoporosis and functional status.

In children the related goal is to optimize bone health and growth: approximately 50% of bone accrual occurs during puberty. Maximizing peak bone mass and establishing a high baseline before the onset of age-related bone loss in adulthood is important. Children should be encouraged to participate in a variety of high-impact activities in their early years. In adults the goal is to maintain bone mass and health with less emphasis on increasing bone mass. However, small increases in bone mass may be achieved by structured weight-training and weight-bearing exercise.

In older adults within RACFs, the goal is to conserve bone mass and avoid fracture. The prevention of injury and maintenance of function is of primary concern to the treating physiotherapist. Recognizing the risks of osteoporosis, modifying risk factors where possible and integrating management with the treating doctor and pharmacist is of importance. Any management of residents with osteoporosis will overlap other treatment ideals associated with risk assessment, falls prevention, balance training and holistic functional goal setting. In RACFs, the aim of physiotherapeutic treatment with residents suffering from osteoporosis or osteopenia in their older adult years is to:

- conserve bone mass
- utilize falls prevention strategies and risk reduction techniques to reduce the likelihood of falls and fractures
- promote good posture and positioning
- manage and reduce pain
- improve mobility and function
- facilitate independence in function, activities of daily living and other activities.

Recognizing risks of osteoporotic fractures

The major determinants of fracture risk are outlined in Table 12.1. It is important to note that each individual will require a case-based, personalized assessment and treatment programme. Single risk factors alone do not reliably predict fracture risk or point to particular treatment methods. Bone mineral density should only be measured if the given result will influence management; it is not used as an ongoing outcome measurement scale to date for residents in aged care.

Table 12.1 *Major determinants of fracture risk and risk modification ability*

Risk factor	Modifiable
Postmenopausal women	No/Yes – ?hormone replacement
Low bone mineral density	Yes
Calcium deficiency	Yes
Vitamin D deficiency	Yes
Previous minimal trauma fracture or family history of such	No/Yes (?early assessment and prevention)
Long-term (>3 months) oral corticosteroid therapy	No/Yes – avoid if possible
Sedentary lifestyle/propensity to fall	Yes
Ageing	No
Cigarette smoking	Yes
Low body weight	Yes

Table 12.2 *Daily requirements of calcium and vitamin D*

Calcium	Vitamin D
Adolescents: 1200–1500 mg/day	Adolescents and adults: 200 IU/daily (when sun exposure is low)
Adults up to 65 years of age: 1000 mg/day	Elderly 600 IU
Postmenopausal women (not on oestrogen) and the elderly: 1500 mg/day	1 μg vitamin D = 40 IU

Modifying risks

The main strategies used to alter the risk factors in osteoporosis management involve exercise, nutrition, lifestyle, falls prevention, the use of hip protectors and drug therapy. Where possible it is obviously beneficial to eliminate or modify risks. Osteoporosis therapy should aim to optimize bone mass, preserve skeletal integrity and prevent falls.

Nutrition

Good nutrition and a balanced dietary intake are important for normal growth and health irrespective of age. Calcium and vitamin D are the two nutritional factors most referred to in relation to osteoporosis although adequate protein intake is also important in frail elderly individuals. Adequate vitamin D and calcium are required for healthy bones. Vitamin D is essential for the intestinal absorption of calcium; blood levels of both decline with age. Supplements will only alleviate deficiency states; there is no current evidence which suggests doses above daily requirements reduce fracture risk. The daily requirements for vitamin D and calcium are indicated in Table 12.2.

Lifestyle/Exercise

Stopping smoking, moderating consumption of alcohol and increasing physical activity can all improve bone health and reduce the risk of falls and fractures. Exercise will be examined in greater detail following the general details in this section. It is important to note that some research suggests that little is known about the effects of physical activity on the risk of hip fracture among those living in care homes or those over 80 years of age. The level of physical activity amongst those living within facilities has been shown to be extremely low (<15% participated in >2 hours/week) (Norton et al 2001). The potential protective effects of exercise always need to be weighed against the increased risk of falling or injury during activities. Therefore there is some evidence to suggest that passive interventions (vitamin D, calcium, hip protectors) are more likely to prevent hip fracture than active ones in the very frail residents living in residential institutions. A decision based on good clinical reasoning and a professional evaluation will provide best practice in this regard. Suitable exercises are suggested and examined in further detail towards the end of this chapter.

Falls prevention

There are a number of risk factors that increase a person's likelihood of falling including age, medications, vision, hearing, continence, mobility levels, strength, gait and cognitive function. These factors are all considered in discussions within the chapters dealing with falls prevention and balance in this text (Chapters 8, 9 and 10; please refer to these chapters for more information). Whilst assessing each resident individually may guide specific interventions, often a multifaceted approach (usually referred to as a 'falls prevention programme') is more effective. This approach will target individual factors such as those mentioned above, yet also include external and internal environmental aspects, medication reviews, case conferences, education of carers, families and residents, and exercise sessions for individuals and groups.

Hip protectors

One strategy used for injury prevention within facilities is the prescription and use of hip protector pads (HPPs). These are prescribed to be worn by residents who have been assessed as having a high risk of falling and thereby sustaining hip fractures. There are many different brands now available with slight variations in components and style. However, the intention is the same. A pad is worn laterally over the hip joint and kept in place by pants or belts of various materials. These pads work to minimize the impact forces felt at the hip joint in a fall by absorbing and dispersing energy created by a fall.

Hip protector pads come in various shapes and sizes and are made of several different materials. Figure 12.1 illustrates a typical type of HPP.

The results of two recent controlled studies based in RACFs have shown that the risk of hip fracture could be reduced by as much as 50–60% by the use of energy-absorbing external hip protectors (Kannus et al 2000, Lauritzen et al 1993).

Merilainen and colleagues (2002) suggest a number of features indicating that HPPs would be useful:

- low body weight
- tall stature
- presence of respiratory disease
- tendency to fall indoors
- inability to walk independently outdoors.

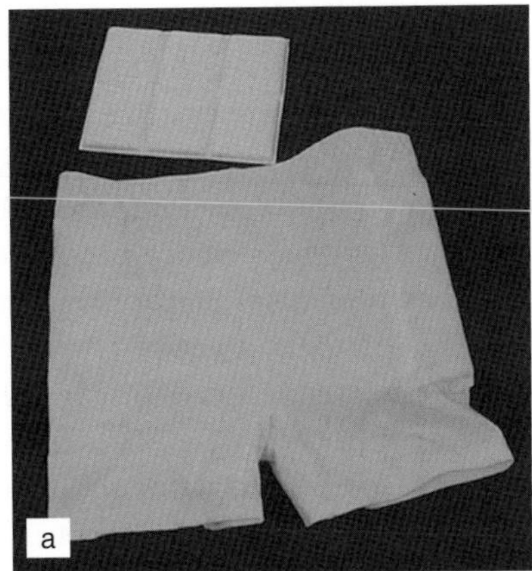

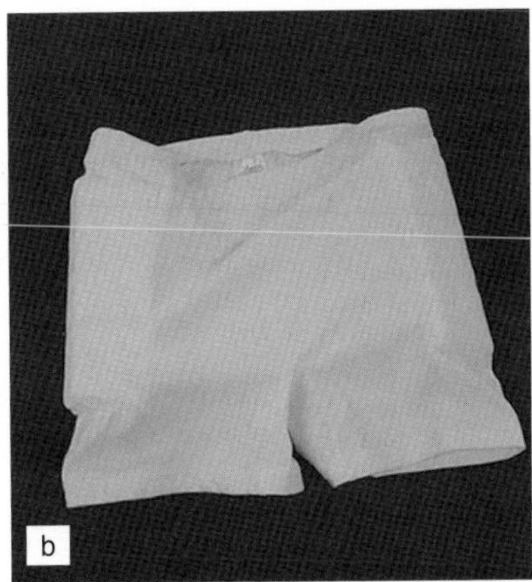

Figure 12.1a & b *A typical hip protector pad.*

These are common features in many older persons living in RACFs, lending support to the argument for mobile residents using hip protectors. However, patient acceptability remains a distinct problem due to skin irritations, lack of insight, and a perception that the pads are uncomfortable (Cameron et al 2001, Hubacher & Wettstein 2001). Other problems identified relate to laundering difficulties, cost, fit, style, infection control and movement of the pad in situ. Education of both residents and staff would seem highly appropriate due to scepticism shown by both key stakeholder groups.

Colon-Emeric et al (2003) have shown the cost-effectiveness of providing hip protectors by comparing the cost of this to the financial expense of medical care needed in the event of hip fracture. This provides a good argument for some residents to use hip protectors as part of their injury prevention strategy.

Drug therapy

The drugs which have been most rigorously tested and shown to reduce spinal fractures in osteoporotic/osteopenic individuals include alendronate, risedronate and raloxifene (Delmas 2002). The most thoroughly tested drugs reported to reduce non-vertebral fractures are calcium and vitamin D for residents in RACFs, and alendronate and risedronate in the community-dwelling older population. Alendronate reduces bone turnover, increasing bone mass by 8% in the spine and 6% in the hip versus placebo in both (Lieberman et al 1995). Parathyroid hormone (PTH) has an ability to reduce both vertebral and non-vertebral fractures and should also provide an alternative intervention approach for patients with severe osteoporosis once it becomes readily available. PTH is normally responsible for controlling the extracellular calcium ion (Ca^{2+}) concentration. It does this by controlling the Ca^{2+} absorption from the gut, renal excretion of Ca^{2+} and release of Ca^{2+} from the bones (Guyton 1991).

Hormone therapy (HT) has associated benefits and risks and the decision to use this therapy, like all others, should be weighed in relation to current research and with consideration to the individual case at hand.

Early evidence was made available suggesting that HT may prevent bone loss in postmenopausal women, and also fractures and chronic heart disease. There is retrospective information suggesting a possible increase in cognitive function and prevention of Alzheimer's disease. The risks of HT include vaginal bleeding, breast tenderness, deep vein thrombosis, pulmonary embolism, as well as a moderate increased risk of breast cancer, endometrial cancer and ovarian cancer. Another recent study which received considerable media coverage showed increased risk of coronary artery disease and ischaemic heart disease; the trial concluded that HT was not the treatment of choice for primary prevention of coronary heart disease and should not be initiated or continued for this effect (WHI 2002). Recent debate has questioned the results in light of the statistical analyses and parameters utilized. As is often the case, further research will need to be undertaken to provide more concrete conclusions, although ethical approval would no doubt be of concern given early indications of increased risk of side effects. Some practitioners believe HT should only be used to control menopausal symptoms and that osteoporosis should be managed by medications such as alendronate, risedronate and raloxifene.

Radiography

The technique of choice to measure bone density is currently dual energy X-ray absorptiometry (DEXA). Levels of bone density measured from DEXA scans can help to guide patient management and intervention although this is more often done within the community and not prioritized with residents in RACFs, especially those residing within a high-care setting. The two-dimensional image which is developed allows the measurement of both cortical and trabecular bone density. Repeat scans are performed at intervals of not less than 12 months as changes in bone density have been shown to require some time for adaptation to be illustrated.

Interpretation usually relies on a comparison of the resident to others in the same matched age group (Z-score) and to the mean peak density of a young, healthy, sex-matched group (T-score). Bone mineral density (BMD) scores recorded have been shown clinically to predict fracture risk within the vertebrae and hip. With each standard deviation below the mean decrease in BMD, there is a 1.9-fold increase in risk of fracture within the vertebrae and a 2.6-fold increase in risk of hip fracture (Cummings et al 1993).

Physiotherapy assessment

As always, a comprehensive assessment precedes treatment and exercise prescription. In regard to osteoporosis more specifically it is important to assess posture and range of motion, muscle strength and endurance, aerobic capacity, balance, pain and function (Bennell et al 2000). Appropriate tests for these measures were outlined in previous chapters. However examples are illustrated below which may provide more useful data for the resident with osteoporosis. Some useful assessment tools appropriate for measuring presentation aspects of osteoporosis are shown in Table 12.3.

Table 12.3 *Useful tools for the assessment of residents with osteoporosis*

Factor	Measurement tool	References
Posture and range of motion	Serial height measurements	Gordon et al 1991
	Distance between tragus and wall	Laurent et al 1991
	Shoulder range and elevation	Bennell et al 1998
	Cervical spine movement	
	Ankle range (especially dorsiflexion)	
	Spinal kyphosis (kyphometer, or flexicurve ruler)	
	Photos	
Strength/ Endurance	Sit to stand	
	Spring gauge	
	Handheld dynamometer	Bohannon 1986
Aerobic capacity	6 minute walk	Steele 1996
	6 metre walk	Hageman & Blanke 1986
	Timed 'up and go'	Podsiadlo & Richardson 1991
Balance	Step test	Hill et al 1996
	Functional reach	Duncan et al 1990
	Clinical test of sensory interaction	Shumway-Cook & Horak 1986
Pain and function	Timed 'up and go'	Podsiadlo & Richardson 1991
	Timed 6 metre walk	Hageman & Blanke 1986
	Visual Analogue Scale (VAS) for pain	Gagliese & Melzack 1997
	McGill Pain Questionnaire	
Quality of life	Osteoporosis Functional Disability Questionnaire	Helmes et al 1995
	Quality of Life Questionnaire of the European Foundation of Osteoporosis (QUALEFFO)	Lips et al 1999
	Osteoporosis Targeted Quality of Life Survey Instrument for use in the community (OPTQoL)	Lydick et al 1997
	Medical Outcomes Study Short Form 36-item Questionnaire (SF-36)	Ware & Sherbourne 1992

Prescribed exercise programmes/ suggested physiotherapy exercises

Exercise is increasingly recognized as a means of reducing risk of osteoporotic fracture and for managing the condition of osteoporosis even in old age. However, the correct choices must be made since not all forms of exercise are suitable; indeed some actually may increase the risk of fracture (Bassey 2001). A general activity programme emphasizing strength, flexibility, coordination and cardiovascular fitness may indirectly reduce the risk of osteoporotic fractures by decreasing the risk of falling and by enabling older persons to remain active, thereby reducing the loss of bone through inactivity (ACSM 1995). The primary benefit of exercise for adult bones is conservation, not acquisition. In elderly individuals, improved fitness and muscle strength contribute to the prevention of falls and a lower risk of fracture. Physical activity may also slow the rate of bone loss. Exercise goals for osteoporosis should include pain reduction, increased mobility and improvements in muscle endurance, balance and stability. These are worthwhile end-points because not only may they prevent falls but they may also improve quality of life. In conjunction with advice to increase dietary calcium, exercise plays a significant part in a lifestyle prescription for reducing fractures in later life.

Resistance training/weights

Although the best exercises for building bones are those involving impact loading of the skeleton (in children), some studies suggest that this is not very effective in adults, especially given the negative effects of increasing risk of osteoarthritis in the older adult and the need for injury prevention. A study on mice further suggested that the ability of bone to respond to mechanical loading is under genetic control (Kodama et al 1999).

The skeleton appears to remain trainable (i.e. responsive to the appropriate stimuli) into at least the 8th decade. Osteogenic loading activities need to be site-specific; for example, jumping has been used as an activity to improve hip BMD. There is no reason to believe that jumping would assist wrist BMD but every reason to be concerned about prescribing this exercise to the elderly, who are already at risk of injury and who often have established disease processes such as osteoarthritis initially. Resistance programmes need to be carefully prescribed and taught well to the elderly. The principles of exercise prescription outlined in the chapter dealing with programming (Chapter 11) should always be followed. A graded resistance programme which begins gently and targets muscle groups surrounding risk areas such as the hip, back and shoulders should be utilized. The evidence regarding load and repetition regimes leans more towards using higher loads with fewer repetitions - this should be kept in mind when developing the target programme. Closed chain exercises are often the safest form of weight training and programmes which use the person's own body weight as resistance are good examples of this, e.g. yoga, Pilates, tai chi. Other aids such as elastic bands and free weights may also be used. The focus should sensibly be on the development of low-impact exercises which improve strength and balance and reduce the risk of falls and subsequent fractures (Turner 2000).

Table 12.4 *Suggested exercises and strategies for residents with osteoporosis*

Strategy	Examples	
Aerobic exercise	Walking 3+ per week, 15–60 minutes Cycling, swimming	
Strengthening exercises	Walking with weights Resistance band exercises Closed chain resistance using own body weight *Lower limb:* hamstring curls squats lunges leg extensions gluteal press quadriceps exercise hip abduction hip adduction calf press rotations* *Upper limb:* biceps curls tricep push-ups latissimus dorsi pectoral squeezes arm raises pull backs wrist curls ball games	Protocol (lower and upper limbs): 8–10 reps 40–60% 1 RM, progress to 80% of 1 RM 8–10 exercises major muscle groups 3 times a week (NB: care must be taken to ensure posture is erect and that a flexing moment is not being transferred to the thoracic and lumbar spine during any of these exercises)
Postural exercises/thoracic extension	Arm raises with deep breathing, trunk extension Chin retraction, deep neck flexors recruitment Lower trapezius setting, scapular retractor training Postural taping (lower trapezius) Stretching and flexibility	
Balance exercises	Walking forwards/backwards/sideways/grapevine stepping/heel and toe walking/skipping/standing on one leg (eyes open/closed) (see Chapter 10 for more ideas)	
Pain management	TENS Gentle heat Hydrotherapy/aquatic physiotherapy Massage Gentle joint mobilization (only applicable in some cases)	
Education	Lifting advice Posture Health promotion (smoking advice, nutrition advice) Information on osteoporosis itself	

table continues

Strategy	Examples
Falls risk assessment and management	Visual and hearing checks Pharmaceutical review Medical review Environmental assessment Shoe prescription Hip protector pads Mobility aid prescription, training and maintenance

* Rotational exercises may be important in order to strengthen bony trabeculae in all directions for improved microarchitectural bony strength. A focus on multi-directional and rotationally based exercises may be of more benefit for both function and injury prevention.
1 RM = repetition maximum, maximum weight which can be lifted once only.

Walking

There is some evidence that the increase in activity needed to achieve the highest level of protection is only very slight. This is encouraging for the frail elderly and their carers. Some research suggests a 5 minute walk daily may be the key to the conservation of bone mass, with levels in excess of this not providing increased protection (Krall & Dawson-Hughes 1994). In general, however, results from research examining walking intervention programmes alone demonstrate that this activity, commonly prescribed to postmenopausal women, does not prevent bone loss alone and needs to be combined with other management strategies such as medication, other exercises such as resistance training and balance activities, and education. While walking has numerous health benefits, it is not primarily prescribed as a skeletal loading (resistance) exercise, probably due to its low magnitude, repetitive and customary qualities. Interestingly, research into its use in this manner in a population with restricted mobility (such as in an RACF) has not been undertaken and may well show positive skeletal effects related to increased loading. Table 12.4 provides some suggestions for exercises suitable for residents with osteoporosis.

See Chapter 11 for more specific principles related to the type, intensity and duration of exercises prescribed.

Exercises to avoid when osteoporosis is established

Any exercise which uses large amounts of force pivoting around weak support structures (bony areas with fracture risk), especially with a long lever, should be avoided in order to prevent injury and fracture. Fast movements, risk-taking activities, excessively ballistic patterns of movement and jumping may all be well avoided. Dynamic abdominal exercises should also be avoided in the aged population due to the increased risk of musculoskeletal damage. Some specific exercises to avoid include sit-ups, twisting exercises, trunk flexion exercises, abrupt or explosive loading and high impact loading (Forwood & Larsen 2000).

Summary

- Osteoporosis is characterized by a reduction in bone mass and subsequent fragility of bone.
- Osteoporosis is one of a number of factors which increase the likelihood of a fracture amongst elderly people.
- There are a number of risk factors for osteoporosis and osteoporotic fractures most of which are modifiable.
- Nutrition plays an integral role in bone maintenance.
- Lifestyle factors can improve bone health and reduce the likelihood of injury.
- Falls protection is of paramount importance.
- Hip protectors may prevent hip fractures; recent studies show positive results.
- Treatment aims to conserve bone mass, reduce the risk of falls, promote an extended posture, reduce pain and improve mobility and function – thereby preventing fractures and improving quality of life.
- In the elderly prevention of fracture is most important. The best advice and expertise will ensure residents keep active and take all steps necessary to avoid falls. Exercises and management suggestions were explored to aid in the treatment given to residents of RACFs with identified or suspected osteopenia and/or osteoporosis.

References

ACSM 1995 ACSM Position Stand on Osteoporosis and Exercise. Medicine and Science in Sports and Exercise 27(4):i–vii

Bassey E J 2001 Exercise for prevention of osteoporotic fracture. Age and Ageing 30-S4:29–31

Bennell K, Talbot R, Wajswelner H, Techovanich W, Kelly D 1998 Intra-rater and inter-rater reliability of a weight-bearing lunge measure of ankle dorsiflexion. Australian Journal of Physiotherapy 44:175–180

Bennell K, Khan K, McKay H 2000 The role of physiotherapy in the treatment and prevention of osteoporosis. Manual Therapy 5(4):198–213

Bohannon R W 1986 Test retest reliability of hand-held dynamometry during a single session of strength assessment. Physical Therapy 66(2): February.

Braunwald E, Fauci A S, Kasper D L et al (eds) 2002 Harrison's principles of internal medicine, 15th edn, vol 2. McGraw-Hill, New York, p 2226–2227

Cameron I D, Venman J, Kurrle S E et al 2001 Hip protectors in aged care facilities: a randomised trial of use by individual high-risk residents. Age and Ageing 30(6):447–481

Colon-Emeric C S, Datta S K, Matchar D B 2003 An economic analysis of external hip protector use in ambulatory nursing facility residents. Age and Ageing 32(1):47–52

Cummings S R, Black D M, Nevitt M C et al 1993 Bone density at various sites for prediction of hip fractures. Lancet 341:72–75

Delmas P D 2002 Treatment of postmenopausal osteoporosis. Lancet 359:2018–2026

Duncan P, Weiner K, Chandler J, Studenski S 1990 Functional reach: a new clinical measure of balance. Journal of Gerontology 45:M192–M197

Forwood M, Larsen J 2000 Exercise recommendations for osteoporosis. A position statement of the Australian and New Zealand Bone and

Mineral Society. Australian Family Physician 29(8):761–764

Gagliese L, Melzack R 1997 Chronic pain in elderly people. Pain 70:3–14

Gordon C C, Cameron Chumlea W C, Roche A F 1991 Stature, recumbent length, and weight. In: Lohman T G, Roche A F, Martorell R (eds) Anthropometric standardisation reference manual. Human Kinetics, Champaign, p 3–8

Guyton A C 1991 Textbook of medical physiology, 8th edn. W B Saunders, Philadelphia

Hageman P, Blanke 1986 Comparison of gait of young women and elderly women. Physical Therapy 66:1382–1387

Helmes E, Hodsman A, Lazowski D et al 1995 A questionnaire to evaluate disability in osteoporotic patients with vertebral compression fractures. Journals of Gerontology Series A – Biological Sciences and Medical Sciences 50:M91–M98

Hill K, Bernhardt J, McGann A, Maltese D, Berkovitis D 1996 A new test of dynamic standing balance for stroke patients: reliability, validity, and comparisons with healthy elderly. Physiotherapy Canada 48:257–262

Hubacher M, Wettstein A 2001 Acceptance of hip protectors for hip fracture prevention in nursing homes. Osteoporosis International 12(9):794–799

Kannus P, Parkkari J, Niemi S 2000 Prevention of hip fracture in elderly people with use of a hip protector. New England Journal of Medicine 343: 1506–1513

Kodama Y, Dimai H P, Wergedal J et al 1999 Cortical tibial bone volume in two strains of mice: effects of sciatic neurectomy and genetic regulation of bone response to mechanical loading. Bone 25:183–190

Krall E A, Dawson-Hughes B 1994 Walking is related to bone density and rates of bone loss. American Journal of Medicine 96:20–26

Laurent M R, Buchanon W W, Ballamy N 1991 Methods of assessment used in ankylosing spondylitis clinical trials. A review. British Journal of Rheumatology 30:326–329

Lauritzen J B, Petersen M M, Lund B 1993 Effect of external hip protectors on hip fractures. Lancet 341:11–13

Lieberman U A, Weiss S R, Bröll J et al 1995 Effect of oral Alendronate on bone mineral density and the incidence of fractures in postmenopausal osteoporosis. New England Journal of Medicine. 333(22):1437–1444

Lips P, Cooper C, Agnusdei D et al 1999 Quality of life in patients with vertebral fractures: validation of the Quality of Life questionnaire of the European Foundation for Osteoporosis (QUALEFFO). Osteoporosis International 19:150–160

Lydick E, Yawn B, Love B et al 1997 Development and validation of a discriminative quality of life questionnaire for osteoporosis (OPTQoL). Journal of Bone and Mineral Research 12:456–463

Merilainen S, Nevalainen T, Luukinen H, Jalovaara P 2002 Risk factors for cervical and trochanteric hip fracture during a fall on the hip. Scandinavian Journal of Primary Health Care 20(3):188–192

Norton R, Galgali G, Campbell A J et al 2001 Is physical activity protective against hip fracture in frail older people? Age and Ageing 30:262–264

Podsiadlo D, Richardson S 1991 The timed 'up and go': a test of basic functional mobility for frail elderly persons. Journal of the American Geriatric Society 39:142–148

Shumway-Cook A, Horak F 1986 Assessing the influence of sensory interaction on balance. Physical Therapy 66:1548–1550

Stedman's Medical Dictionary, 26th edn. 1995. Williams & Wilkins, Baltimore

Steele B 1996 Timed walking tests of exercise capacity in chronic cardiopulmonary illness. Journal of Cardiopulmonary Rehabilitation 16:25–33

Turner C H 2000 Exercising the skeleton: beneficial effects of mechanical loading on bone structure. The Endocrinologist 10:164–169

Ware J E, Sherbourne C D 1992 The MOS 36-item Short Form Health Survey (SF-36). 1: Conceptual framework and item selection. Medical Care 30: 473–483

WHI 2002 Women's Health Initiative Investigators. Writing Group. Risks and benefits of estrogen plus progestin in healthy postmenopausal women. Principal results from the Women's Health Initiative randomised controlled trial. JAMA 288(3):321–333

13 Aquatic physiotherapy for residents in aged care facilities

Ann Rahmann

This chapter aims to:

- identify the types of exercise undertaken in water
- consider the indications and contraindications for exercise in water
- discuss the hydrodynamic principles and physiological responses utilized when exercising in water
- discuss the benefits of managing various impairments with water exercise.

Introduction

The therapeutic benefits of immersion in water have been known for thousands of years (Edlich 1987). By using a clinical reasoning approach, the positive advantages of exercise in water can be combined with the best of current scientific knowledge to maximize the outcomes for older people from this enjoyable activity.

It is useful to first consider the different types of water activity currently available and safety issues related to the use of aquatic therapy with elderly people.

Types of exercise in water

Recent guidelines published by the Australian Physiotherapy Association (APA) clearly describe the different types of exercise in water (Larsen et al 2002).

- **Hydrotherapy** – is used as a general description and covers the wide variety of activities undertaken in a heated pool.
- **Aquatic physiotherapy** – has been defined by the APA as the specific practice of physiotherapy in water carried out by a physiotherapist. This can include individual treatments, group programmes, aquatic physiotherapy classes and physiotherapy prescribed exercise programmes.
- **Water exercise** – is exercise carried out in water to maintain and upgrade body strength, flexibility, conditioning and general fitness and to promote a sense of wellbeing, and is usually performed or instructed by exercise professionals. This includes such activities as community-run water exercise classes.

- **Aquatic fitness activities** - covers aqua fitness, aquarobics, deep water running and should be run by an exercise professional with suitable training, e.g. exercise physiologist or aquatic fitness leader.
- **Swimming activities** - includes learn to swim, therapeutic swimming and swimming for those with disabilities.

Because of the potential for multiple health problems in the elderly, most people living in residential care facilities will require specific aquatic physiotherapy programmes rather than the more general approach of water exercise.

Contraindications and precautions

Prior to entering the pool, everyone including helpers should complete a screening questionnaire in order to determine if they suffer from any health conditions that may be affected by immersion. This should cover aspects such as the current status of:

- cardiovascular and respiratory systems
- central nervous system - particularly epileptic fits
- gastrointestinal and genitourinary system
- infectious conditions (tinea and plantar warts)
- eyes and ears (vision or hearing problems might reduce safety due to reduced ability to communicate)
- skin integrity
- psychiatric conditions, behavioural or cognitive problems
- acute inflammatory conditions
- swimming ability or fear of water
- general mobility, assistance required to walk or dress
- physical ability to determine mode of pool entry/exit.

The APA guidelines clearly explain that each potential client must be individually assessed. The assessment findings should then be used to determine treatment goals and procedures through a clinically reasoned process that takes the physiological effects of immersion into consideration. Factors that contraindicate or require extra precautions to be taken by the physiotherapist when taking a particular resident into the pool must be considered and acted on. Consultation with peers working with similar clients or other informed professionals may be required. In particular, regarding infection control, staff and medical specialists might be consulted. Never put yourself or the client at risk if unsure of safety (Larsen et al 2002).

Contraindications

There are few absolute contraindications for hydrotherapy. Examples of situations where entry to the pool is contraindicated include:

- unreliable faecal incontinence
- skin tears or wounds that cannot be covered with a waterproof dressing or sleeve (e.g. Seal-Tight, Brisbane, Australia)

- infected discharges
- methicillin-resistant *Staphylococcus aureus* (MRSA) in an open wound or present in the gastrointestinal or urinary tract.

However, many medical conditions common in older people require care and caution when the person is being treated in the pool. For example, there is an increased risk of a hypotensive episode when exiting the pool because of the effect of immersion on the cardiovascular system. People with low blood pressure need to be carefully supervised when exiting and showering after a pool session. A water temperature of above 35.5°C can also increase the risk of a hypotensive episode. For the elderly, it is therefore necessary to consider not only the effect of immersion on the cardiovascular system but also the temperature of the pool water itself.

Another important factor to consider with the elderly is fragile skin. It is necessary to make sure any skin tears have appropriate dressings applied before entering the water. Some types of waterproof dressings need to be applied several hours before immersion to ensure the best adhesion and sealing. In addition, skin tends to soften in the water so it is easy for fragile skin to be damaged without the person realizing. Potential sources of damage can be equipment or even the pool surfaces themselves. Footwear such as foot socks or surf shoes can be worn in the pool as a preventive measure, particularly for people with poor distal sensation such as diabetics with peripheral neuropathy. The physiotherapist must be aware of potential problems and take precautions accordingly.

A thorough and clearly explained list of conditions and precautions is contained in The APA Guidelines, Appendix II: Management of precautions for activity/treatment in a hydrotherapy pool (Larsen et al 2002). It is important for all therapists working in hydrotherapy, particularly with older people, to familiarize themselves with these conditions and management suggestions.

Non-swimmers and independent pool exercise

Just because a person cannot swim, does not mean he or she is unable to safely exercise independently in the pool. To assess water safety, the physiotherapist should check that the person can:

- enter the water independently
- roll from prone to supine and regain a safe breathing position
- if unable to walk or touch the bottom (i.e. if they are out of their depth), propel themselves to the edge of the pool and a position of safety while maintaining a safe breathing position
- exit the pool safely or get into pool hoist independently (Larsen et al 2002).

If the person is not safe and competent in completing these tasks independently, the physiotherapist should recommend that the resident attend individual sessions or have a trained carer who can come into the pool and assist them. It is important to note that 'independent' means that the person does not rely on a buoyancy device to achieve the competencies.

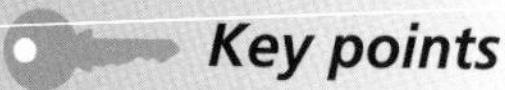

Key points

There are few absolute contraindications to aquatic therapy for older people. However, because the elderly in residential care often have multiple medical problems, the physiotherapist must carefully consider safety issues when deciding who is appropriate for pool therapy and whether a group or individual setting is the best option. Safety of all concerned should be the paramount consideration. The physiotherapist also needs to decide whether a particular facility has sufficient staff, access and safety equipment to meet all the needs of their particular clients.

Hydrodynamic principles

An understanding of hydrodynamic principles and the way they affect movement in water is important in designing an effective water-based exercise programme (Thein & Thein Brody 1998). The basic concepts are most easily understood by considering what occurs when water is still and then when it is moving (Becker 1997).

When water is still, the main principles are:

- density
- buoyancy
- hydrostatic pressure.

When water is moving, they are:

- water flow – laminar and turbulent
- drag forces.

These concepts are thoroughly discussed in most general hydrotherapy texts to which the reader is referred but will be briefly outlined here to highlight the clinical considerations when taking elderly people into the pool.

Density

The density of an object is simply its mass per unit volume and is commonly reported in kilograms per cubic metre. Relative density or specific gravity is the ratio of an object's density compared to water (Becker 1997). The relative density of the human body compared to water varies throughout life and is dependent on the amount of lean muscle and adipose tissue. On average the body's relative density is 0.974. That is, the body is a little less dense than water and will tend to float (Becker 1997). The gradual decrease in muscle mass later in life means that for older people, the relative density drops to about 0.86 (Reid Campion 1997a). This means that older people will float more easily and also that generally women float more easily than men. Clinically, it is important to consider a person's density in the water. For example, someone who is plump and short or with a higher body mass index (BMI) may tend to float more easily. If the person also cannot swim, he/she will require close supervision to ensure the risks associated with losing footing or getting out of his/her depth are minimized.

Buoyancy

When a person is in water, two opposite forces are acting. Gravity acts in a downward direction and the force of buoyancy acts upwards, with the buoyant force being equal to volume of water displaced by the submerged part (Edlich 1987). For the clinician, this simply means that people weigh less in water (Harrison et al 1992). This can be extremely beneficial in situations where, for example, reduced weight-bearing is medically necessary such as healing pelvic fractures or a recent total hip replacement.

Safety in the water is also related to the metacentric principle. When the opposing forces of gravity and buoyancy are the same, the person is stable and balanced in the water. If the forces are unequal, for example if a person is floating and lifts one arm out of the water, rotation of the body will occur until balance is again achieved (Reid Campion 1997b). Because of this principle, it will be much more difficult for a person who has an asymmetrical posture due for example to hemiplegia to maintain balance in the pool, particularly when floating. Fluctuating muscle tone can also make it difficult for a person to control his/her position in the water independently. Appropriate supervision is a necessity for these people when in the water.

Hydrostatic pressure

Water exerts a constant pressure at the same depth on a submerged object. This pressure also increases with depth and with increasing density of the liquid (Reid Campion 1997b). In practical terms, this means that the water pressure around the feet of a person standing in waist deep water is about 89 mmHg (Becker 1997). This is probably one of the ways immersion can help to reduce swelling in the tissues although there is controversy in the literature about the exact mechanism. People with respiratory limitation such as asthma or chronic obstructive pulmonary disease may actually find that the water pressure around their chest is uncomfortable and increases breathlessness. However, an interesting study involving emphysema patients was reported recently. Subjects breathed in while their head was out of water, and then squatted so their nose was under water and breathed out. This was done for 30 minutes, three times a week for 2 months. The results showed significant improvements in both cardiac output and FEV_1 (forced expiratory volume in 1 second) (Kurabayashi et al 1998). Positive pressure breathing is often used in land-based physiotherapy for respiratory patients so there is no reason to suppose that the water-based equivalent should be any less beneficial. People with shortness of breath need to be carefully monitored while they are in the pool and the treatment position and depth of water carefully chosen. Physiotherapists should also remember that there can be significant benefits from activities in the pool for older people with these conditions.

Laminar and turbulent water flow

Objects moving through water are affected by the water flow. Laminar flow is where an object is streamlined through the water. Turbulent flow, as the name suggests, is where the water makes currents and eddies and smooth movement is more difficult (Becker 1997). For the clinician, these forces can be used to make exercises in water easier or harder. Streamlined movements with little turbulence in the water are smooth and effortless. Turbulence created by moving more quickly can make movement through the water more difficult and is an easy way to increase the difficulty of an exercise (Reid Campion 1997b). However, turbulence can be a problem for older people in the pool. A frail elderly person whose balance in the water is poor may be almost swept off his/her feet either by someone walking past quickly or if there are a lot of people in the pool and the water is moving a lot.

Drag forces

Drag forces are related to the shape of an object and the speed of its movement through water and so are less with laminar flow and greater with turbulent water flow (Becker 1997). Two types of drag forces are relevant to hydrotherapy. Pressure drag is created by the turbulence behind a moving object and surface drag is the resistance of the water flowing over the surface of an object (Poyhonen et al 2000).

The effect of pressure drag means that the larger and less streamlined an object is, the more difficult it will be to move through the water. The faster the speed of the movement, the greater the drag forces will be because there will be more turbulence in front of the object and greater drag forces behind it (Hillman et al 1987). Clinically this effect can be used to make exercises harder by adding paddles or flippers to increase the forces the neuromuscular system has to overcome in order to move in the water.

It is harder to move through water than air due to surface drag (Poyhonen et al 2000). Because of the density of water, it is 790 times more difficult to move through water than air (Reid Campion 1997b). The benefit of this resistance is obvious because, for example, it takes about four times as much energy to swim than to run an equal distance (Edlich 1987). Another less well-known advantage is that if someone loses balance in the pool, he/she will not fall as quickly as on land and may have time to regain balance using appropriate strategies (Josephson et al 2001).

Thermodynamic principles

Keeping a constant core temperature is important and the body uses a complex combination of mechanisms to maintain it (Becker 1997). When exercising in a heated hydrotherapy pool, it is more difficult for the body to maintain homeostasis (Reid Campion 1997d). As Reid Campion (1997d) highlights, there is considerable controversy in the literature about what is a suitable temperature for a hydrotherapy pool. Temperatures of around 28 to 30°C are suitable for active exercise such as swimming or aquarobics (Edlich 1987), whereas lower temperatures of 26 to 28°C are more suitable for the intensive training of elite athletes (Thein & Thein Brody 1998). Thermoneutral water is at skin temperature, or around 33 to 34°C (Reid Campion 1997d). This is the most comfortable temperature for less active exercise and older people because it minimizes stress on the body's thermoregulatory system (Golland 1981). Selection of a facility with a pool at the appropriate temperature is particularly important with the elderly because they find it more difficult than younger people to cope with temperature changes (Evans et al 1993).

Physiological effects of immersion and exercise in water

A basic understanding of the physiological effects of exercising and being in water is necessary because of the multiple health problems common in the elderly. It must be noted that most research has used young adults as subjects and only a few studies have examined the effect of immersion in the elderly. There are also differing views in the literature about the nature of the changes with immersion and exercise in water. Much depends on the water temperature and intensity of exercise. In older people, the two systems most affected by immersion are the cardiovascular and the renal systems and they will be considered here.

Cardiovascular effects

Immersion in water increases the amount of blood centrally in the thorax by about 700 ml and an increase in stroke volume and cardiac output results (Pendergast et al 1993). This mechanism is thought to be one of the reasons why heart rate at a given intensity of exercise is lower in water than on land. However, exercise intensity and type as well as water depth and pool temperature can all affect the relationship between heart rate and oxygen consumption (Cureton 1997). Bradycardia occurs on immersion. This can be greater in people taking beta-blockers, a common medication given to elderly patients (Levin 1997). It is also important to remember that hydrostatic pressure is equal to venous pressure in the legs so that, on getting out of the water, venous pooling in the limbs may rapidly occur, causing a drop in blood pressure (Bookspan 1997). Residents whose ability to move about on land is very limited should also be carefully supervised until accustomed to activities in the pool, simply because they are able to do more exercise in the water than their cardiovascular system is used to. While elderly people may be quite safe exercising in the pool, the therapist must be aware of the variety of cardiovascular changes that can occur when exercising in water, as well as when entering and exiting the pool.

Renal effects

The overall effect of immersion in warm water is diuresis but it is a result of the interaction of many factors. Bookspan (1997) summarized the mechanisms of immersion diuresis as follows:

- Hydrostatic pressure – causes blood to be shunted centrally in the thorax, increasing cardiac output.
- Temperature – colder water increases the effect, less important in thermoneutral water.
- Hydration – if already dehydrated, the body decreases output to conserve fluids.
- Age – diuresis occurs more quickly and in a greater volume in the elderly.

In older people, the positive effect of this diuresis is that it is a very efficient mechanism for reducing oedema (Reid Campion 1997b). However, care must be taken to ensure the elderly drink fluids during and after hydrotherapy treatment because they are often already dehydrated. The treating physiotherapist must also be aware if anyone has kidney dysfunction because, as mentioned previously, water temperature is an important factor affecting the degree of diuresis from immersion. Careful monitoring of the time spent in the pool may be also necessary initially until the tolerance to immersion is determined. Staff must ensure that everyone adequately rehydrates by drinking water after getting out of the pool to minimize the adverse effects of dehydration, such as headaches.

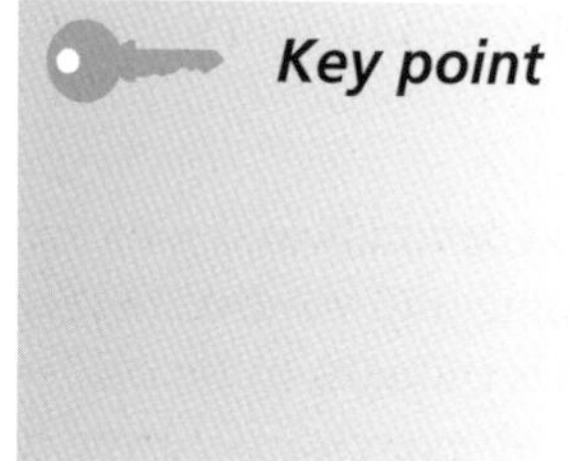

A variety of physical principles and physiological effects need to be understood in order for older people to safely utilize the pool. Moving and being in water provide a unique environment for the elderly to exercise. Using clinical reasoning to combine both the hydrodynamic principles and goals for the individual client, a stimulating and beneficial treatment programme can be developed.

Aquatic physiotherapy

Over the years, anecdotal evidence has increased regarding the benefits of water-based therapy. A systematic review of the literature was recently published (Geytenbeek 2002). The outcome was that, although much research remains to be done, there is evidence to support its use in pain management, improvement of functional ability, flexibility, strength and balance as well as self-efficacy. Diagnostic groups that benefit include rheumatic conditions and chronic low back pain in people of all ages.

The following discussion will use a clinical reasoning focus to discuss the practical aspects of aquatic physiotherapy for elderly people with problems related to:

- postural stability and balance
- strengthening
- maintaining functional abilities
- pain and psychological factors
- general fitness
- neurological conditions.

Postural stability and balance

Balance involves postural stability and the dynamic control of the body while moving to achieve a functional goal. Maintenance of postural alignment and stability of the trunk is important for function and balance in the elderly, particularly those with osteoporosis (Larsen 1998). The structural changes occurring with age that affect posture include an alteration of the normal spinal curves with generally an increase in thoracic kyphosis and a loss of the lumbar lordosis (Kirkegard et al 1998). These changes are likely to be more marked in residents of aged care facilities who are generally less mobile than older people still living in the community.

The ability to independently move and balance tends to deteriorate with age and this results in an increased risk of falling (Woollacott 1993). Maintenance of independent and functional balance relies on the integration of multiple sensory and motor systems (Josephson et al 2001).

However, the ability to control balance is complex and is dependent on the nature of the task as well as the environment in which the activity is to be undertaken (Huxham et al 2001). Elderly people who have fallen or fear falling can enter a downward spiral. They move less to try and prevent falls, which then leads to weakness and reduced ability to balance and then they are more reluctant and less able to move and the cycle continues (Simmons & Hansen 1996).

Balance is integral to all movement; it is therefore important to train by developing successive skill levels and then the skills learned are able to be transferred across into different activities (Huxham et al 2001). The water environment is an ideal place to retrain or maintain the ability to balance, particularly for those who have entered the downward spiral of decreased activity. The benefits of exercise in water to improve balance have been shown in several studies (Alexander et al 2001, Josephson et al 2001, Lord et al 1993, Simmons & Hansen 1996). The positive effect may be due to a number of factors. A wide variety of activities at various speeds and ranges of movement can be easily included. Also, the effect of surface drag in the water means that dynamic movements, such as reaching to the limits of stability, can be done more slowly and with greater confidence in water than on land. This allows those residents whose reactions are not as rapid as they should be to practise without the fear of falling. As a caution though, it is important to remember that frail elderly people can easily lose their footing in the pool if the water becomes too turbulent. People who have poor balance and a history of falls usually require close supervision in the pool. Combinations of activities in a group setting can be easily organized, but must take into account the varying functional abilities and water safety of all participants. The speed and type of exercise as well as the depth of water should be tailored to suit each person's abilities.

A clinically important but often overlooked advantage of balance activities in water is the fact that people exercise in water with bare feet. The ankle joint tends to lose range with ageing and this can have a marked effect on balance (Vandervoort 1999). Josephson and colleagues (2001) noted that subjects in their water exercise group had greater range of ankle dorsiflexion than those in the non-water treatment group. In younger athletes with a sprained ankle, the addition of aquatic exercise improved single leg balance more than land-based exercise alone (Geigle et al 2001). Clinically it seems logical that balancing and exercising in bare feet in the water could help the older person to activate muscles around the ankle more effectively, improve movement in stiff joints of the feet and also increase the proprioceptive input from the feet and ankles.

Land-based exercise has been shown to improve both strength and balance in older people (Lord & Castell 1994) . Similarly, regular aquatic exercise has been shown to significantly improve functional mobility, flexibility and balance in the elderly (Josephson et al 2001, Lord et al 1993). Pool exercise is an evidence-based alternative method of balance training and postural re-education for the elderly.

Strengthening

An understanding of the importance of maintaining and improving muscle strength in the elderly to retain function and quality of life has been growing in recent years (Latham et al 2002). However, it appears that not just any exercise will do. The most important factor in gaining muscle strength is the intensity of the exercise and not the age or frailty of the person (Fiatarone & Evans 1993). A second crucial factor is that in order to continue to improve strength, the resistance of exercises needs to be progressed over time (Barrett & Smerdely 2002). Both principles are just as important in water-based activities as they are for land-based exercises (Thein & McNamara 1997). There has been little published research regarding the effect of aquatic exercise on strength in the elderly. One recent study showed significant improvements in strength and fitness among older women after 12 weeks of water exercise (Takeshima et al 2002).

Strengthening activities in the aquatic environment can start in the range and at the rate that the person can comfortably manage (Speer et al 1993). This is an obvious advantage for the less physically able elderly people from residential aged care settings who may be quite restricted in their ability to move and therefore exercise on land. Exercises can be made more difficult using the principles of hydrodynamics. Working against buoyancy, moving faster or moving something larger like paddles or flippers will all increase the work of an exercise. A metronome can be a very useful piece of equipment to encourage people to progress the speed of movement in the water. Rates should be set with both the individual's ability and the specific exercise in mind because a set rate will not be suitable for all exercises. The physiotherapist skilled in aquatic treatment will be able to select the most appropriate way to progress particular exercises for each individual.

The pool is also an excellent environment for beginning to activate and strengthen very weakened muscles, such as in the frail elderly, early after surgery or after an injury. Buoyancy in the water allows more gentle active movements than conventional dry-land therapy and can build strength to enable a safe transition to active dry-land therapeutics (Speer et al 1993). As these authors highlight, exercises in the water can be an extremely beneficial adjunct to more traditional physiotherapeutic techniques.

With a thorough understanding of the principles of exercise in water, effective strengthening programmes can be undertaken in the pool, particularly for the very frail and debilitated.

Maintaining functional abilities

Difficulty living independently due to declining balance, strength or mobility is commonly the reason elderly people will move into a residential care setting (Kirkegard et al 1998). Physiotherapists who work with the elderly know that, for example, the ease of getting out of a chair often has more to do with the height of the chair than with the person's specific static quadriceps strength. What is often overlooked when considering the functional abilities of the elderly in research is that the relationship between strength and function is task specific (Chandler et al 1997). Movement normally takes place at a variety of speeds depending on the context of the activity (Moy 2003). Without realizing it, elderly people will often slow down their voluntary movements in order to try and control their balance and over time this leads to a reduced ability to move quickly (Woollacott & Manchester 1993). When looking at muscle activation patterns during a stepping task, it was found that patterns varied both within and between subjects (Mercer & Sahrmann 1999). This highlights the need for elderly people to practise balance and functional tasks in a variety of settings and at a range of different speeds (Carr et al 2002). The pool is an ideal environment where strength and balance activities can be easily combined into functional activities that may not be possible on land for the frail aged (Levin 1997). Sit to stand and stepping up and down are two examples of exercises that can be practised easily in the water. The types of activities and the variations of speed and the control required are only limited by the physiotherapist's imagination.

Negotiating stairs is a particularly difficult locomotor task for many elderly people and they will often have moved into residential care because of problems with this activity (Cavanagh et al 1997). The importance of eccentric muscle strength in such functional activities is well known (Carr et al 2002). However, the effect of ageing on eccentric muscle strength has not often been investigated. One small study found that women seemed to have a significantly greater loss of eccentric strength with age than men (Bellew et al 1998). Most aquatic exercises involve predominantly concentric muscle activity (Thorpe & Reilly 2000). Eccentric exercise is possible with an understanding of hydrodynamics by using muscle activation to counteract the effect of buoyancy.

Functional activities such as walking are extremely beneficial activities for the elderly but those in residential care are often limited in their ability to walk any distance or at speed. Walking in the pool can be a way of retraining or maintaining this ability in those who normally find walking difficult (Simmons & Hansen 1996). When walking through water at a level that is 50% of a person's height, the patterns of electromyographic muscle activation were found to be the same as when walking on land (Petrofsky et al 2002). The authors found that muscle activity changed with increasing depth of water so the optimum depth of water for re-educating a normal gait pattern is 50% of the person's height. Different speeds and changes in directions add to the challenge and variety of the task. The therapist needs to weigh up the advantages of normal muscle activation patterns in shallower water, with the pain relief gained in deeper water. A suitable depth for each person should be chosen, depending on his/her goals, abilities and treatment aims.

Speer and colleagues (1993) in discussing shoulder rehabilitation identified the contribution hydrotherapy plays in restoring muscle activation and coordination to enable normal function of the entire pectoral girdle. Considering the often multiple health problems of the elderly, the ability to move and function normally in the water is an important benefit, not only around the shoulder girdle but for the whole neuromuscular system. Complex functional activities not possible on land can also be accomplished more independently in the water environment.

Pain and psychological factors

Back pain is a common problem encountered in elderly residents and is often associated with joint degeneration and osteoporosis. Efficient trunk stability and good posture is needed to prevent pain. This is provided by a combination of action from global, torque-producing muscles such as latissimus dorsi and local muscles such as multifidus that attach closely onto the spinal vertebra to provide stability for the spinal segments (Richardson & Jull 1995). The ability of the motor system to control posture and stability appropriately is dependent on an efficient central nervous system (Hodges 2000). Alterations to the normal structure of the spine and trunk in the elderly must affect the ease with which global and local muscles can be activated. Pain is known to alter the activation of the muscles which normally provide stability for the trunk (Hodges & Richardson 1996). In an elderly person with poor posture, the addition of pain from a vertebral crush fracture must further compromise the normal patterns of activity of these stabilizing muscles. Reducing pain to allow normal muscle patterns to be reactivated is crucial in rehabilitation after such an event and the support provided by water is useful in attaining this aim (Fig. 13.1).

Relief of pain is often reported as a benefit of aquatic therapy (Alexander et al 2001, Lee 1997, Smit & Harrison 1991). The mechanism for this is considered to be simply the reduction in weight-bearing due to buoyancy, allowing the unloading of painful structures (Wyatt et al 2001).

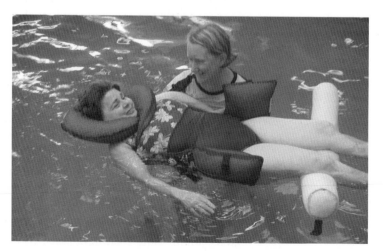

Figure 13.1
Supported supine float is a useful position for people with problems such as back pain or crush fractures. Pain is significantly reduced and this allows facilitation of postural and deep stabilizing trunk muscles.

However, current research from the field of chronic pain neurobiology provides a much broader and potentially more exciting explanation for the effect of immersion for someone who is in pain. Pain processing is often thought of as a simple input/output mechanism but this view is being increasingly challenged as brain imaging techniques improve. The mature organism model considers the way, in a painful state, the brain samples input not only from the tissues but also from the environment as well as thoughts and previous experiences (Gifford 1998). What this means in clinical terms is that pain should not be considered simply a 'tissue-based' process but one that can be influenced by many different factors. 'Movements that are feared, avoided and context dependent will have to be presented to the brain in different ways, for example in different environments, or the movement "broken down" or paced ... Clearly, the more functional the movement and the more it links into the desired activity and achievable goals, the better' (Butler 2000). The pool is therefore a powerful rehabilitation tool for people with pain because they are able to accomplish functional movements without the overlay of pain. Areas within the brain that would normally be activated by the thought of or commencement of a painful activity can be modified or 'turned down' and the perception of pain altered (Butler 2003). Normal patterns of muscle activity are then, logically, easier to achieve.

Frequent pain is reported by one-third of older adults and 20% restrict their activities because of significant levels of pain (Reyes-Gibby et al 2002). The study also showed that higher levels of pain were closely related to poorer self-perceived health. However, other studies have found that the elderly tend to underestimate their pain levels so the real figure may be closer to 50% (Weiner 2002). Interestingly, the 'old-old' also tend to rate their health more favourably than the 'young-old' despite having a far greater risk of dying simply because of their age (Idler 1993). What this means in relation to the aged in residential care is that more than half are likely to have significant pain, but in spite of this, they are likely to be quite positive about their general state of health.

For those who are less happy about their health, exercise in the pool can have additional benefits. Older people who regularly swam were found to have a more positive body image, better bone density and felt they were stronger than community-centre attendees who did not exercise regularly (Benedict & Freeman 1993). Exercise is thought to help in the management of anxiety and depression through its effect on brain monoamines (Chaouloff 1989) and pain through the stimulation of beta-endorphin release (Schwarz & Kindermann 1992). Several studies looking at arthritic conditions have demonstrated reduced pain and increased self-efficacy with aquatic exercise programmes (Ahern et al 1995, Wyatt et al 2001). Another important psychological influence to consider is the positive social nature of pool treatment. People having aquatic physiotherapy are not treated alone in a single cubicle but rather in a pool with other people of varying abilities. The importance of support and positive feedback from others in facilitating improvement in chronic pain patients has recently been highlighted (Gifford 2002, Muncey 2002). It has been suggested that the positive reinforcement of exercising in a class with others may be even more important than the content of the class itself (Minor et al 1989). Physiotherapists should not underestimate the benefit of this particular aspect of aquatic therapy.

Dementia and impaired cognition should briefly be mentioned because they are often thought to be a contraindication to aquatic exercise. Safety in the water is the predominant issue because people with these conditions will often lack the insight and concentration to exercise with a group (Levin 1997). As discussed earlier, it is the responsibility of the supervising physiotherapist to decide whether the person is safe or not to attend a group programme. If group activities are not suitable, the most appropriate form of water activity would then be either individual 'one on one' sessions with the physiotherapist or to train a carer to specifically look after that one person in the pool. It is also important to remember that it may be more beneficial for people with cognitive impairments to come to the pool when it is relatively quiet rather than when it is busy.

When the current knowledge of pain processing is combined with the ease of movement in water, as well as the realization that about half of all elderly people have significant pain, the benefits of aquatic therapy for older people with pain are clear. The psychological benefits for people should also be remembered.

General fitness

It is being realized that, particularly for the elderly, some activity is better than none at all. A walking programme just twice a week was shown to improve fitness in elderly, sedentary women (Hamdorf et al 1992). Because it is possible to move more easily in the water, general fitness and cardiovascular exercise is made possible for the elderly who cannot easily move on land. Many studies have been undertaken on younger subjects that show it is possible to maintain cardiovascular fitness through pool exercise (Bishop et al 1989, Cassady & Nielsen 1992, Kirby et al 1984, Whitley & Schoene 1987). Positive improvements have also been shown in the fitness of older people by using water exercise (Danneskiold-Samsoe et al 1987, Ruoti et al 1994, Sanford Smith et al 1998, Takeshima et al 2002). Even people with late-onset poliomyelitis were able to reduce their training heart rate after a twice weekly, 8-month water exercise programme (Willen et al 2001).

Basic outlines of aquatic fitness classes for older people are common (Levin 1997). Water-based exercise can be a particularly effective way to improve the cardiovascular fitness of the elderly from all levels of residential aged care settings, provided the activities are tailored to suit the abilities of the particular people involved and adequate supervision and assistance is available. One important point to remember is that due to the hydrodynamic effects of immersion, when exercising in water, the heart rate can be between six and fifteen beats per minute lower than when exercising on land (Hamer & Morton 1990). The relationship between heart rate and VO_2 (oxygen consumption) is dependent on the exercise intensity and type, as well as the water depth and temperature, so it can be confusing to try and determine appropriate levels from the literature. Using heart rate is probably a less reliable method of measuring exercise intensity, particularly with the elderly. A convenient and easy-to-use alternative is Borg's perceived rate of exertion (PRE) where the person simply rates on a scale up to 20 how hard they feel they are working (Borg 1982). The moderately hard level of around 12 to 14 has been correlated with training heart rates of 70% of maximum training heart rate (Hamer & Slocombe 1997). However, while many of the elderly in residential aged care may not be able to manage the amount of exercise that younger more able people can, the perceived rate of exertion is still a useful measure clinically to encourage them to work a little harder in the water. As they get stronger and fitter, they will be able to achieve more repetitions or a longer period of exercise at the same level of exertion.

Maintaining cardiovascular fitness is no less important for the residents of aged care facilities than for the well elderly living in the community. Effective pool programmes can be developed using the combination of hydrodynamic principles and clinical reasoning to benefit even the most debilitated of people because they can move more easily in the water than on land.

Neurological conditions

Treatment in the water of people with neurological impairments is considered controversial. 'Many neurological physiotherapists are wary of treating their patients in the water, reserving hydrotherapy for the later stages when not too much harm can be done and the patient enjoys doing something a bit different' (Gray 1997). Most of the debate within the literature is related to the varying approaches used to treat neurological patients (Reid Campion 1997c). One point of view is that the unusual environment and way muscles work in water is not the best way to relearn function. The opposing view is that functional activities are possible in the pool with less manual assistance and can therefore provide earlier normal movement input and motivation for the patient. Much of the success of aquatic treatment for these patients depends on the clinical skills of the treating physiotherapist in understanding hydrodynamic principles and how they can affect or assist the neurologically impaired person. The benefits of aquatic exercise for this group of patients have been tone reduction, maintenance of joint range, static and dynamic balance, earlier and more effective strengthening, cardiovascular benefits, motivation, recreation and social integration (Morris 1997).

Principles of aquatic treatment for acute neurological conditions will not be covered here as residents are usually into the subacute or chronic phase when they reach aged care settings. The rehabilitation goals of balance re-education, cardiovascular fitness, functional activity and strengthening previously discussed are just as relevant for those with neurological conditions (Carr et al 2002). Several aspects specific to treating neurological dysfunction in the elderly in the pool will be briefly reviewed here.

Abnormal tone

There are few published studies looking at the effect of aquatic exercise in neurological subjects. One study showed that the gait characteristics of people with spastic hemiplegia improved after aquatic exercise (Zamparo & Pagliaro 1998). It was thought this could be due to a reduction in spasticity. A subsequent study then showed that hypertonicity was no worse after the pool treatment (Pagliaro & Zamparo 1999). Subjects for the second study included 26 people from age 26 to 81, with diagnoses of hemiplegia, paraplegia, tetraplegia or multiple sclerosis. Although this study did not demonstrate reduction in tone, the fact that tone was not made worse in any of the diverse groups is important to note.

Maintaining or regaining normal muscle length is often a treatment aim in people with increased tone. Standing in the shallow end of the pool with weight down through the feet or walking up a pool ramp are effective ways to regain or retain ankle flexibility where there is increased tone in the calf. Those who are unable to stand easily out of the water can often accomplish this in the pool (Fig. 13.2). The benefits of stretching can then be easily combined with functional activities such as sit to stand or step-ups as a progression in the water, just as it would be in a land-based programme.

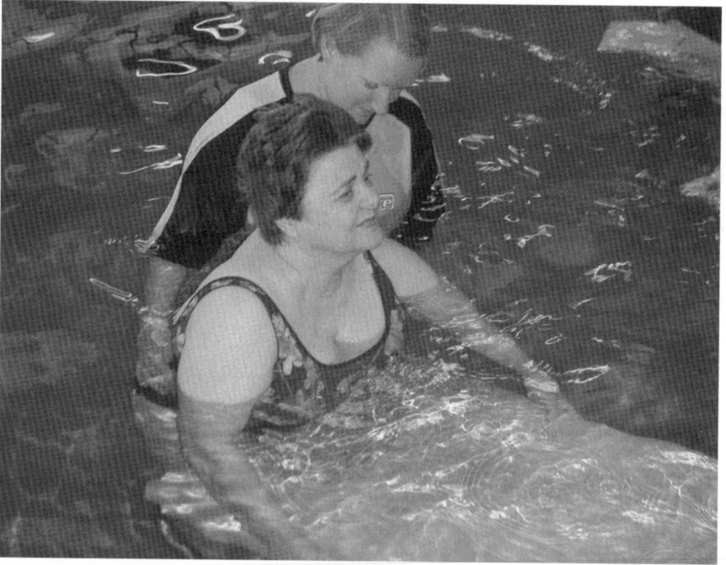

Figure 13.2
This woman who is unable to stand independently out of the pool, can stand at the plinth with even weight-bearing through her legs. This position also allows weight-bearing and positioning of her affected left arm at a more normal muscle length. She has minimal active movement in the left arm but this position also allows her to do modified push-ups independently while still maintaining pelvic and trunk stability.

Clinically, the most important issue to be aware of with someone who has increased tone is that a sudden change in tone can make him/her rapidly roll or lose balance and therefore risk drowning if unable to return to a safe breathing position. A cough or sneeze or even getting cold can be enough to cause a rapid increase in tone. Close supervision by a physiotherapist or carer is generally always the safest option for those with unpredictable hypertonicity.

Hypotonicity or low muscle tone presents a different problem. For example, someone with a dense hemiplegia can find that his/her leg tends to float due to the effect of buoyancy combined with limited active movement. Using an ankle weight can provide enough proprioception and 'counterbalance' to the effect of buoyancy to allow more functional activities such as standing and walking. Particular care should be taken that buoyancy is not carrying the limb into a painful range at the glenohumeral joint even though a painful, hemiplegic shoulder can be comfortably supported and moved in the water, often more easily than on land. Muscles unable to work against gravity can begin to move a limb in the supported environment of the water.

Exercises to address the rigidity of Parkinson's disease can be easily incorporated into a water-based programme. Because movement in water is slower, people are able to reach to the limits of their stability and range comfortably in the pool and therefore often feel safer going further into range. Activities such as those focusing on trunk rotation in standing and rolling from prone to supine can be particularly effective in the water environment.

Proprioceptive dysfunction

It has been suggested that hydrostatic pressure surrounding the limbs in the water can provide proprioceptive input that enhances active movement (Speer et al 1993). Many activities in the water can be used to increase proprioceptive input. For example, lying prone on elbows on a pool plinth while kicking with the legs provides proprioceptive input for the shoulder girdle and upper limbs, as well as trunk and lower limb stability and strengthening (Fig. 13.3). Standing and pushing down on a kickboard is another example.

These examples highlight the fact that one water-based exercise can achieve several different treatment aims so treatment can be very efficient. Walking in water reduces the amount of weight-bearing through the feet but adding ankle weights can increase the proprioceptive input and improve walking ability of those with poor control. Residents with truncal ataxia also find a scuba-diving weight-belt worn around the waist can give added stability and input when walking in the pool. The amount of weight can be varied and reduced when control improves.

Walking in water

Recently, the use of walking on a treadmill with bodyweight support on land has become a common therapeutic technique for neurological patients (Hesse et al 1995, Shepherd & Carr 1999). Treadmill walking with 30% of

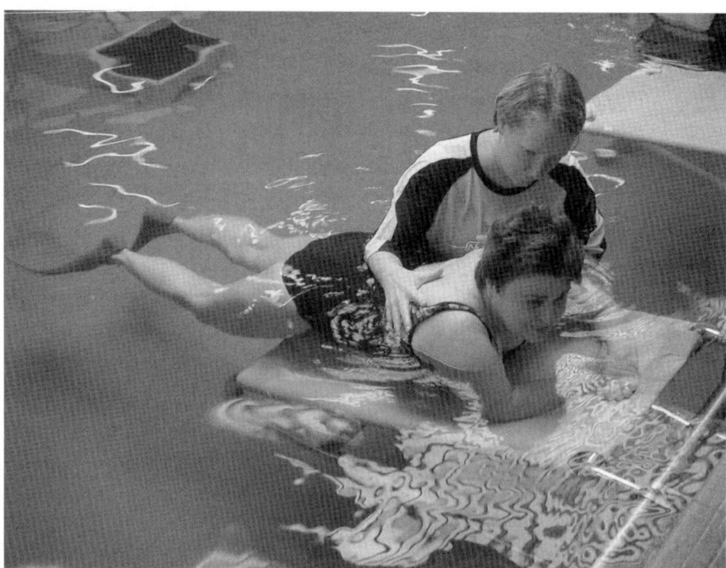

Figure 13.3
This photograph shows how one activity in the water can achieve several therapeutic aims at the same time. This woman has had a stroke and is wheelchair dependent out of the pool. While strengthening her knee and hip extensors using flippers, she is also getting proprioceptive input through her affected left arm as well as activating trunk and neck extensors.

the body weight supported demonstrated significant improvements in activation of pelvic stabilizing muscles as well as providing a dynamic stimulus to the hemiplegic gait pattern (Hesse et al 1997). In the pool, immersion to 30% body weight occurs at about the level of the xiphisternum in quiet standing (Reid Campion 1997a). There is no reason to presume that walking in the pool at that level is any less beneficial than walking on a treadmill. In addition, in the pool it is possible to include functional tasks such as stepping and squats which cannot be done safely on a treadmill. It is important to remember that when walking through water, increasing the speed of walking can enhance the strengthening, cardiovascular and weight-bearing benefits of the activity (Harrison et al 1992).

One of the common reasons given for not walking people with neurological problems in the pool is that it is more difficult to facilitate the correct gait pattern, e.g. foot placement. A recent study (Petrofsky et al 2002) demonstrated that when walking in water at 50% of body height, patterns of muscle activation were the same as land-based walking. It is therefore possible to re-educate normal gait patterns in the water. There is no reason why such things as straps that loop around the foot and ankle and are then held by the therapist or plastic splints such as ankle-foot orthoses cannot be used with an old pair of sandshoes in the pool to facilitate gait re-education and aerobic endurance. Walking people with neurological problems in the pool has many more advantages than disadvantages, not the least of which is that fewer people are needed to walk a heavily dependent person in the water than on land.

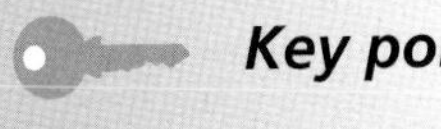

Key point

With careful thought about the individual's problems and how they may be affected by moving in water, combined with the best of current neurology practice, creative and therapeutic aquatic programmes can be developed. Gray (1997) gives an excellent overview of practical treatment ideas and aquatic therapists treating people with neurological conditions are encouraged to read her suggestions.

Conclusion

Aquatic physiotherapy is an exciting tool for physiotherapists caring for older people. Movements or exercises that are impossible on land can often be performed in water. As the treatments are performed in small groups, the opportunity to communicate with other people is beneficial and the treatment is enjoyable and relaxing. Residents gain confidence in their ability to cope both physically and socially as a result of participation in a pool programme (Jackson 1996). Surely these positive outcomes summarize the goals of physiotherapy intervention for the elderly in residential aged care settings.

Summary

- Exercise in water has a unique set of risks and physiological effects that must be considered before commencing a programme of activities.
- Safety issues relating to therapist/patient numbers in the pool, adequate supervision, each individual's competence in the water and the suitability of a particular facility must be carefully assessed and documented.
- By understanding and applying the hydrodynamic principles of density, buoyancy, hydrostatic pressure, water flow and drag forces, the variety of exercises possible in water is virtually limitless.
- A particular advantage of aquatic exercise for the elderly is its efficiency because a single exercise can address a variety of treatment goals at the same time.
- Just as on land, exercises must be tailored to an individual's needs and details of depth of water, speed and range specified.
- The enjoyment and social environment of aquatic exercise makes it an exciting addition to the treatment options for elderly residents of aged care facilities. People with almost all types of medical conditions are able to take part in some form of activity in the pool.

References

Ahern M, Nicholls E, Simionato E, Clark M, Bond M 1995 Clinical and psychological effects of hydrotherapy in rheumatic diseases. Clinical Rehabilitation 9:204–212

Alexander M J L, Butcher J E, MacDonald P B 2001 Effect of a water exercise program on walking gait, flexibility, strength, self-reported disability and other psycho-social measures of older individuals with arthritis. Physiotherapy Canada Summer: 203–211

Barrett C, Smerdely P 2002 A comparison of community-based resistance exercise and flexibility exercise for seniors. Australian Journal of Physiotherapy 48(3):215–219

Becker B E 1997 Aquatic physics. In: Ruoti R G, Morris D M, Cole A J (eds) Aquatic rehabilitation. Lippincott, Philadelphia

Bellew J M, Nitz A, Hart A 1998 Gender specificity in the age-related decline of strength: concentric versus eccentric. Isokinetics and Exercise Science 7:1–9

Benedict A, Freeman R 1993 The effect of aquatic exercise on aged person's bone density, body image, and morale. Activities, Adaptation and Aging 17(3):67–85

Bishop P A, Frazier S, Smith J, Jacobs D 1989 Physiologic responses to treadmill and water running. The Physician and Sports Medicine 17(2): 87–94

Bookspan J 1997 Physiologic effects of immersion at rest. In: Ruoti R G, Morris D M, Cole A J (eds) Aquatic rehabilitation. Lippincott, Philadelphia

Borg G V 1982 Psychophysical basis of perceived exertion. Medical Science and Sports Exercise 14:377

Butler D S 2000 The sensitive nervous system. Noigroup Publications, Adelaide

Butler D S 2003 The representation – a new paradigm in rehabilitation? Paper presented at the 2nd Annual Gerontology Conference, Brisbane, Australia

Carr J H, Ow J E G, Shepherd R B 2002 Some biomechanical characteristics of standing up at three different speeds: implications for functional training. Physiotherapy Theory and Practice 18:47–53

Cassady S, Nielsen D 1992 Cardiorespiratory responses of healthy subjects to calisthenics performed on land versus in water. Physical Therapy 72(7): 532–538

Cavanagh P R, Mulfinger L M, Owens D A 1997 How do the elderly negotiate stairs? Muscle and Nerve Supplement 5:S52–S55

Chandler J, Duncan P, Studenski S 1997 Choosing the best strength measure in frail older persons: Importance of task specificity. Muscle and Nerve Supplement 5:S47–S51

Chaouloff F 1989 Physical exercise and brain monoamines: a review. Acta Physiologica Scandinavica 137:1–13

Cureton K J 1997 Physiologic responses to exercise in water. In: Ruoti R G, Morris D M, Cole A J (eds) Aquatic rehabilitation. Lippincott, Philadelphia

Danneskiold-Samsoe B, Lyngberg K, Risum T, Telling M 1987 The effect of water exercise therapy given to patients with rheumatoid arthritis. Scandinavian Journal of Rehabilitation Medicine 19:31–35

Edlich R F 1987 Burn Rehabilitation Forum Editorial. Journal of Burn Care and Rehabilitation 8(6):579

Evans E, Rendell M, Bartek J et al 1993 Thermally-induced cutaneous vasodilation in aging. Journal of Gerontology 48(2):M53–M57

Fiatarone M, Evans W 1993 The etiology and reversibility of muscle dysfunction in the aged. Journal of Gerontology 48:77–83

Geigle P, Daddona K, Finken K et al 2001 The effects of supplemental aquatic physical therapy on balance and girth for NCAA Division 3 athletes with a grade 1 or 2 lateral ankle sprain. Journal of Aquatic Physiotherapy 9(1):13–20

Geytenbeek J 2002 Evidence for effective hydrotherapy. Physiotherapy 88(9):514–529

Gifford L 1998 Pain, the tissues and the nervous system: a conceptual model. Physiotherapy 84(1):27–36

Gifford L 2002 An introduction to evolutionary reasoning: diets, discs, fevers and the placebo. In: Gifford L (ed) Topical issues in pain, vol 4. CNS Press, Falmouth, Cornwall

Golland A 1981 Basic hydrotherapy. Physiotherapy 67(9):258–262

Gray S 1997 Neurological rehabilitation. In: Reid Campion M (ed) Hydrotherapy: principles and practice. Butterworth-Heinemann, Oxford

Hamdorf P A, Withers R T, Penhall R K, Haslam M V 1992 Physical training effects on the fitness and habitual activity patterns of elderly women. Archives of Physical Medicine and Rehabilitation 73:603–608

Hamer P, Morton A 1990 Water-running: Training effects and specificity of aerobic, anaerobic and muscular parameters following an eight-week interval training programme. Australian Journal of Science and Medicine in Sport 22(1):13–22

Hamer P, Slocombe B 1997 The psychophysical and heart rate relationship between treadmill and deep water running. Australian Journal of Physiotherapy 43:265–271

Harrison R A, Hillman M, Bulstrode S 1992 Loading of the lower limb when walking partially immersed: implications for clinical practice. Physiotherapy 78(3):164–166

Hesse S, Bertlet C, Jahnke M et al 1995 Treadmill training with partial body weight support compared with physiotherapy in nonambulatory hemiparetic patients. Stroke 26(6):976–981

Hesse S, Helm B, Krajnik J, Gregoric M, Mauritz K 1997 Treadmill training with partial body weight support: influence of body weight release on the gait of hemiparetic patients. Journal of Neurological Rehabilitation 11:15–20

Hillman M R, Matthews L, Pope J M 1987 The resistance to motion through water of hydrotherapy table-tennis bats. Physiotherapy 73(10): 570–572

Hodges P 2000 The role of the motor system in spinal pain: Implications for rehabilitation of the athlete following lower back pain. Journal of Science and Medicine in Sport 3(3):243–253

Hodges P W, Richardson C A 1996 Inefficient muscular stabilization of the lumbar spine associated with low back pain. Spine 21(22):2640–2650

Huxham F E, Goldie P A, Patla A 2001 Theoretical considerations in balance assessment. Australian Journal of Physiotherapy 47(2):89–100

Idler E L 1993 Age differences in self-assessments of health: age changes, cohort differences or survivorship? Journal of Gerontology 48(6):S289–S300

Jackson A 1996 Hydrotherapy as experienced by outpatients in a general hospital. British Journal of Therapy and Rehabilitation 3(11):601–608

Josephson S R, Josephson D L, Nitz J C 2001 Evaluation of a long-term water exercise program for the elderly: focusing on balance. Australasian Journal on Aging 20(3):147–152

Kirby R L, Sacamano J T, Balch D E 1984 Oxygen consumption during exercise in a heated pool. Archives of Physical Medicine and Rehabilitation 65:21–23

Kirkegard Y, Sapsford R, Howard J, Markwell S 1998 The aged. In: Sapsford R, Bullock-Saxton J, Markwell S (eds) Women's health: A textbook for physiotherapists. W B Saunders, London

Kurabayashi H, Machida I, Kubota K 1998 Improvement in ejection fraction by hydrotherapy as rehabilitation in patients with chronic pulmonary emphysema. Physiotherapy Research International 3(4):284–291

Larsen J 1998 Osteoporosis. In: Sapsford R, Bullock-Saxton J, Markwell S (eds) Women's health: A textbook for physiotherapists. W B Saunders, London

Larsen J, Pryce M, Harrison J et al 2002 Guidelines for physiotherapists working in and/or managing hydrotherapy pools. Australian Physiotherapy Association Policy Documents

Latham N, Anderson C, Bennett D, Stretton C 2002 Progressive resistance strength training for physical disability in older people (Cochrane Review). The Cochrane Library, Issue 2, 2003. Oxford: Update Software

Lee C 1997 Orthopaedics. In: Reid Campion M (ed) Hydrotherapy: principles and practice. Butterworth-Heinemann, Oxford

Levin A 1997 Water fitness for the older adult and frail aged. In: Reid Campion M (ed) Hydrotherapy: principles and practice. Butterworth-Heinemann, Oxford

Lord S, Castell S 1994 Effect of exercise on balance, strength and reaction time in older people. Australian Journal of Physiotherapy 40(2): 83–88

Lord S, Mitchell D, Williams P 1993 Effect of water exercise on balance and related factors in older people. Australian Journal of Physiotherapy 39(3):217–222

Mercer V S, Sahrmann S A 1999 Postural synergies associated with a stepping task. Physical Therapy 79(12):1142–1152

Minor M A, Hewett J E, Webel R R, Anderson S K, Kay D R 1989 Efficacy of physical conditioning exercise in patients with rheumatoid arthritis and osteoarthritis. Arthritis and Rheumatism 32(11): 1396–1405

Morris D M 1997 Aquatic rehabilitation of the neurologically impaired client. In: Ruoti R G, Morris D M, Cole A J (eds) Aquatic rehabilitation. Lippincott, Philadelphia

Moy D 2003 The science behind functional training. Network February:65–67

Muncey H 2002 Explaining pain to patients. In Gifford L (ed) Topical issues in pain, vol 4. CNS Press, Falmouth, Cornwall

Pagliaro P, Zamparo P 1999 Quantitative evaluation of the stretch reflex before and after hydro kinesy therapy in patients affected by spastic paresis. Journal of Electromyography and Kinesiology 9:141–148

Pendergast D R, Fisher N M, Calkins E 1993 Cardiovascular, neuromuscular and metabolic alterations with age leading to frailty. Journal of Gerontology 48(Special Issue):61–67

Petrofsky J S, Connel M, Parrish C, Lohman E, Laymon M 2002 Muscle use during gait on land and in water. British Journal of Therapy and Rehabilitation 9(1):6–14

Poyhonen T, Keskinen K, Hautala A, Malkia E 2000 Determination of hydrodynamic drag forces and drag coefficients on human leg/foot model during knee exercises. Clinical Biomechanics 15:256–260

Reid Campion M 1997a Assessment and recording. In: Reid Campion M (ed) Hydrotherapy: principles and practice. Butterworth-Heinemann, Oxford

Reid Campion M 1997b Basic physics: shape and density. In: Reid Campion M (ed) Hydrotherapy: principles and practice. Butterworth-Heinemann, Oxford

Reid Campion M 1997c Neurosurgical and neurological conditions. In: Reid Campion M (ed) Hydrotherapy: principles and practice. Butterworth-Heinemann, Oxford

Reid Campion 1997d Key features of pool design and caring for the pool. In: Reid Campion M (ed) Hydrotherapy: principles and practice. Butterworth-Heinemann, Oxford

Reyes-Gibby C, Aday L, Cleeland C 2002 Impact of pain on self-rated health in the community-dwelling older adults. Pain 95(1–2):75–82

Richardson C A, Jull G A 1995 Muscle control – pain control. What exercises would you prescribe? Manual Therapy 1:2–10

Ruoti R G, Troup J T, Berger R A 1994 The effects of non-swimming water exercises on older adults. Journal of Orthopaedic and Sports Physical Therapy 19(3):140–145

Sanford Smith S, MacKay-Lyons M, Nunes-Clement S 1998 Therapeutic benefit of aquaerobics for individuals with rheumatoid arthritis. Physiotherapy Canada Winter:40–46

Schwarz L, Kindermann W 1992 Changes in β-endorphin levels in response to aerobic and anaerobic exercise. Sports Medicine 13(1): 25–36

Shepherd R, Carr J 1999 Treadmill walking in neurorehabilitation. Neurorehabilitation and Neural Repair 13:171–173

Simmons V, Hansen P 1996 Effectiveness of water exercise on postural mobility in the well elderly: an experimental study on balance enhancement. Journal of Gerontology 51A(5):M233–M238

Smit T E, Harrison R 1991 Hydrotherapy and chronic lower back pain: a pilot study. Australian Journal of Physiotherapy 37(4):229–234

Speer K P, Cavanaugh J T, Warren R F, Day L, Wickiewicz T L 1993 A role for hydrotherapy in shoulder rehabilitation. American Journal of Sports Medicine 21(6):850–853

Takeshima N, Rogers M E, Watanabe E et al 2002 Water-based exercise improves health-related aspects of fitness in older women. Medicine and Science in Sports and Exercise 34(3):544–551

Thein J M, Thein Brody L 1998 Aquatic-based rehabilitation and training for the elite athlete. Journal of Orthopaedic and Sports Physical Therapy 27(1):32–41

Thein L, McNamara C 1997 Aquatic rehabilitation of clients with musculoskeletal conditions of the extremities. In: Ruoti R G, Morris D M, Cole A J (eds) Aquatic rehabilitation. Lippincott, Philadelphia

Thorpe D E, Reilly M 2000 The effect of an aquatic resistive exercise program on lower extremity strength, energy expenditure, functional mobility, balance and self-perception in an adult with cerebral palsy: a retrospective case report. Journal of Aquatic Physiotherapy 8(2):18–24

Vandervoort A A 1999 Ankle mobility and postural stability. Physiotherapy Theory and Practice 15(2): 91–103

Weiner D K 2002 Improving pain management for older adults: an urgent agenda for the educator, investigator, and practitioner. Pain 97(1–2):1–4

Whitley J, Schoene L 1987 Comparison of heart rate responses: water walking versus treadmill walking. Physical Therapy 67(10):1501–1504

Willen C, Stibrant Sunnerhagen K, Grimby G 2001 Dynamic water exercise in individuals with late poliomyelitis. Archives of Physical Medicine and Rehabilitation 82:66–72

Woollacott M H 1993 Age-related changes in posture and movement. Journal of Gerontology 48 (Special Issue):56–60

Woollacott M H, Manchester D L 1993 Anticipatory postural adjustments in older adults: are changes in response characteristics due to changes in strategy? Journal of Gerontology 48(2):M64–M70

Wyatt F B, Milam S, Manske R C, Deere R 2001 The effects of aquatic and traditional exercise programs on persons with knee osteoarthritis. Journal of Strength and Conditioning Research 15(3):337–340

Zamparo P, Pagliaro P 1998 The energy cost of level walking before and after hydro-kinesy therapy in patients with spastic paresis. Scandinavian Journal of Medicine and Science in Sport 8:222–228

14 Physiotherapy for pelvic floor dysfunction in the aged care setting

Ruth Sapsford

This chapter aims to:

- give an overview of pelvic organ and pelvic floor muscle (PFM) function
- explain the normal age-related changes in these organ systems
- describe the conditions, causes and symptoms of bladder and bowel dysfunction that commonly occur in the elderly
- outline the management of each condition, and indicate what physiotherapy intervention is appropriate
- provide a detailed description of physiotherapy techniques suggested for the specific conditions.

Introduction

Pelvic organ function, like all body systems, deteriorates with age. However, the recent onset of symptoms may be the result of changes in a patient's medical condition, or pharmacological or dietary intake. Physiotherapists need to be cognizant of this and ensure that these factors are addressed before instituting treatment.

Pelvic floor muscles and their function

The pelvic floor must provide support for the pelvic organs at rest and with activity. It contributes to urinary and anal continence and releases for elimination. The predominance of slow twitch muscle fibres enables continuous tonic muscle activity. It is a musculoskeletal unit with the passive subsystem limiting range of organ descent, the active subsystem providing muscular support, outlet closure and release, and the neural subsystem ensuring that the tonic muscles are active at rest with recruitment of strength occurring at the appropriate time and speed. Details of the muscle complex are provided in Table 14.1.

Pelvic floor and abdominal muscle co-activation

It has now been established that the PFMs are part of the local abdominal muscle capsular system. Like other components – the diaphragm, transversus abdominis and the deep fibres of multifidus – the PFMs have been shown to have an anticipatory or feedforward activation prior to a rapid

Table 14.1
The pelvic floor muscles

Layers	Muscles	Attachments	Function
Superficial	Bulbospongiosus	Perineal body to clitoris Perineal body to penile bulb	Sexual arousal Urethral emptying and sexual arousal
	Ischiocavernosus	Ischial tub. to clitoris Ischial tub. to penile body	Sexual arousal Penile erection
	Superficial transverse perineum	Ischial tub. to perineal body	Perineal stability
	External anal sphincter	Coccyx to perineal body	Anal continence
Intermediate (NB: gender variations occur)	Intrinsic urethral sphincter	Intramural urethra	Resting urethral pressure and rapid urethral closure before ↑ intra-abdominal pressure
	Compressor urethrae	Ischiopubic ramus to urethra	
	Urethrovaginal sphincter	Urethra to perineal body	
Deep (levator ani)	Puborectalis	U-shaped muscle from pubic bone around anorectal junction	Maintains anorectal angle for continence
	Pubococcygeus (PC)	Pubic bone and arcuate line to tip of coccyx	Compresses and supports vagina and rectum
	Iliococcygeus	Arcuate line and ischial spine to sides of coccyx	Rectal support
	(Ischio)coccygeus	Ischial spine and sacrospinous ligament to sides of lower sacral segments	Rectal support

arm movement (Hodges & Richardson 1996, Hodges et al 1997, 2002, Moseley et al 2002). Co-activation of the abdominal and pelvic floor muscles during voluntary exercise has been shown in recent research. During a maximal PFM contraction the abdominal obliques and transversus abdominis are activated (Neumann & Gill 2002, Sapsford et al 2001). The abdominal muscle response varied depending on the position of the lumbar spine - whether in flexion, extension or a neutral position. The reverse response has also been demonstrated with pubococcygeus (the main PFM) and the external anal sphincter contracting during isometric abdominal holds. As the strength of the abdominal hold increased, the PFM activity increased (Sapsford & Hodges 2001).

Relaxation of the abdominal wall also affects the activity in the PFM, with pubococcygeal EMG activity falling below its resting baseline when the abdominal wall was allowed to relax and sag forward (Sapsford & Hodges 2001).

Urethrovesical function

The bladder is the only smooth muscle hollow organ under voluntary control. Its interlacing muscle layers, which constitute the detrusor muscle, allow extensibility during filling with a minimal increase in pressure. The pressure in the filling phase is generally $<10\,cmH_2O$. The bladder has a capacity of 500–600 ml in healthy people, though there is no finite limit and larger volumes are frequently noted. Emptying generally occurs at 70–75% of capacity, leaving a residual of zero. The rate of filling, which is a continuous process, depends on fluid intake, ambient temperature, alcohol and certain drugs. Fluid intake is extremely variable and so influences voiding frequency. Urine is produced in a circadian pattern with antidiuretic hormone, produced by the posterior pituitary gland, reducing production at night. Thus the frequency of daytime voiding with a fluid intake of 1.5–2 litres is between 5 and 8 times. Nocturia, defined as waking from sleep to void, occurs once in 22% of females and 12% of males aged between 14 and 69 years (Boedker et al 1989). The term polyuria is applied to urine production >2500 ml in 24 hours.

The bladder neck, at the apex of the bladder base (the trigone), should be closed during filling. The bladder neck is the proximal part of the urethra and is embedded within the detrusor muscle. In males it is the site of the smooth muscle internal urethral sphincter, which prevents retrograde ejaculation. This sphincter is under autonomic control and has no equivalent in the female.

The female urethra is 3–4 cm in length. Its closing pressure at rest is dependent on the mucosa, which is oestrogen sensitive, the vascular submucosa, also oestrogen sensitive, elastic fibres which resist distension, smooth muscle layers and the intrinsic striated muscle urethral sphincter. The urethra has no direct attachment of the PFM, but is embedded in the lower third of the anterior vaginal wall, which provides its support. Thus when the vagina loses its support so does the urethra. In the male the urethral smooth muscle component extends through the prostate with the striated sphincter distal to the prostatic apex.

Urethral pressure increases occur with voluntary pelvic floor contractions and with strong isometric abdominal contractions (Sapsford et al 1998). However, the urethral pressure must increase automatically prior to increases in intra-abdominal pressure that occur with lifting, sneezing, coughing and laughing. Increases in urethral closing pressure during a cough occur in the distal part of the urethra and precede the increase in bladder pressure by 200–250 milliseconds (Constantinou & Govan 1982, Thind et al 1990). These changes, measured in females, are attributed to the periurethral sphincter muscles in the intermediate layer of the pelvic floor (DeLancy 1990).

Urinary continence – what maintains it?

Continence depends on a number of factors and like other systems within the human body can still function effectively even if there is some degree of impairment. Urethral pressure must be greater than bladder pressure except during micturition. This is dependent on:

- bladder pressure that remains low during filling
- urethral closing pressure that is stable
- appropriate recruitment of the periurethral sphincter mechanism during increases in intra-abdominal pressure.

Urethral instability has been noted in 25% of incontinent women referred to an assessment clinic. With the sound of running water urethral pressure was noted to fall by 30% or more in these women, giving a sensation of urge (Skehan et al 1990). Appropriate urethral pressure increases, prior to the bladder pressure increase, did not occur in women with stress urinary incontinence (Thind et al 1990).

Micturition – the process

Voiding generally occurs in sitting in females and standing in males.

- On sitting the pelvic floor and the abdominal muscles relax.
- The PFM, bladder neck and vagina descend.
- Vaginal dorsal movement with descent allows the urethrovesical angle to widen and the bladder neck to open.
- Urine can then flow into the proximal urethra.
- This triggers the detrusor to contract, thus shortening and widening the urethra.
- The bladder keeps contracting until it is empty.
- At the end of voiding the urethra closes and the pelvic floor is elevated into its resting position.
- In men the abdominal wall must be relaxed in standing to allow pelvic floor relaxation and urethral opening.

Neurological control of voiding

The control of voiding occurs in the pons and is relayed through the sacral micturition reflex centre (S2–4). Studies have shown increased regional cerebral blood flow in the right dorsomedial pontine tegmentum, the periaqueductal grey matter, the hypothalamus and the right inferior frontal gyrus during voiding (Blok et al 1997a). These areas control detrusor activity. The forebrain area may be associated with the decision to commence voiding. In study subjects who tried vigorously to void but were unable to do so despite a full bladder, blood flow increased in the right ventral pontine tegmentum. It seemed that this area controlled the urethral sphincter and pelvic floor muscles and may play a role in storage of urine. The area may also be involved in tonic pelvic floor muscle activity. Further studies on cerebral blood flow showed that the superomedial precentral gyrus, the most medial part of the motor cortex, was activated during voluntary pelvic floor muscle exercises. The area seemed to be involved in conscious withholding of urine, but had no connection with the pontine area responsible for automatic control of micturition (Blok et al 1997b).

Normal changes with ageing

The following changes may affect bladder function as people age.

Decreases

- Bladder capacity.
- Detrusor contractility.
- Urine flow rate.
- Urethral closing pressure at rest.
- PFM support.
- Oestrogen.
- Fluid intake (old people frequently lose their sense of thirst).
- Response to antidiuretic hormone.
- Cerebral inhibition of voiding.

Increases

- Frequency of daytime voiding.
- Nocturia.
- Bladder overactivity.
- Residual urine.
- Urethral and vaginal mobility related to parity and straining at stool.
- Atrophic urethritis and vaginitis.
- Benign prostatic hypertrophy.
- Night-time urine production.

These changes of bladder overactivity, decreased bladder contractility and increased residual urine have been shown in approximately half of a healthy, continent 80- and 90-year-old mixed gender population group (Resnick et al 1995).

Problems of urinary control with ageing

Pelvic floor functional systems are divided into urethrovesical, anorectal and in females uterovaginal. While changes with ageing occur in all functional and support systems, it is vaginal delivery in women, with stretch to passive structures and partial pelvic floor neuropathy, which is generally considered the catalyst for problems in later life. These problems may be latent for many years.

Menopausal effects with the withdrawal of oestrogen compound the problems. However, problems in old age are not confined to parous women, so other muscle factors, e.g. abdominal muscle recruitment, may also be implicated. In men, benign prostatic hypertrophy (BPH) is universal with ageing and contributes to urinary dysfunction.

While the prevalence of all types of pelvic floor dysfunction increases with age, a recent community-based survey across all ages (MacLennan et al 2000) showed that 46.2% of women and 11.1% of men acknowledged some form of major pelvic floor dysfunction at the time of the survey. Urinary incontinence was the most common condition. Women in the 70–74-year age bracket had a prevalence of 51.9% and men over 75 years 17.6%. Significant associations with pelvic floor dysfunction included increasing age, higher parity and the mode of delivery, increasing body mass index, respiratory problems and coughing, diabetes, osteoporosis and arthritis. Neurological conditions present their own set of problems.

Prevalence of frequent urinary incontinence in elderly nursing home patients was 50% (Ouslander et al 1982), with 16–25% amongst those in residential homes for the elderly (Tobin & Brocklehurst 1986a). Faecal incontinence also occurred in 41% of those with urinary incontinence in those residential homes. These figures increase with increased dependency of the resident.

Lower urinary tract dysfunction

The main types of problems related to the urethrovesical system as they affect the ageing population are outlined below. Definitions are based on the 'The standardisation of terminology of lower urinary tract function: report from the standardisation sub-committee of the International Continence Society' (Abrams et al 2002). In older literature different terminology will be found.

Voiding-related problems

These include slow stream, difficulty in commencing, stream starts and stops, need to strain, post-micturition dribble, incomplete emptying (with resultant urinary tract infections).

Storage-related problems

- Increased daytime frequency: complaint of voiding too often.
- Nocturia: being woken from sleep to void.
- Urgency: sudden compelling desire to pass urine.
- Stress urinary incontinence: involuntary leakage on effort or exertion, sneeze or cough.
- Urge urinary incontinence: involuntary leakage accompanied by or preceded by urgency.
- Mixed urinary incontinence: a combination of both stress and urge incontinence.
- Nocturnal enuresis: loss of urine occurring during sleep.
- Continuous urinary incontinence: continuous leakage.

Conditions of urinary dysfunction are explained in more detail in the following sections. Advice and some management strategies are also included. Physiotherapeutic interventions are described in detail later in the chapter.

Voiding dysfunction

Voiding dysfunction implies that there is a reduced urine flow rate or reduction of volume voided. Voiding frequency may be increased as the bladder is only partially emptied each time.

Causes

1. Underactive detrusor contractility occurs in many older persons (Resnick et al 1995). In elderly women (mean age > 80 years), normal bladder contractility was associated with a vaginal oestrogen effect in almost 70% of those studied. In those with impaired bladder contractility an oestrogen effect was found in only half as many. The authors suggested that oestrogen deficiency should be considered as a potential factor in impaired bladder contractility in women (Kuchel & Resnick 1997).
2. Outlet obstruction. There is a strong relationship between large cystoceles and urodynamically proven voiding dysfunction in females. However, there was no evidence that other forms of uterovaginal prolapse caused voiding dysfunction (Manning et al 1998). In males urethral outlet obstruction is related to prostatic enlargement.
3. Urinary tract infections (UTI) are another consequence of residual urine and are common amongst elderly women in retirement communities. If, however, the bacteriuria is asymptomatic there seems to be little benefit from investigation and treatment (Abrutyn et al 1994). Bacteriuria occurs in 25–40% of non-catheterized patients in long-term residential care. Pyuria is common in this group, and may not be associated with bacteriuria (McMurdo & Gillespie 2000). Overuse of antibiotic medication provides opportunities for antimicrobial resistance to develop. Thus judicious use is advised.
4. Post-micturition dribble describes an involuntary loss of urine immediately after finishing passing urine. In men it usually occurs after leaving the toilet and is associated with pooling of urine in the bulbar part of the urethra. In women it occurs after rising from the toilet and may be associated with a cystocele. Management for men includes 'milking' of the residual urine from the bulbar urethra at the end of the void. Upward pressure with three or four fingers behind the scrotum and dragging the fingers forward should help to empty the residual urine.

Physiotherapy interventions for voiding dysfunction include use of a voiding position and pattern and double voiding PFM exercise.

Urinary incontinence

'While it is often stated that urinary incontinence is a major factor in referral for institutional care, there are few convincing data to support this assertion' (Fonda et al 1998, p 280). Thom et al (1997), though, determined that the risk of hospitalization was 30% higher in women and 50% higher in men following medically recognized urinary incontinence. It also substantially increased the risk of admission to a nursing home.

Older frail people include those in long-term care, with dementia, and the house-bound who need assistance for some aspects of daily living. Co-morbid conditions with urinary incontinence within this group include faecal impaction, confusional states, functional disabilities and medication. While the types of problems amongst this group of people have been documented, validated research into the long-term efficacy of treatment for their urinary incontinence has been limited (Fonda et al 1998). Much of the information results from studies on community-dwelling, cognitively intact, old people.

In frail nursing home residents the causes of urinary incontinence are:

- bladder overactivity
- effort activities which increase intra-abdominal pressure above the urethral pressure
- urethral obstruction
- bladder underactivity
- bladder overactivity with impaired contractility (Griffiths et al 2002, Resnick et al 1996).

Quality of life (QOL) in response to changing continence status has been investigated in 90 000 nursing home residents (Dubeau et al 1999). Incontinence seems to have the greatest impact on QOL in those with moderate impairment of activities of daily living, but even affected those with functional and cognitive impairment. These findings seem to indicate that interventions to improve continence would be worthwhile.

Thus many nursing home residents are toileted 2-hourly (timed voiding) to improve their continence status, usually without consulting the resident, even though it is intrusive, costly and labour intensive. Prompted voiding, in which nursing home patients were asked whether they would try to void and were offered assistance to do so, resulted in significant reduction in incontinent episodes (Schnelle 1990). This may be a preferable alternative to timed voiding.

In a recent study mentally competent residents were questioned about their treatment preferences to attain a 50% or 100% improvement in continence (Brandt et al 2002). The majority of residents did not want day/night toileting and more than one-third did not desire 2-hourly day voiding. Not all would take a pill to improve their continence status. Incontinent residents were less ready to accept these treatment options than those who were continent. The authors suggest that residents should be consulted about the treatment interventions that are acceptable rather than treating them all alike.

However, even in the old (>90 years) with severe frailty and multiple pathologies, detailed assessment and active management of their incontinence resulted in overall improvement in more than half those investigated (Gautum et al 1999).

Increased daytime frequency

This is the complaint of voiding more frequently than usual and is based on previous voiding patterns for that individual. While frequency of voiding in younger people is dependent on fluid intake, level of physical activity and ambient temperature, in the aged other factors are added to this list.

Causes Increased daytime frequency may be due to urinary tract infection, bladder overactivity, incomplete bladder emptying, anxiety or medication such as diuretics.

Management The traditional method of assessment uses a frequency/volume chart in which the number of voids and the volume per void are recorded. This record needs to be kept for at least 24 hours and preferably 48 hours. Fluid intake and types of fluid should be recorded at the same time. However, many community-based patients find such monitoring tedious and this would be compounded in the aged care setting. Recording the number of voids per 24 hours and the times of voiding as well as the fluid intake (mugs of fluid per day) can be an easier alternative.

Advice regarding modifying fluid intake and strategies to defer voiding can then be provided.

Physiotherapy interventions include use of a voiding position and pattern, deferred voiding, and tonic PFM re-education.

Nocturia

This is defined as the number of voids preceded and followed by sleep. It is considered pathological if it occurs more than twice a night. This frequency has been noted in 50% of those older than 80 years (Swithinbank et al 1998a).

Causes

1. Nocturnal polyuria This occurs when >35% of total 24-hour urine output is produced in the sleeping hours. This was noted in 71% of 80-year-olds with nocturia (Swithinbank et al 1998a). This change in the usual circadian pattern of urine production occurs in normal, continent and urodynamically assessed elders (Morgan et al 2000).

Factors associated with disordered circadian urine output (Weiss et al 1998) include:

- diuretic medication, alcohol, caffeine, and excessive fluid intake late before retiring
- congestive heart disease, peripheral oedema (accumulation of water in extracellular space)
- stroke, diabetes
- renal insufficiency
- decreased plasma vasopression levels.

An increased oedema ratio before sleep has been noted in the elderly with nocturia – that is the ratio of extracellular water to total body water volume (Sugaya et al 2001).

2. Sleep apnoea Significant associations have been found between nocturia and sleep apnoea, irritable bladder symptoms and apnoea, and nocturia and body mass index in adults of both genders older than 55 years (Umlauf et al 1999).

3. Nocturnal detrusor overactivity (NDO) This was the most common cause of nocturia – in more than half the subjects studied. Mixed nocturnal polyuria and NDO occurs in about one-third of the cases (Weiss et al 1998).

Effects Nocturia causes sleep disturbance in the frail and increased risk of traumatic injury from falls. Many women consider it bothersome if it occurs more than two times a night.

Management Strategies suggested for nocturia, after medical aspects have been addressed, include:

- Evening fluid restriction. Those who complain of thirst during the night may ease this by sucking an ice cube rather than consuming a full glass of water.
- Timed diuretics. These may be taken in the late afternoon and this may help clear peripheral oedema accumulated during the day.
- An afternoon nap. Resting with legs horizontal or elevated for an hour or two may assist extracellular fluid return, rather than all of this occurring at night.
- Topical vaginal oestrogen. This is more effective than systemic oestrogen in decreasing urgency and frequency (Cardozo et al 2001).

Oral desmopressin (vasopressin), an antidiuretic agent, has been used in the treatment of nocturnal polyuria. However, side effects of headache, nausea, dizziness and abdominal pain have occurred. In patients over 65 years, hyponatraemia, where the serum sodium levels fall below normal, is a significant problem and generally rules out this form of treatment in the older age groups of both genders (Abrams et al 2001).

Physiotherapy interventions include PFM tonic re-education, use of a voiding position and pattern and daytime deferment to increase bladder capacity.

Urgency and urge incontinence

This is experienced as a strong desire to void that cannot be deferred. It frequently results in immediate urine loss at the onset of urge, or as approaching or undressing at the toilet. Loss is often a large volume that necessitates a change of clothing. In many cases it is perceived as a penile or perineal sensation which can trigger a response of perineal pressure by hand or crossing of legs in females. Males may compress the penis. These actions mimic those used by young children who are gaining bladder control. These strategies have been shown to have an inhibitory effect on bladder pressure, via afferents of the dorsal nerve of penis and clitoris and afferents from the hip adductor muscles (Lindstrom & Sudsuang 1989). Urge urinary incontinence, but not stress urinary incontinence, has also been implicated in non-spinal, non-traumatic falls and fractures (Edwards 2000).

Symptoms

- Perineal or penile sensation of urge to void.
- Inability to defer voiding, worse as the person nears the toilet.
- Increased day frequency.
- Nocturia.
- Large volume urine loss.
- Urge often occurs on rising from bed or chair.

- Urge can be triggered by the sound of running water, homecoming, key in the door.

Prevalence Urge incontinence occurs in 23.9% of males and 36.4% of females over 70 years.

Those with weak or intermittent stream are more likely to report a sense of urge. Age and female gender increase the risk of urge with or without incontinence (Nuotio et al 2001).

Causes

1. Decreased bladder inhibition due to:
   - ↓cerebral blood flow, particularly underperfusion of the right superior frontal lobe (Griffiths et al 1994)
   - neurological conditions (stroke, parkinsonism), which can interfere with normal inhibitory pathways
   - ↓PFM support of the bladder (Gunnarsson & Mattiasson 1999).
2. Decreased urethral closing pressure:
   - ↓periurethral oestrogen results in ↓urethral closing pressure (oestrogen nourishes the urethral mucosa and vascular submucosa)
   - ↓periurethral muscle activity
   - spontaneous fall in maximal urethral pressure (urethral instability) prior to unprovoked detrusor contraction (Wise et al 1993).
3. Bladder overactivity due to mechanical factors:
   - prolapse drag ± urethral kinking
   - uterine fibroid pressure
   - BPH outlet obstruction (Rosier et al 1995)
   - Bladder stones, tumour.
4. Decreased bladder contractility with or without bladder overactivity (Griffiths et al 2002).
5. Medication - diuretics, anticholinergics, antipsychotics, sedatives, hypnotics (Kirschner-Hermanns et al 1997).
6. Anxiety.

Management As existing medication can contribute to urgency and urge incontinence, a review of medication is important before any treating medications are added. Response to treatment of urinary urge incontinence in the elderly varies.

Use of oxybutynin chloride, an antispasmodic, in those with bladder overactivity ± impaired detrusor contractility (mean age of 79 years) resulted in side effects of a dry mouth and increased post-void residuals. Constipation occurred rarely. Treatment was successful in both groups, but cure rates were less in those with impaired contractility (Miller et al 2000). Outcome measures of treatment in women >75 years using oxybutynin + bladder retraining for 6–8 weeks resulted in reduction of day frequency and incontinent episodes (Wagg et al 1999). Topical vaginal oestrogen is also helpful (Cardozo et al 2001).

Physiotherapy interventions include monitoring of urinary output, via a frequency/volume chart, and fluid intake, urge control techniques and retraining tonic and strong PFM support.

Factors predicting urine loss prior to treatment in the elderly include fluid intake, voiding frequency, impaired orientation in time on cognitive testing. Factors that predicted persistent loss, after treatment, were underperfusion of the cerebral cortex, reduced bladder sensation, and impaired orientation in time on cognitive testing. The latter two are consistent with underperfusion of the right superior frontal lobes (Griffiths et al 1994, 1996).

Stress urinary incontinence

Stress incontinence occurs when the bladder pressure (due to an increase in abdominal pressure) is greater than the urethral closing pressure. It affects women predominantly, but may be less of a problem in the aged than urge incontinence. This is particularly so if the person coughs or sneezes infrequently. It can occur in men following radical prostatectomy for cancer of the prostate. Urine loss is generally a spot loss at the time of increased intra-abdominal pressure. Also continuous seepage of urine can occur with walking and moving if the resting urethral pressure is low.

Symptoms A spot loss of urine associated with sneeze, cough, laugh, lift, bend.

Causes

- Weak PFM support of the urethra and vagina.
- Weak periurethral sphincter muscles, which are responsible for urethral closure prior to increases in intra-abdominal pressure (IAP) with effort.
- Increased vaginal, urethral and bladder neck mobility due to vaginal deliveries, regular straining at defecation, chronic coughing and obesity.
- Obesity generates higher resting abdominal pressures and higher pressures on coughing than occur in those within a normal weight range (Sullivan et al 2000).
- Weak abdominal tonic and phasic activity. When women lean forward to bend or lift, the abdominal wall can sag forward. It seems that transversus abdominis does not hold automatically. When the abdomen sags, pubococcygeal resting activity falls below baseline (Sapsford & Hodges 2001). It has been observed clinically in those with weak abdominal muscles, that the abdomen bulges instead of drawing in during coughing. This results in decreased PFM recruitment.

Associated conditions Elderly women with stress urinary incontinence are more likely to have:

- atrophic vaginitis
- cystocele
- rectocele
- hysterectomy

- oestrogen replacement therapy
- greater body mass index
- increased parity
- decreased vaginal muscle tone
- decreased sustained PFM contraction (Burns et al 1993).

Treatment Options for women include a conservative approach of PFM rehabilitation (Berghmans et al 1998), or a surgical intervention such as Burch colposuspension or tension free vaginal tape. Treatment programmes for post-radical prostatectomy incontinence that included pelvic floor exercise ± neuromuscular stimulation found no difference in outcomes 32 weeks post surgery (Moore et al 1998). Recent clinical observations indicate that increasing intensity of abdominal exercise, with pelvic floor holds, has resulted in a marked decrease in urine loss in men with stress incontinence following radical prostatectomy. The added demands of uphill running (which requires increased tonic abdominal activity) have further enhanced continence (P. Dornan 2002, personal communication). Some of those in the aged care setting will be able to cope with increased abdominal muscle activity.

Physiotherapy intervention focuses on PFM rehabilitation.

Nocturnal enuresis

This is the term for loss of urine during sleep.

Causes It was noted in many older subjects (mean age 79 years) that enuresis occurred in close time relationship to an episode of sleep apnoea or hypopnoea (Ouslander et al 1999). Specific sleep disorders may be implicated in the pathophysiology of night-time incontinence. Associated conditions include nocturia >2, urgency and urge incontinence and stress urinary incontinence, but enuresis is not always related to age (Swithinbank et al 1998b).

Management Strategies must first deal with other medical problems. In those who do not wake to void, arousal to bladder sensation does not occur, though bladder sensation may be impaired even in waking hours. People who are mentally competent may be prepared to use an alarm to be woken after 4 hours of sleep to void.

Continuous urinary incontinence

This tends to be a continuous loss of urine both day and night. Loss that only occurs in the upright position is likely to be due to low urethral resting pressure.

Causes

1. Non contracting bladder. In the elderly this is likely to be related to some form of autonomic neuropathy, such as can occur in diabetes. Urine loss occurs when the pressure of urine is greater than the resting urethral pressure. Voiding can occur with an increase in intra-abdominal pressure, e.g. with straining, but seepage will occur in the absence of bladder awareness and regular emptying. Management options include intermittent clean self-catheterization or an indwelling catheter.

2. Bladder outlet obstruction. Prostatic enlargement can obstruct the urethra, leading to straining and overflow. Bladder volumes may reach high levels. This may also result from a cystocele, which kinks the urethra and restricts flow. However, reduction of the cystocele, either by a pessary or surgery, can unmask an incompetent urethral sphincter and this leads to further incontinence.

Urogenital prolapse

Pelvic organs are supported by passive and active systems - fascia and ligaments and striated muscle. Failure in either of these systems can lead to prolapse. However, anterior pubococcygeus histological examination showed no difference in muscle fibre type percentage and fibre diameter in patients with prolapse and/or urinary incontinence when compared to asymptomatic women. Fibre types were 66% slow twitch fibres in comparison with 48% in other human female muscle (Heit et al 1996).

Prolapse is a protrusion of a pelvic organ or structure distal to its normal anatomical level. It can involve the bladder (cystocele), the urethra and bladder (cystourethrocele), the uterus and vagina (uterine descent, vaginal vault prolapse, enterocele) or the rectum (rectocele). Any organ descent within the vagina is termed a 1st degree prolapse. A 2nd degree prolapse reaches the introitus, and a 3rd degree protrudes beyond the introitus. While a cystourethrocele (the anterior compartment) is the most common type of prolapse, the majority of patients demonstrate problems in the middle and posterior compartments as well. These have been demonstrated on dynamic cystoproctography (Maglinte et al 1999). Significant associations have been found between large rectoceles and anal incontinence.

Prevalence

This is very difficult to ascertain as many prolapses are asymptomatic. In a younger population, 20–59 years, 30.8% of the women had a prolapse, but only 2% were 2nd degree. Associated conditions in this group were parity, PFM strength and maximum birth weight (Samuelsson et al 1999). By the age of 80 years the lifetime risk of undergoing surgery for prolapse in America was 11.1% (Olsen et al 1997).

Causes

- Congenital collagen deficits - a decrease in the total collagen content has been observed. Women with these types of problems have been noted to have joint hypermobility (Norton et al 1995).
- Increasing parity plus larger birth weight babies.
- Increases in intra-abdominal pressure such as occur with frequent coughing in chronic obstructive pulmonary disease and smoking. Frequent straining at stool in those with difficult evacuation can contribute to prolapse (Spence-Jones et al 1994).
- Vaginal vault prolapse may occur following hysterectomy, or bladder neck suspension.

Symptoms

- Dragging discomfort and/or a sense of heaviness due to abnormal tension on the stretched passive tissues. This is worse after prolonged standing or at the end of the day.
- A lump protruding from the vagina.
- Urinary symptoms, e.g. stress urinary incontinence, urgency and frequency.
- Incomplete bladder emptying, resulting from urethral kinking, with frequency and urinary tract infection.
- Uterine prolapse is often accompanied by low backache.
- A rectocele often results in incomplete bowel emptying.

Management

Stretched passive structures will not shorten with pelvic floor exercise. However, in cases of heaviness and dragging, improving tonic PFM support can relieve these symptoms as well as those of low backache. Symptomatic prolapses generally require surgical repair. Uterine prolapse can be supported with a pessary that elevates the cervix. This requires adequate PFM tissue to maintain the pessary in position. A pessary can be a long-term option in some women. However, those who strain to evacuate will be likely to push the pessary out. Women with a rectocele may use upward perineal body pressure, or backward pressure on the rectocele per vaginam, to assist evacuation. Upward perineal pressure increases rectal tone (Gosselink & Schouten 2002).

Physiotherapy interventions for these conditions include tonic PFM rehabilitation, and teaching of voiding and defecation positions and patterns. These are beneficial taught prior to surgery to enable optimal function postoperatively.

Anorectal function

Normal anorectal function results in defecation between three times a day and three times a week in more than 90% of a healthy working population (Drossman et al 1982). Ease of emptying depends on fibre and fluid intake, colonic motility, rectal sensitivity and contractility, pelvic floor support and anal release.

Colonic motility

Liquid contents pass into the colon via the ileocaecal valve and traverse the ascending, transverse, descending and sigmoid colon into the rectum. Different types of colonic activity either move the contents back and forth to allow absorption of water and electrolytes, or propel them onwards. This peristalsis is stimulated by food ingestion – gastrocolic reflex – and in some people by moving and walking. Coffee has been observed to trigger rectosigmoid motility, and a subsequent desire to evacuate, in some people, and this occurs with or without caffeine (Brown et al 1990). Ingestion of hot water does not produce the same effect as coffee in this population. A similar stimulating effect of coffee, either with or without caffeine, has been reported recently on blood pressure and nervous system activity (Corti et al 2002). In healthy people increasing physical activity does not generally change the rate of passage of intestinal contents, but the effect in the poorly mobile aged population is likely to differ.

Rectal filling

The rectum begins at the sacral convexity and ends at the anorectal junction just anterior to the tip of the coccyx. The rectal smooth muscle walls, inner circular and outer longitudinal, extend into the anal canal. Here the inner circular muscle thickens to form the internal anal sphincter (IAS), which is under autonomic control and is responsible for 85% of anal resting pressure. The striated external anal sphincter (EAS) encircles the IAS, contributing 15% to the anal resting pressure. Puborectalis is incorporated into the deep part of EAS and acts as one with it. Voluntary contraction of the anal sphincter - squeeze pressure - can double the resting pressure but cannot be maintained for long.

Initial awareness of rectal filling occurs with <30 ml of contents (sensory threshold volume). This awareness triggers the IAS to relax, and there is a simultaneous increase in EAS activity to maintain continence. This IAS relaxation allows the very sensitive anal mucosa to sample the rectal contents, but defecation can still be deferred. The IAS activity recovers quickly with a consequent reduction in EAS activity back to resting levels. Further intermittent rectal filling will result in a desire to evacuate at around 60–100 ml of contents (defecation threshold volume). At this time the IAS remains relaxed and EAS activity is increased to maintain continence until evacuation is imminent. This reflex is termed the rectoanal inhibitory reflex (RAIR) and is mediated by receptors of the enteric nervous system within the rectal wall. If evacuation does not proceed, the rectum accommodates to the contents, the sensation of rectal fullness dissipates, and the IAS and EAS return to their normal resting pressure levels. The desire to empty may not occur again until the next bolus of faecal matter enters the rectum, possibly on the next day. Such a definite RAIR response to rectal filling may not occur if contents pass into the rectum very gradually (Rasmussen 1994).

Anal continence – what maintains it?

For a person to be continent the anal pressure must be greater than the rectal pressure whenever contents are present. Resting rectal pressure is <5 cmH_2O, whereas resting anal pressure may be 75–80 cmH_2O (Akervall et al 1990).

The following factors contribute to anal continence:

- anal pressure that is greater than rectal pressure
- puborectalis maintains the anorectal angle at or <90 degrees
- awareness of rectal contents
- RAIR relaxes the IAS, but EAS activity compensates to maintain continence
- rectal compliance and capacity can accommodate contents
- rate of filling, consistency and volume of contents must be within reasonable limits.

Defecation – the process

The person sits or squats and bowel emptying proceeds in the following order.

- Relaxation of the pelvic floor occurs, in particular puborectalis and the EAS, and the abdominal muscles.
- The pelvic floor descends, the anorectal angle widens and the anal canal widens and shortens.
- The rectum empties due to its intrinsic contractions.
- If effort is required to commence or continue evacuation, the waist widens sideways (bracing) due to the combined action of diaphragmatic descent and activation of the transverse, internal oblique and external oblique abdominal muscles. This increases IAP.
- The PFM hold isometrically in the lowered position to support the rectum against the increased IAP (Lubowski et al 1992).
- The abdominal wall is bulged forward by further descent of the diaphragm and lengthening of the held abdominal muscles (Chiarelli & Markwell 1992, Markwell & Sapsford 1995). This bulging allows release of puborectalis and EAS.
- Evacuation proceeds until the rectum is empty. However, complete emptying does not always occur.
- The pressure in IAS and EAS is restored once the rectum is empty and the pelvic floor ascends to its resting position (Markwell 1998). This is termed the closing reflex.

Changes in anorectal function with ageing (Akervall et al 1990)

Decreases

- Maximal rectal volume.
- Resting anal pressure.
- Maximal anal squeeze pressure.
- Volume of contents to trigger RAIR.
- Pelvic floor support.

Increases

- Threshold pressure to trigger RAIR.
- Threshold pressure for perception of rectal filling.

Rectal contractions were observed in 78% of the normal sampled population. There was an association with gender (less in females), but not age. While increasing parity did not show any effect on anal function in women in the study by Akervall et al (1990), sphincter integrity and pressures, both IAS and EAS, can be affected by vaginal delivery (Sultan et al 1994, Wynne et al 1996). Age seems to affect maximal squeeze pressure more than the resting pressure.

There are also changes in intestinal motility that influence function. These include decreased colonic contractions and decreased gastrocolic reflex. Immobility contributes to delayed colon transit.

Problems of anorectal function with ageing

Constipation, faecal incontinence, faecal impaction and obstructed defecation are the most common problems facing those in aged care. They do not seem to be separate entities as they can be in younger people, for constipation and obstructed defecation lead to faecal impaction in which contents then bypass the impacted faecal mass and result in soiling and incontinence.

Constipation

In true constipation intestinal contents are slow to reach the rectum, hence there is a decreased frequency of evacuation. Slow colonic transit occurs throughout the life spectrum, but in the aged other factors may cause or exacerbate slow transit. The more common causes are listed.

Causes

- Decreased fibre and fluid intake.
- Megacolon/megarectum.
- Decreased neurological functioning affecting autonomic and enteric systems.
- Endocrine changes such as hypothyroidism.
- Pharmacological ingestion – e.g. opiates, antidepressants, diuretics, iron, anticholinergics.
- Immobility.
- Irritable bowel syndrome.
- Faecal impaction and outlet obstruction.

Symptoms (Talley et al 1993)

- Straining >25% of time.
- Hard stool >25% of time.
- Feeling of incomplete evacuation >25% of time.
- Fewer than 2–3 stools per week.
- Postprandial abdominal bloating.
- Haemorrhoids.
- Rectal mucosal prolapse.
- Laxative and enema use are indicative of constipation.

Faecal impaction with decreased frequency of evacuation and consequent faecal incontinence is particularly common in demented patients and those with severe mobility impairments in the nursing home population (Chassagne et al 2000).

Management This is a continual process in this group. Use of osmotic agents, e.g. lactulose, combined with rectal stimulants and weekly enemas resulted in fewer episodes of faecal incontinence in those patients who had complete rectal emptying (Chassagne et al 2000). This resulted in a reduced workload for the carers. In those who participated in prompted voiding for urinary function, there was also an increase in the frequency of bowel movements. Those whose urinary control improved on the prompted voiding regimen also had a greater proportion of continent bowel movements (Ouslander et al 1996). Suggested positive contributing factors were increased mobility for voiding, increased fluid intake at the prompted void (everyone was given fluid at the time of prompting) and possible positive response of faecal impaction to this programme.

Physiotherapy intervention in the management of constipation in nursing home patients is likely to be very limited. Less dependent, motivated residents will benefit from improving tonic PFM activity prior to defecation retraining.

Obstructed defecation

This is the term used when a patient reports the desire to evacuate but is unable to get the contents out. There is a feeling of anal blockage, incomplete emptying and a prolonged defecatory attempt. Use of upward digital perineal body pressure and digital disimpaction are also noted (Talley et al 1993). Obstructed defecation and slow colonic transit often coexist.

Signs noted on defecography are rectocele, enterocele, rectal prolapse, anal incontinence and excessive pelvic floor descent. Those with more vaginal deliveries and a hysterectomy are likely to be at greater risk. A gastrorectal reflex resulting in increased rectal tone occurs in healthy controls after the ingestion of food. It has also been noted in people with obstructed defecation who have normal colon transit times, but is impaired in those with prolonged transit (Gosselink & Schouten 2001).

Causes Poor rectal support results in excessive pelvic floor descent during attempted defecation (Markwell 1998). A rectocele allows rectal contents to be pushed into the lax rectal tissue and a bulge is noted in the vagina. Both of these conditions result in regular straining with later development of haemorrhoids as well as the signs mentioned earlier. Pain, due to repeated pudendal nerve stretch, may develop later.

Management As with constipation, less dependent motivated residents will benefit from:

- encouragement to respond to the desire to defecate after food ingestion – particularly ingestion after a prolonged period without food, e.g. in the morning
- adequate dietary fibre intake, frequently with a fibre supplement as well as fruit and vegetables; those people with coexisting slow colonic transit may find bloating is aggravated by wheat grain fibre products and other high fibre foods
- use of digital perineal support.

Physiotherapy intervention should improve tonic PFM activity prior to defecation retraining.

Anal incontinence

More recently the term anal incontinence has been used, instead of faecal incontinence (FI), as this includes accidental loss of gas, liquid or solid contents. While vaginal delivery has been stated as the precipitating factor in most cases of anal incontinence in a younger population, those in nursing home care present with two main problems. They either have faecal impaction with bypassing of the mass by liquid contents or a neurogenic cause. Symptoms such as diarrhoea must be investigated.

Prevalence In those >75 years living at home 3% reported regular FI (Edwards & Jones 2001). Figures for women were higher than for men. Prevalence figures vary depending on the criteria used – whether loss is occasional or daily or any stated frequency in between. Significant associations with FI were anxiety, depression and increasing disability. Amongst those in residential homes for the elderly 10.3% were incontinent one or more times a week (Tobin & Brocklehurst 1986b). There was an even distribution of those with faecal impaction and neurogenic incontinence. While the majority affected suffered from dementia, poor mobility was also a factor. Higher figures are reported for nursing homes.

Causes Pudendal nerve stretching during vaginal delivery may be the precursor of later neurogenic problems. Occult anal sphincter tears induced by vaginal delivery result in immediate problems of control, but neurogenic damage does not manifest itself until later in life, and is compounded by ageing and disease. These patients tend to pass formed stool. Repair of torn anal sphincters, as diagnosed by anal endosonography, can have benefit even in the elderly.

Faecal impaction and bypassing result from an accumulation of faecal matter in the rectum. These patients tend to have continual soiling. Decreased colon motility and gastrocolic reflexes, as well as an increased threshold for perception of rectal contents, mean that filling does not trigger a defecation response as it did in younger years. If then there is little pelvic floor support of the rectum on attempted evacuation in the presence of reduced rectal contractility, emptying will be infrequent and incomplete, and further rectal filling will add to the mass.

Incomplete rectal emptying with a small loss of residual contents, not associated with impaction, may occur in many of those in all areas of care and in the community. Contributing factors to incomplete emptying are consistency of faecal contents and poor rectal support during evacuation.

Management For nursing home residents with faecal impaction treatment involves ongoing care to relieve the impaction and prevent recurrence. Enemas to clear the impaction, followed by regular osmotic laxatives and enemas were used to keep the rectum empty. Residents with neurogenic incontinence were constipated with codeine phosphate and given twice weekly enemas (Tobin & Brocklehurst 1986b). The cure rate in residents who complied with the chosen regimen was 87% (Tobin & Brocklehurst 1986b).

Physiotherapy intervention of defecation retraining is helpful for those with incomplete emptying and loss some time later. The ingestion of a stool-bulking agent, such as psyllium, creates a bigger stool which empties more completely and this complements the retraining.

Physiotherapy interventions for urogenital and anorectal dysfunction in the aged care setting

Physiotherapists teaching the following strategies will only be able to assist the patient with using patterns of voiding, defecation and urge control for short periods. Thus further assistance and reinforcement of these patterns for the more dependent residents will rely on input from other staff. Thus physiotherapists who share information on functional activities by working together with the patient and staff will find this combined approach enhances patient care. Use of any of these strategies will depend on the mental competency of the individual, motivation, reinforcement of instruction and the ease of incorporating them into daily life.

Voiding position and pattern

This position and pattern is useful for incomplete bladder emptying, post-micturition dribble and in women with vaginal prolapse.

If women sit nearer the front of the toilet seat, they tend to sink back into the hole, resulting in posterior pelvic tilt and lumbar flexion. Some may also hold the grab rail and accentuate the spinal flexion.

Assist/encourage them to sit well back on the seat, sit erect, then lean forward at the hips. The feet need to be well supported. This position allows better anterior pelvic tilt and allows the relaxed abdominal wall to fall forward. This is assisted by gravity. Depending on flexibility, height and foot support they may support the trunk by hands propped on the thighs. Relaxation of the abdominal wall allows relaxation of the pubococcygeus and urethral sphincter.

Urine flow may be slow to start. Time must be allowed for the bladder to begin contracting. When the flow stops, sit upright for 5–10 seconds, then lean forward again. A further amount of urine may be emptied. This pattern can be repeated accompanied by the sound of running water, which may trigger a further bladder contraction. Thus the patient may do a double or even a triple void. Ideally straining should be avoided. However, when detrusor contractility is compromised, straining may be the only way, other than catheterization, that people can empty.

Defecation position and pattern

The following position and pattern are helpful in faecal incontinence due to incomplete emptying, obstructed defecation and in women with prolapse. In fact it seems to reduce the effort required for evacuation in many asymptomatic persons.

Rectal emptying requires rectal support, anal release and an effective expulsive effort (Markwell & Sapsford 1995). People who strain may not maintain rectal support as they push, and find it hard to empty or to empty completely. They frequently return to the toilet one or more times, to complete evacuation. Prior to learning an emptying pattern patients need to improve the PFM support by rehabilitating tonic muscle activity.

Sinking into the toilet seat results in lumbar flexion. Pushing to empty from this position increases lumbar flexion, tightens the anal outlet and pushes the perineum down. Sitting back on the seat provides thigh support and allows forward leaning at the hips. This forward lean opens the anus (Tagart 1966). Toe support provides trunk stability. The upper body

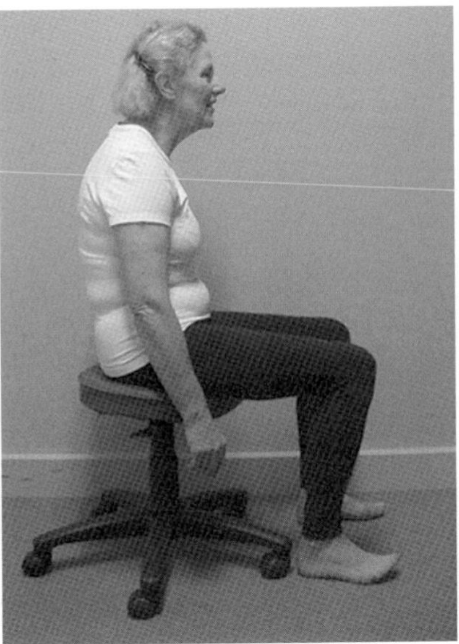

Figure 14.1
A flexed lumbar spine and slumped sitting position can lead to incomplete bladder and bowel emptying. Many older patients may be perched on a high seat with legs dangling. Foot support is needed for trunk stability.

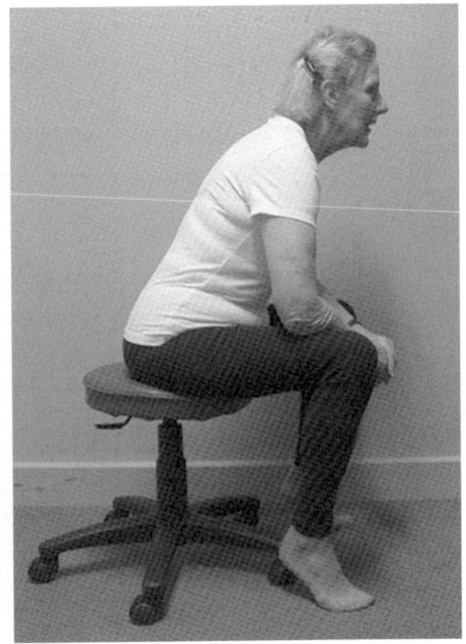

Figure 14.2
In forward lean sitting, while maintaining a good lumbar curve, it is easy to relax the abdominal wall for voiding. This is useful for all women, but is particularly helpful for those who suffer from post-micturition dribble.

can be supported through the arms with hands or forearms propped on the thighs. A good lumbar curve encourages a better pushing pattern. Assuming this position may be difficult for those who use a raised toilet seat. See Figures 14.1, 14.2, 14.3 and 14.4.

As the person pushes, the spine should not move, the lower ribs widen sideways (this action provides rectal support) and the abdomen bulges forward (this action opens the anal outlet) (Markwell & Sapsford 1995). If there is pelvic floor laxity, perineal descent will still occur using this pattern. Digital support of the perineum or ischiorectal fossa region (between the anus and the ischial tuberosity) may help in these cases. Digital support of the perineal body region during defecation has been shown to increase rectal tone in healthy controls and to a lesser extent in those with obstructed defecation (Gosselink & Schouten 2002). Upward pressure in the ischiorectal fossa region supplements or provides rectal support against the increased IAP. This support is normally provided by iliococcygeus. Frequently, initial emptying requires effort or digital support, then the rest of the contents are passed easily. This is more likely to occur if adequate fibre in the diet results in a soft, formed and textured stool. Contents that are pasty are harder to empty completely and require prolonged wiping attempts. Use of this defecation pattern, at the end of

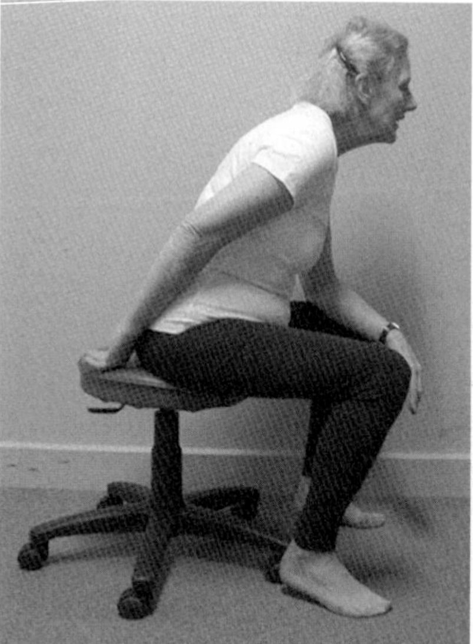

Figure 14.3
The position for defecation is similar to that used for voiding. Forward leaning at the hips opens the anal outlet. Forearms resting on thighs (one arm has been straightened for the purposes of the photograph), heels raised with weight resting on toes and eyes looking ahead, not down, all assist in maintaining a lumbar curve. This lumbar curve facilitates an effective evacuation pattern of abdominal bulging (see text).

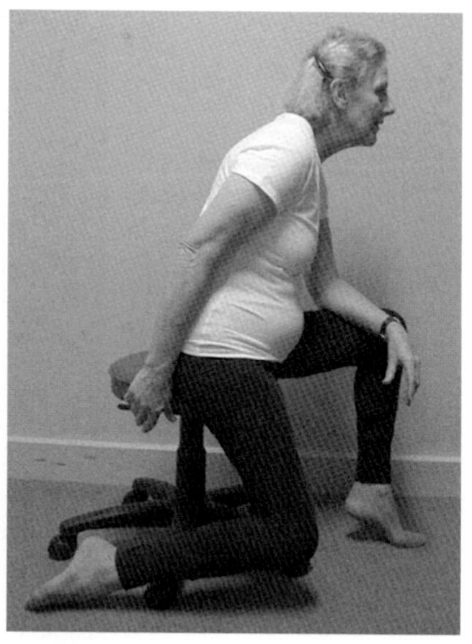

Figure 14.4
Those people using a raised toilet seat due to limited hip flexion after hip replacement may still be able to assume a forward lean position if the affected hip is in a more extended position with either knee flexion or extension.

the initial part of evacuation when the person feels that emptying is not complete, may empty any residual faecal matter, and avoid soiling.

Retraining, involving activation of support first followed by anal release while the support is maintained, can result in more effective emptying, when there is perineal descent. However, this is a complex pattern and may be beyond the ability of this group of patients to achieve. Referral to a physiotherapist who works with pelvic floor dysfunction may be an option for suitable patients.

Urge prevention and urge control

Urgency is often perceived as a perineal or penile sensation, which is probably related to urethral relaxation. Urge is more of a problem when moving from lying and sitting into standing, or when walking and bending. In forward lean the abdominal wall often sags forward with consequent relaxation of the PFM. To prevent urge occurring in the above situations the lower abdominal wall should be held gently firm before moving (Sapsford & Hodges 2001). The hold should be sustained while walking to the toilet or until the bladder overactivity quietens. Gentle lower abdominal holds should be used during vacuuming or bending, but should never impact on breathing. See section on tonic PFM activity, below.

Some women have found that wearing an abdominal support garment is beneficial in inhibiting urgency (Pietzsch et al 2001). Lifting the lax lower abdomen by hand and holding it lifted as they walk to the toilet has been helpful in maintaining bladder control for some women. These two strategies are probably more beneficial in those with an obese abdomen.

When the urge begins certain strategies can be used to quieten it. However, the earlier the strategy is implemented the more successful it will be. Once the detrusor muscle is contracting and urine is escaping, there is little hope of controlling it. The following actions have been found helpful:

- hand pressure over clitoris and to give vaginal support
- pressure on the glans or compressing the penis
- sitting on the edge of a firm chair with pressure over the vaginal/perineal region
- crossing legs – hip adductor afferents have an inhibitory effect on the bladder when standing
- a firm PFM hold – though this does not have an inhibitory effect on the bladder (Lindstrom & Sudsuang 1989)
- strong gluteal contraction (buttock squeeze) combined with curling the toes down when standing.

Each of these interventions needs to be maintained until the urge sensation fades. It may take 10–12 seconds. The last two are the only ones that are socially acceptable. When the urge quietens, the person can then walk to the toilet to void. However, the urge often returns while walking unless the person shifts their mental focus to something other than the bladder. Counting every step as they walk and while undressing can provide another focus. Gentle lower abdominal holds, which result in tonic PFM activity, while walking and undressing may help too.

Once the patient has learnt to subdue the urge they should be encouraged to defer voiding. This deferment should commence with one or two minutes and should gradually increase. This is called bladder training. The bladder slowly adapts to greater volumes and does not signal the need to empty so soon. This retraining may take 3 to 6 months and is often conducted with help from an antispasmodic medication, e.g. oxybutynin chloride. However, many older people may never be able to defer, but they may reach the toilet without loss. Daytime deferment with consequent increase in bladder capacity may benefit those with nocturia.

Tonic pelvic floor muscle activity

This strategy is useful in preventing urinary urgency, to decrease the discomfort of a prolapse, to initiate pelvic organ support prior to lifting, coughing and sneezing, and as the initial phase of a PFM rehabilitation programme.

The pelvic floor muscles have a predominance of slow twitch fibres to maintain tonic activity for sustained antigravity support and outlet closure. Loss of tonic activity has been demonstrated in some women with stress urinary incontinence, and even in some nulliparous females (Deindl et al 1994). Thus retraining of tonic activity prior to strengthening seems warranted. Activation of slow twitch PFM fibres to retrain tonic activity requires a slow and gentle onset and a sustained hold at low intensity. This can be approached in two ways.

Gentle isometric lower abdominal muscle holds have been shown to activate pubococcygeus and the external anal sphincter (Sapsford & Hodges 2001). In standing with a normal lumbar curve and without moving the spine, the patient very slowly and gently draws in the lower abdomen towards the spine, without using any respiratory effort. The muscle is then held, and light breathing recommences. A subjective awareness of slight perineal tension, either urethral, vaginal or anal, should be reported on abdominal in-drawing or release of tension on relaxation. This abdominal action can be palpated and observed, and is more obvious on release. Women who have had vaginal repair surgery may have limited or no perineal awareness in response to lower abdominal activation. Sustained holds should be built up to 10, 15, 20 and more seconds, repeating five in a row, five times a day. When the action has been mastered they can then be incorporated into daily activities in standing, e.g. cleaning teeth, showering, ironing, talking and later walking and sitting. Use before and during bending and lifting activities can prevent loss of urine in many women.

An alternative approach is to use a very gentle cognitive periurethral muscle hold. In upright unsupported sitting with a good lumbar curve, the patient gently holds an imagined flow of urine. As the flow is held, lower abdominal palpation will note an increase in tension, or a slight drawing-in of the deep abdominal muscles. Release of the abdomen on release of the imagined urine flow may be more obvious than the tensioning effect.

Pelvic floor muscle strengthening

Once the tonic activity has been mastered, strengthening of the PFM can be added. However, tonic exercise should not cease when strength work begins. Coughing and sneezing require a stronger PFM activation. Strengthening can be achieved either by cognitive PFM holds, or by strong isometric abdominal holds (Sapsford & Hodges 2001). Even without building up much strength a cognitive PFM hold prior to and during a cough has been shown to significantly decrease urine loss in women with mild to moderate stress urinary incontinence (Miller et al 1998). Focusing the hold around the urethral and vaginal area is more beneficial. A correct cognitive PFM hold can be detected by placing the hand over the vagina and perineum. A correct action should draw the perineum up and the vagina up and closed a little. An incorrect action is felt as a downward and outward bulging. Patients can check this for themselves through their underwear.

When the abdominal route is to be used for PFM strengthening in women with a perineal awareness of activation, the same pattern is used to initiate the hold as is used for tonic activity. The focus is on the lower abdomen, beginning with a slow and gentle action and then continuing to draw the lower abdomen in towards the spine and hold it there hard for up to 6 seconds. The spine should not move. There should be an awareness of increasing vaginal or perineal tension with the increased abdominal hold. Breathing patterns are somewhat restricted during the strong abdominal hold, but the breath should not be held. Usual strengthening programmes may include 5–8 repetitions twice a day. Feedback from patients has indicated that many women find it easier to perform and remember to do the abdominal holds both for tonic and strength work, than to do a formal pelvic floor exercise programme. PFMs do not gain their optimum strength unless the abdominal muscles are also strengthened.

Cough and sneeze patterns

These actions require a rapid and strong PFM response. They are also more respiratorily effective if the abdominal muscles produce a strong and rapid in-drawing action (DeTroyer & Estenne 1988, Estenne & Gorini 1992). Strong abdominal isometric activation induces strong pubococcygeal activation (Sapsford & Hodges 2001). In many women with lax muscles the abdomen bulges out as they cough. If the abdomen bulges pubococcygeus activity is decreased (Sapsford & Hodges 2001). A stronger muscle contraction can be achieved if muscles are put on a stretch prior to contraction. Diaphragmatic breathing as physiotherapists know it will put the abdominal muscles on more of a stretch than if inspiration occurs as a rib cage widening and elevation action. Those people using the strong abdominal activation for increasing PFM strength may find it easier to develop continent cough and sneeze patterns.

Prior to teaching coughing and sneezing patterns diaphragmatic breathing should be checked and corrected as necessary. Lying should be the first position used, progressing to sitting and standing. Practice of nose blowing can precede coughing. The pattern is practised initially in sitting and later in standing using a diaphragmatic breath in, followed immediately by the nose blow or cough with a strong cognitive abdominal in-drawing. Viewing the action in a mirror can be very helpful. These patterns are practised daily. Activation of the nose blow and cough patterns should give a subjective awareness of vaginal or perineal support or lift. There should not be a sense of vaginal bulging. It may be that regular practice of the correct pattern develops an automatic response as occurs in motor relearning. Similar retraining can be applied to sneeze and laugh patterns. However, when respiratory conditions or infections cause repeated severe coughing which fatigues muscle support, firm hand support over the vagina and perineum will restrict downward bulging and this reduces urine loss. Obviously this can only be used in appropriate situations.

Conclusion

Almost all physiotherapy interventions require a self-help approach from the patient to achieve a successful outcome. Community-dwelling elderly people are often well motivated to maintain or improve their quality of life and are prepared to undertake an exercise programme. But old people, even in the community, find it harder and harder to make the effort required. Urinary and faecal incontinence are distressing conditions that should spur the sufferer to participate in a programme. But taking a pill or wearing a pad are easier options in many cases. And this is more so for those in residential aged care. Hence exercise programmes must be simple and involve the least number of the most effective exercises, and be functionally based. If patients cannot see some benefit within a very short time they will be deterred. Exercises such as gentle lower abdominal holds to prevent urge on rising from sitting or urine loss on forward bending are very easy to achieve. All that is then needed is to remember to use them at the appropriate time. Coughing patterns require a more dedicated approach.

It is hoped that the treatment strategies outlined in this chapter provide some interventions that physiotherapists can use for the benefit of residents in the aged care setting.

Summary

- Signs and symptoms can indicate the type of problem affecting the resident.
- Other medical conditions and prescribed medication can impact on bladder and bowel function.
- Medical investigations are required for some conditions.
- Each problem requires a specific physiotherapy intervention.
- Use the simplest strategy first.
- Keep the exercise programme to a minimum.
- Incorporate exercises and strategies into functional tasks and positions.
- Refer more complex problems to pelvic floor physiotherapists.

References

Abrams P, Weiss J, Mattiasson et al 2001 The efficacy and safety of oral desmopressin in the treatment of nocturia in men. Neurourology and Urodynamics 20:456–457

Abrams P, Cardozo L, Fall M et al 2002 The standardisation of terminology of lower urinary tract function. Neurourology and Urodynamics 21:167–178

Abrutyn E, Mossey J, Berlin J A et al 1994 Does asymptomatic bacteriuria predict mortality and does antimicrobial treatment reduce mortality in elderly ambulatory women? Annals of Internal Medicine 120:827–833

Akervall S, Nordgren S, Fasth S et al 1990 The effects of age, gender, and parity on rectoanal function in adults. Scandinavian Journal of Gastroenterology 25:1247–1256

Berghmans L C M, Hendriks H J M, Bo K et al 1998 Conservative treatment of stress urinary incontinence in women: a systematic review of randomised clinical trials. British Journal of Urology 82:181–191

Blok B F M, Willemsen A T M, Holstege G 1997a A PET study on brain control of micturition in humans. Brain 120:111–121

Blok B F M, Sturms L M, Holstege G 1997b A PET study on cortical and subcortical pelvic floor musculature in women. Journal of Comparative Neurology 389:535–544

Boedker A, Lendorf A, H-Neilsen A et al 1989 Micturition pattern assessed by frequency/volume chart in a healthy population of men and women. Neurourology and Urodynamics 8:421–422

Brandt L, Griffiths D, Resnick N 2002 Nursing home residents' preferences for urinary continence treatment: what are they and are they consistent? Neurourology and Urodynamics 21:430–431

Brown S R, Cann P A, Read N W 1990 Effect of coffee on distal colon function. Gut 31:450–453

Burns P A, Nochajski T H, Pranikoff K 1993 Predictors of incontinence in elderly women. Neurourology and Urodynamics 12:432–434

Cardozo L, Lose G, McClish D et al 2001 Oestrogen treatment for symptoms of an overactive bladder: results of a meta-analysis. Proceedings of IUGA conference abstract 67

Chassagne P, Jego A, Gloc P et al 2000 Does treatment of constipation improve faecal incontinence in institutionalised elderly patients? Age and Ageing 29:159–164

Chiarelli P, Markwell S 1992 Let's get things moving. Gore and Osment, Sydney

Constantinou C E, Govan D E 1982 Spatial distribution and timing of transmitted and reflexly generated urethral pressures in healthy women. Journal of Urology 127:964–969

Corti R, Binggeli C, Sudano I et al 2002 Coffee acutely increases sympathetic nerve activity and blood pressure independently of caffeine content. Circulation 106:2935–2940

Deindl F M, Vodusek D B, Hesse U et al 1994 Pelvic floor activity patterns: comparison of nulliparous continent and parous urinary stress incontinent women. A kinesiological EMG study. British Journal of Urology 73:413–417

DeLancey J O L 1990 Anatomy and physiology of urinary continence. Clinical Obstetrics and Gynecology 33:298–306

DeTroyer A, Estenne M 1988 Functional anatomy of the respiratory muscles. Clinics in Chest Medicine 9:175–193

Drossman D A, Sandler R S, McKee D C et al 1982 Bowel patterns among subjects not seeking health care. Gastroenterology 83:529–534

Dubeau C E, Simon S, Morris J N 1999 The impact of urinary incontinence and changing continence status on quality of life in nursing home residents. Neurourology and Urodynamics 18:389

Edwards N 2000 Urinary incontinence: does it increase risk of falls? Journal of the American Geriatrics Society 48:721–725

Edwards N I, Jones D 2001 The prevalence of faecal incontinence in older people living at home. Age and Ageing 30:503–507

Estenne M, Gorini M 1992 Action of the diaphragm during cough in tetraplegic subjects. Journal of Applied Physiology 72:1074–1080

Fonda D, Resnick N M, Colling J et al 1998 Outcome measures for research of lower urinary tract dysfunction in frail older people. Neurourology and Urodynamics 17:273–281

Gautam P C, Jamieson A D, Donald S 1999 Do the very frail, oldest old benefit from active management of urinary incontinence? Neurourology and Urodynamics 18:390

Gosselink M J, Schouten W R 2001 The gastrorectal reflex in women with obstructed defecation. International Journal of Colorectal Disease 16:112–118

Gosselink M J, Schouten W R 2002 The perineorectal reflex in health and obstructed defecation. Diseases of Colon and Rectum 45:370–376

Griffiths D J, McCracken P N, Harrison G M et al 1994 Cerebral aetiology of geriatric urge incontinence. Age and Ageing 23:246–250

Griffiths D J, McCracken P N, Harrison G M et al 1996 Urge incontinence in elderly people: factors predicting severity of urine loss before and after pharmacological treatment. Neurourology and Urodynamics 15:53–57

Griffiths D J, McCracken P N, Harrison G M et al 2002 Urge incontinence and impaired detrusor contractility in the elderly. Neurourology and Urodynamics 21:126–131

Gunnarsson M, Mattiasson A 1999 Female stress, urge, and mixed urinary incontinence are associated with a chronic and progressive pelvic floor/vaginal neuromuscular disorder. Neurourology and Urodynamics 18:613–621

Heit M, Benson J T, Russell B et al 1996 Levator ani muscle in women with genitourinary prolapse: indirect assessment by muscle histopathology. Neurourology and Urodynamics 15:17–29

Hodges P W, Richardson C A 1996 Inefficient muscular stabilization of the lumbar spine associated with low back pain. Spine 21:2640–2650

Hodges P W, Butler J E, McKenzie D K et al 1997 Contraction of the human diaphragm during rapid postural adjustments. Journal of Physiology 505: 539–548

Hodges P W, Sapsford R, Pengel L 2002 Feedforward activity of the pelvic floor muscles precedes rapid upper limb movements. Australian Physiotherapy Association Conference, Sydney, abstract 21

Kirschner-Hermanns R, Scherr P, Resnick N M 1997 Relationship of medication use to urinary urgency and incontinence in the elderly: a population based study. Neurourology and Urodynamics 16: 437–438

Kuchel G A, Resnick N M 1997 Does estrogen deficiency contribute to impaired bladder contractility in older women? Neurourology and Urodynamics 16:443–444

Lindstrom S, Sudsuang R 1989 Functionally specific bladder reflexes from pelvic and pudendal nerve branches: an experimental study in the cat. Neurourology and Urodynamics 9:393

Lubowski D Z, King D W, Finlay I G 1992 Electromyography of the pubococcygeus muscle in patients with obstructed defecation. International Journal of Colorectal Disease 7:184–187

MacLennan A H, Taylor A W, Wilson D H et al 2000 The prevalence of pelvic floor disorders and their relationship to gender, age, parity and mode of delivery. British Journal of Obstetrics and Gynaecology 107:1460–1470

McMurdo M E T, Gillespie N D 2000 Urinary tract infection in old age: over-diagnosed and over-treated. Age and Ageing 29:297–298

Maglinte D D, Kelvin F M, Fitzgerald K 1999 Association of compartment defects in pelvic floor dysfunction. American Journal of Roentgenology 172: 439–444

Manning J, Korda A, Benness C 1998 Does uterovaginal prolapse cause voiding dysfunction? Neurourology and Urodynamics 18:327

Markwell S 1998 Functional disorders of the anorectum and pain syndromes. In: Sapsford R, Bullock-Saxton J, Markwell S (eds) Women's health: a textbook for physiotherapists. W B Saunders, London, p 366

Markwell S J, Sapsford R R 1995 Physiotherapy management of obstructed defecation. Australian Journal of Physiotherapy 41:279–283

Miller J M, Ashton-Miller J A, DeLancey J O L 1998 A pelvic muscle precontraction can reduce cough-related urine loss in selected women with mild SUI. Journal of the American Geriatrics Society 46: 870–874

Miller K L, DuBeau C E, Bergmann M A et al 2000 Dose titration key to oxybutynin efficacy for geriatric incontinence even with DHIC. Neurourology and Urodynamics 19:538–539

Moore K N, Griffiths D J, Hughton A 1998 A randomised controlled trial of pelvic muscle exercises or pelvic muscle exercises plus electrical stimulation for post radical prostatectomy urinary incontinence. Neurourology and Urodynamics 17:424–426

Morgan K, Bergmann M, Kiely D et al 2000 The voiding pattern of normal elders. Neurourology and Urodynamics 19:536–537

Moseley G L, Hodges P W, Gandevia S C 2002 Deep and superficial fibres of lumbar multifidus muscle are differently active during voluntary arm movements. Spine 27(2):E29–E36

Neumann P, Gill V 2002 Pelvic floor and abdominal muscle interaction: EMG activity and intra-abdominal pressure. International Urogynecology Journal 13:125–132

Norton P A, Baker J E, Sharp H C et al 1995 Genitourinary prolapse and joint hypermobility in women. Obstetrics and Gynecology 85:225–228

Nuotio M, Jylha M, Luukkaala T et al 2001 Urgency and urge incontinence and voiding symptoms in men and women aged 70 and over. Neurourology and Urodynamics 20:496–497

Olsen A L, Smith V J, Bergstrom J O et al 1997 Epidemiology of surgically managed pelvic organ prolapse and urinary incontinence. Obstetrics and Gynecology 89:501–506

Ouslander J G, Kane R L, Abrass I B 1982 Urinary incontinence in elderly nursing home patients. Journal of the American Medical Association 248: 1194–1198

Ouslander J G, Simmons S, Schnelle J et al 1996 Effects of prompted voiding on fecal incontinence among nursing home residents. Journal of the American Geriatrics Society 44:424–428

Ouslander J, Adelman C, Khan N et al 1999 Does night-time incontinence disrupt sleep in geriatric patients? Neurourology and Urodynamics 18:386

Pietzsch A, Sapsford R, Bullock-Saxton J 2001 Use of an abdominal support garment in the management of urgency and urge incontinence. Physiotherapy Honours research project. The University of Queensland

Rasmussen O O 1994 Anorectal function. Diseases of Colon and Rectum 37:386–403

Resnick N M, Elbadawi A, Yalla S V 1995 Age and the lower urinary tract. What is normal? Neurourology and Urodynamics 14:577–579

Resnick N M, Brandeis G H, Baumann MM et al 1996 Misdiagnosis of urinary incontinence in nursing home women: prevalence and a proposed solution. Neurourology and Urodynamics 15:599–618

Rosier P F W M, de la Rosette J J M C H, Wijkstra H et al 1995 Is detrusor instability in elderly males related to the grade of obstruction? Neurourology and Urodynamics 14:625–633

Samuelsson E C, Victor A F T et al 1999 Signs of genital prolapse in a Swedish population of women 20 to 50 years of age and possible related factors. American Journal of Obstetrics and Gynecology 180:299–305

Sapsford R R, Hodges P W 2001 Contraction of the pelvic floor muscles during abdominal maneuvers. Archives of Physical Medicine and Rehabilitation 82:1081–1088

Sapsford R R, Markwell S J, Clarke B 1998 The relationship between urethral pressure and abdominal muscle activity. Abstracts from 7th National CFA Conference on Incontinence, Australian Continence Journal 4:102–110

Sapsford R R, Hodges P W, Richardson C A et al 2001 Co-activation of the abdominal and pelvic floor muscles during voluntary exercises. Neurourology and Urodynamics 20:31–42

Schnelle J F 1990 Treatment of urinary incontinence in nursing home patients by prompted voiding. Journal of the American Geriatrics Society 38: 356–360

Skehan R, Moore K H, Richmond D H 1990 The auditory stimulus of running water: its effect on urethral pressure. Neurourology and Urodynamics 9:351–353

Spence-Jones C, Kamm M A, Henry M M et al 1994 Bowel dysfunction: a pathogenic factor in uterovaginal prolapse and stress urinary incontinence. British Journal of Obstetrics and Gynaecology 101:147–152

Sugaya K, Nishijima S, Oda N et al 2001 Biochemical analysis of nocturia in the elderly. Neurourology and Urodynamics 20:458–460

Sullivan J, Lewis P, Howell S et al 2000 Abdominal pressure, obesity and incontinence in women. International Continence Society conference, Tampere, Abstract 170

Sultan A H, Kamm M A, Hudson C 1994 Pudendal nerve damage during labour: prospective study before and after childbirth. British Journal of Obstetrics and Gynaecology 101:22–28

Swithinbank L V, Vestey S, Abrams P 1998a Nocturnal polyuria in community dwelling women. Neurourology and Urodynamics 17:314–315

Swithinbank L V, Donovan J, Rogers C et al 1998b Nocturnal enuresis in adult women: a hidden problem. Neurourology and Urodynamics 17:315–316

Tagart R E B 1966 The anal canal and rectum: their varying relationship and its effect on anal continence. Diseases of Colon and Rectum 9:449–452

Talley N J, Weaver A L, Zinsmeister A R et al 1993 Functional constipation and outlet delay: a population-based study. Gastroenterology 105:781–790

Thind P, Lose G, Jorgensen L et al 1990 Variations in urethral and bladder pressure during stress episodes in healthy women. British Journal of Urology 66: 389–392

Thom D H, Haan M N, Van Den Eeden S K 1997 Medically recognised urinary incontinence and risks of hospitalisation, nursing home admission and mortality. Age and Ageing 26:367–374

Tobin G W, Brocklehurst J C 1986a The management of urinary incontinence in local authority residential homes for the elderly. Age and Ageing 15:292–298

Tobin G W, Brocklehurst J C 1986b Faecal incontinence in residential homes for the elderly: prevalence, aetiology and management. Age and Ageing 15:41–46

Umlauf M, Burgio K, Bliwise D et al 1999 Mechanisms of nocturia in older adults: preliminary results of clinical interviews. Neurourology and Urodynamics 18:385

Wagg A, Cumming K, Malone-Lee J G 1999 Age and the measurement of outcome of treatment of the overactive bladder. Neurourology and Urodynamics 18:388

Weiss J P, Blavais J G, Stember D S et al 1998 Nocturia in adults: aetiology and classification. Neurourology and Urodynamics 17:467–472

Wise B G, Cardozo L D, Cutner A et al 1993 Prevalence and significance of urethral instability in women with detrusor instability. British Journal of Urology 72:26–29

Wynne J M, Myles J L, Jones I et al 1996 Disturbed anal sphincter function following vaginal delivery. Gut 39:120–124

SECTION 4 SPECIAL CONSIDERATIONS OF PAIN AND PALLIATIVE CARE

15 Pain in the elderly

Tina Souvlis and Venerina Johnston

This chapter aims to:

- outline the prevalence of pain in the older population
- provide an understanding of neurophysiological mechanisms of nociception, development of chronic pain and modulation of pain
- provide an understanding of musculoskeletal pain mechanisms
- provide an overview of pain assessment methods
- provide an overview of management of pain by physiotherapy techniques.

Introduction

Chronic pain can be a disabling problem for the older adult. It is often thought that pain may be a natural consequence of ageing. However, pain is most often related to disease and pathology and not solely due to the process of ageing. The incidence of diseases associated with pain and the likelihood of having multiple health problems increases with age (Farrell et al 1996). The definition of pain that has been developed by the International Association for the Study of Pain (IASP) is 'an unpleasant sensory and emotional experience associated with actual or potential tissue damage, or described in terms of such damage'. They note that 'the inability to communicate verbally does not negate the possibility that an individual is experiencing pain and is in need of appropriate pain relieving treatment' (Merskey & Bogduk 1994). Thus pain is a complex phenomenon encompassing physiological and emotional elements. It is recognized that special problems such as depression, anxiety, decreased mobility and increased risk of drug interactions may influence the poor management of pain (Ferrell 1991, Popp & Portenoy 1996).

Physiotherapists play a key role in the management of pain for the older patient in residential care as the prevalence of pain of musculoskeletal origin increases with age. As well, physiotherapists manage patients who have pain and movement impairments as a result of disease that is not of musculoskeletal origin. Therefore, knowledge of the physiology of pain as well as assessment and management strategies are necessary to provide optimal care.

In this chapter, the prevalence of pain in the elderly will be discussed. A section on the neurophysiology of nociceptive processing and the changes that occur in the nervous system that contribute to the development of chronic pain will provide a background for discussion of assessment and management strategies for this patient group.

Prevalence of pain in the adult population

In Australia, the majority of people aged 65 years and over (66%) rated their own health as being good, very good or excellent. However, the percentage of people who describe their health as fair or poor increases with age. Ten per cent of people aged 65–75 years and 13.5% of people aged 75 years and over describe their health as poor (Department of Families 2003). The prevalence of physical conditions also increases with age, with 21% of adults between 25 and 34 years and 77% of adults over 65 years reporting a physical condition such as visual impairment, hearing impairment or arthritis. Many of these impairments are of a chronic nature, and cause functional deficits and pain. Some authors believe that as many as 85% of people over 65 years have at least one health problem which predisposes to pain (Harkins et al 1994).

Many studies have investigated the overall frequency of pain in society. The estimates show a great variability from 7% (Bowsher et al 1991) to 40% (Brattberg et al 1989). Among institutionalized elderly, the prevalence of pain has been reported to range from 49 to 83% (Fox et al 1999). These disparities in reported prevalence may be due to methodological variations.

- There were variations in the definitions of pain and nature of questions asked (Bassols et al 1999, Gagliese et al 1999, Helme & Gibson 1999). Some researchers assessed for any type of pain in the previous 2 weeks (Bredkjaer 1991), pain 'on and off' for more than 3 months (Bowsher et al 1991), some for fleeting, minor or 'obvious pain' (Brattberg et al 1989) or 'often troubled by pain' (Crook et al 1984).
- The samples from which the study population was drawn could be electoral roles, telephone books, workers, nursing homes or medical practices (Gagliese et al 1999, Simmonds & Scudds 2001).
- The method of assessment varied from telephone interviews (Bassols et al 1999, Bowsher et al 1991), postal questionnaires (Bergman et al 2001, Roy & Thomas 1986) to physical examination by a rheumatologist (Carmona et al 2001).

Types of pain

Acute pain

Acute pain is primarily a symptom of disease or injury whereas chronic pain represents a disease in itself (Sternbach 1986). It was said by Harkins et al (1994) that 'acute pain associated with cutaneous structures, most fractures and muscle, joint and tendon strain probably do not change in a clinically significant manner with age in otherwise healthy, elderly people'. Helme & Gibson (1999) likewise believe that acute pain occurs at much the same rate across all age groups but older people experience more chronic pain.

Chronic pain

Harkins et al (1994) define chronic pain as pain persisting at least one month beyond the usual course of an acute disease. It is considered that older people are more susceptible to the experience of pain than other sectors of the population (Cowan et al 2003). This is considered related to the high prevalence of musculoskeletal disorders, phantom pain and cancer pain in this age group (Ferrell 1991). Although it is believed that age does not decrease pain perception, there is evidence that emotional suffering related to pain may be less in the older than younger chronic pain patient (Harkins et al 1994).

Chronic pain in the elderly varies with location, age and gender

A study by Crook et al (1984) was one of the first to show that pain prevalence increased with increasing age for persistent pain described as longer than 2 weeks' duration. The prevalence of temporary pain was found to be unrelated to age. Other studies suggest the prevalence of pain peaks in the middle years (Bergman et al 2001, Brattberg et al 1989, Helme & Gibson 1999) and declines thereafter to a steady rate. However, Roy & Thomas (1986) found 83% of nursing home residents aged over 65 years had reported musculoskeletal pain with 18% saying is was at a high to intolerable level.

A longitudinal study by Brattberg et al (1997) spanning 24 years included 321 subjects with a baseline age of 53 years, and the authors found that only 6.2% of the sample did not report any pain in any location over the entire period. They found that the prevalence of pain differs with location, with chest and abdominal pain increasing with age (Brattberg et al 1997). The increase in chest pain was thought to be due to cardiovascular disease. They also found the prevalence of musculoskeletal pain in the back and hips decreased with age, thought to be due to retirement from work-related risk factors. Harkins et al (1994) found the prevalence of headaches and low back pain decreased with age after peaking in middle years of 45–50 (Gagliese et al 1999, Helme & Gibson 1999).

However, the majority of studies indicate that musculoskeletal pain is a significant problem for the older population, with musculoskeletal illness representing 50% of all painful aetiologies in subjects over 70 years of age (Bassols et al 1999) and every fifth individual over 60 years of age reported a musculoskeletal illness (Bredkjaer 1991). Other studies have found pain of musculoskeletal origin is the most common type of pain in older adults (Afable & Ettinger 1993, Bowsher et al 1991, Brattberg et al 1997, Bredkjaer 1991, Gagliese et al 1999), with Simmonds & Scudds (2001) reporting that prevalence of articular joint pain in the over-65s is twice that of younger adults.

Most epidemiological studies have found that women have a significantly higher prevalence of pain than men of similar age (Crook et al 1984) but Brattberg et al (1997) found no significant gender differences regarding the number of occasions pain was reported over 24 years. However, for musculoskeletal pain, women reported more severe pain more often and in more locations than men.

It is thought that pain remains a neglected phenomenon in older people (Closs 1994) due to under-reporting (Gagliese et al 1999, Herr 2002a) and inadequate assessment. Hence, pain in the elderly is considered to be under-treated and inadequately managed (Chibnall & Tait 2001, Cowan et al 2003, Crook et al 1984, Simmonds & Scudds 2001).

What factors contribute to the under-reporting of pain in the elderly?

- The elderly may de-emphasize pain due to other significant life events such as death of a spouse or loss of independence (Helme & Gibson 1999). This phenomenon was highlighted by Seitsamo & Klockars (1997), who studied 30- to 64-year-old workers over 11 years. They found that although the number of diseases increased with age, the workers considered themselves in good health. This was explained by the reference group theory, whereby people assess their own situation by comparing themselves with a peer group.
- Many older adults may fear the meaning of pain (Simmonds & Scudds 2001), believing it may be related to impending death or loss of independence or need for hospitalization (Herr 2002a) or the presence of co-morbidities that compete for the attention of health care staff (Chibnall & Tait 2001).
- Cultural variations in pain reporting may lead some elderly to under-report pain if stoicism is part of their cultural background (Helme & Gibson 1999).
- There is a tendency for health care personnel, family and older patients themselves to discount the levels of reported pain due to ageist attitudes. Very often, pain is accepted as a natural part of the ageing process and hence not reported (Chibnall & Tait 2001, Cowan et al 2003).

What factors contribute to the inadequate assessment of pain in the elderly?

- Tools used for pain assessment have been mainly validated and used in young populations and extrapolation to the elderly is difficult and may not be valid (Chibnall & Tait 2001).
- Variability in the cognitive awareness and communication levels in the elderly are major barriers to adequate assessment and management of pain (Cohen-Mansfield & Lipson 2002, Ferrell 1995, Herr 2002b).
- There is significant discussion in the literature about the lack of knowledge of health care providers in the assessment of pain (Cowan et al 2003, Simmonds & Scudds 2001).

What factors contribute to the under-treatment of pain in the elderly?

- Physicians' and nurses' fears regarding the use of drugs is a significant reason for the under-treatment of pain (Herr 2002a). Their fears surround the possible side effects of respiratory depression, increased risk of falling and addiction (Ardery et al 2003, Chibnall & Tait 2001).
- It has been suggested that older people feel less pain than younger adults due to altered perception of pain (Harkins et al 1994). However, a review by Gagliese et al (1999) and a study by Harkins & Price (1992) found no significant age differences in pain intensity or unpleasantness ratings.

Neurophysiology of pain

The nociceptive system normally becomes activated to signal damage or impending damage to the body. However, there exists a variable link between injury, disease and pain. This is evident following ankle sprain when pain, swelling and inability to walk on the leg rapidly follow damage to the ligament. In contrast, patients with severe damage to lungs due to cancer may not experience any pain. Pain can be referred to remote sites, e.g. angina pain may also be experienced as left arm pain. Phantom limb pain following limb amputation can be severe and debilitating. Whilst the value of pain following an injury can be understood - to decrease behaviours that may cause further injury - the value of chronic and referred pain is less obvious. It does illustrate, however, that changes that occur following injury and disease can upregulate the activity within the nervous system to produce chronic pain.

Nociception

Nociceptors are receptors that are responsive to noxious or damaging stimuli. The skin has a dense innervation of nociceptors (Galea 2002). There are also nociceptors in tissues including muscle, bone, joint capsules, viscera and blood vessels and in the nervous system (e.g. meninges and peripheral nerve sheaths). In contrast, no nociceptors have been located in the brain and spinal cord, articular cartilages, synovium, lung parenchyma and visceral pleura (Galea 2002). The receptor has been described as a free nerve ending which subserves the reception of noxious and other stimuli (Bessou & Perl 1969, Burgess & Perl 1967).

Two types of afferent fibres are associated with the conduction of the nociceptive stimuli (Bessou & Perl 1969, Burgess & Perl 1967). Small thinly myelinated fibres (Aδ) conduct at a velocity of 5–30 metres/second and provide well-localized sharp sensation or 'first pain' whereas non-myelinated (C) fibres conduct more slowly (0.5–2 metres/second) and provide a dull, less well-localized sensation also known as 'second pain' (Melzack & Wall 1996).

Cutaneous nociceptors may have a specific response to mechanical stimuli such as strong pressure or they may be polymodal, responding to a variety of stimuli including mechanical, heat, cold and chemical. There are also a group of mechanically insensitive or 'silent' nociceptors which respond to chemical stimuli and may become sensitized to mechanical stimulation in the presence of injury and inflammation (Galea 2002).

Nociceptors from deep structures such as muscles and joints share similar properties to cutaneous receptors in that they can be described as mechanosensitive or polymodal. The classification of these afferents is group III fibres for the small diameter, thinly myelinated fibres while group IV fibres are non-myelinated. In muscle, nociceptors respond to excessive stretch, rapid contraction (group III) and during contraction in the presence of ischaemia (group IV) (Mense 1993). In the joint, noxious pressure or extremes of joint movement can stimulate the nociceptors (Schaible & Grubb 1993). As in cutaneous structures, silent nociceptors can be activated in the presence of inflammation. For viscera, inflammation and distension of muscular walled organs such as the bladder are stimuli that are capable of producing pain. Inflammation of organs such as the uterus can lead to the development of referred pain and distal muscle changes (Giamberardino et al 1999).

Afferent fibres cluster to form spinal nerves to convey information from the periphery to the central nervous system. The cell bodies of the afferent fibres are located in the dorsal root ganglia where there exists a correlation between the size of the cell body and the afferent fibre. In general, large cell bodies are associated with larger diameter fibres transmitting predominantly non-noxious mechanical information, with smaller cells and their fibres relaying nociceptive stimuli (Galea 2002).

The spinal nerves split into dorsal and ventral roots prior to entering the spinal cord. The dorsal horn is the area where primary processing of sensory information takes place. There exists a functional differentiation for processing depending on where afferents terminate within the dorsal horn. It is generally accepted that the nociceptive afferents terminate predominantly in laminae I and II with some termination of the myelinated fibres only going into lamina V (Rexed 1954). Lamina II, also known as the 'substantia gelatinosa', is the site of potential modulation or 'gating' of nociceptive information by inhibitory influences of large myelinated afferents and inhibitory interneurons described in the 'Gate Control Theory' postulated by Melzack & Wall (1965). Large myelinated afferent fibres terminate in laminae III, IV and V (Galea 2002, Melzack & Wall 1996).

The afferent fibres can synapse with dorsal horn neurons of the nociceptive specific (N-S) type or with wide dynamic range (WDR) neurons. N-S cells are activated by high threshold noxious stimuli whereas WDR cells are activated by both innocuous and noxious stimuli, with the firing rate of the cells dependent on the stimulus intensity. Lamina I contains both types of neurons. However, lamina II and V cells are primarily of the WDR type (Galea 2002, Sluka & Rees 1997).

Ascending transmission

Each of the laminae, except for lamina II, sends projections supraspinally to centres such as the thalamus, the reticular activating system and the midbrain. The anterolateral system consisting of the spinothalamic, spinoreticular and spinomesencephalic tracts relays information about nociception and temperature. The dorsal column pathways, which convey information about touch and proprioception, have also been reported to relay information from unmyelinated afferent fibres that synapse with dorsal column nuclei (Galea 2002).

In the thalamus, there are two subdivisions of nuclei that receive nociceptive input from the projection neurons. These divisions are the lateral and medial groups. There is a direct projection from the primary somatosensory cortex for localization of sensory stimuli. Projections from the medial nuclei appear to have a wider distribution network including the anterior cingulate gyrus. This network is thought to be associated with arousal and affective states related to the painful stimulus (Galea 2002, Sluka & Rees 1997). Projections to the midbrain periaqueductal grey area, basal ganglia, limbic system and of course the cortex have also been described and all have a role in the discrimination and modulation of nociception (Coghill et al 1994).

Pain

While the mechanisms described above illustrate the physiological process of nociception, the experience of pain is a subjective one. It is the net result of ascending input, and the influence of descending controls. Nociceptive system function can be upregulated in the presence of injury or disease so that the system is said to exhibit plasticity, that is changes depending on a number of influences rather than being static in nature. Chronic pain may be the result of changes to the processing of sensory information by the nociceptive system in addition to the ongoing disease and pathology.

There are a number of peripheral and central nervous system mechanisms that contribute to the development of chronic or persistent pain. Altered sensitivity within the nociceptive system can lead to the development of hyperalgesia, defined as an increased response to a stimulus that is normally painful, or allodynia, described as pain due to a stimulus that does not normally provoke pain (Merskey & Bogduk 1994).

Hyperalgesia may be related directly to the tissue involved in the injury – primary hyperalgesia – or may develop at a distant site. This is known as secondary hyperalgesia and may be a mechanism for referred pain. Primary hyperalgesia develops as a result of peripheral sensitization of the nervous system. Following injury, hyperalgesia, allodynia and spontaneous pain can become apparent. For example, in the simple case of a sprained ankle, there is increased tenderness around the ankle, pain at rest and pain on movement. A number of mechanisms can contribute to the development of peripheral sensitization. In inflammation after injury, there is a release of chemicals such as prostaglandins, bradykinin, serotonin and histamine causing a change in the pH of the tissues, which in turn, causes stimulation of the polymodal nociceptors – particularly the C or group IV fibres. In addition, activation of the C-fibre afferents also causes the release of substance P and calcitonin gene related peptide (CGRP) which further increase the release of inflammatory mediators (Dray 1996, Sluka & Rees 1997, Sluka et al 1995). This process is known as neurogenic inflammation.

Changes in sodium and potassium ion channel permeability of the cell can result in the increased response to stimulus that characterizes hyperalgesia (Dray 1995). Hyperpolarization of the nerve fibre that normally occurs after nerve firing can be inhibited by the action of 'inflammatory soup' chemicals such as bradykinin, serotonin and prostaglandins. This allows the afferents to fire more frequently. Recruitment of 'silent nociceptors' that then become sensitized and responsive to mechanical stimulation occurs following tissue injury, thereby further increasing afferent barrage to the central nervous system.

Central sensitization also occurs in the spinal cord and supraspinal cells after injury. It is a complex phenomenon and changes in the spinal cord dorsal horn, particularly in the superficial laminae, are brought about by tonic input from sensitized nociceptors (Mayer et al 1999). Central mechanisms subserving this process involve the NMDA receptor, which consists of an ion channel and several sites for activation by a number of substances. These include excitatory amino acids such as glutamate, which is co-released with substance P from peripheral afferents to produce a cascade of intracellular effects that increase the excitability of the cell and cause spread sensitization in spinal cord neurons (Mao et al 1995, Mayer et al 1999, Price et al 2000).

Another mechanism that is important particularly in the presence of nerve injury is the reorganization that can occur at the spinal cord level. Myelinated afferents that would normally terminate in laminae III or IV now grow into lamina II, where there is potential for these axons to synapse with neurons involved in the transmission of nociceptive stimulation (Woolf & Mannion 1999). Thus a number of changes in the organization and function of the central nervous system are brought about by afferent barrage following injury in the periphery (Melzack & Wall 1996).

These changes in spinal cord neuron excitability can also alter the output of the motor system. There are a number of theories that describe the effect of pain on the motor function. Enhanced flexor withdrawal reflexes are evident as a consequence of pain and may persist following resolution of injury (Wall & Woolf 1984). The 'vicious cycle' model or the pain/spasm/pain cycle proposed by Johansson & Sojka (1991) and the 'pain adaptation' model (Lund et al 1991) are examples of such hypotheses. Limitations to both these theories have been highlighted in that in some cases, a decrease in muscle activity can be observed in the presence of acute muscle pain which may in turn lead to a coordination change in the performance of a motor task (i.e. pain adaptation). In other situations, accumulation of metabolites due to overactivity in motor units may sensitize the nociceptive system, producing a pain/spasm/pain cycle. Although there are anecdotal clinical reports in support of this 'vicious cycle' model, little conclusive evidence currently exists. More recently another model has emerged which describes changes in motor recruitment patterns between larger global muscles and smaller intersegmental muscles that might more adequately explain the complex relationship between pain and motor control (Hides et al 1994, Hodges & Richardson 1996, Hodges 2001). Sterling et al (2001) suggest that a key effect of pain is to disrupt control of synergistic muscle functions in addition to potential influences on agonist and antagonist functions as suggested by the pain adaptation theory.

There is also evidence of the influence of altered nociceptive processing on the autonomic nervous system. Changes in the structure of the sympathetic fibres in the dorsal root ganglion have been demonstrated following nerve constriction injury (Janig & McLachlan 1992) and development of sensitivity by afferents to circulating noradrenaline released from sympathetic fibres may increase pain (Janig et al 1996). Development of complex regional pain syndrome following injury demonstrates, at the extreme, the possible interrelationship of the sympathetic nervous and nociceptive systems (Stanton-Hicks et al 1998).

Thus change in nociceptive processing can have wide-ranging and important influences on behavioural responses to pain-provoking stimuli. Evident as increased withdrawal reflexes or alterations in motor control, changes in the motor system are the key signs that a therapist can use in the assessment of painful conditions and the sequelae. Severe debilitating symptoms can result from changes to autonomic (particularly sympathetic nervous system) system changes.

Descending inhibitory systems

Activation of pain inhibitory systems can also influence the nature of pain following injury. As mentioned above, the pain experience is complex and dependent on the state of the nociceptive system and the activity within the descending pain inhibitory system. It is evident that both direct and external stimulation of the central nervous system can cause activation of the descending inhibitory circuitry. The premise that endogenous mechanisms exist within the nervous system to inhibit or modulate pain has been the subject of extensive research using brain stimulation, stress and morphine induced analgesia models. These studies are relevant and significant in that they have provided us with a number of important observations that have formed the broad theoretical construct upon which continuing research into analgesia related to physiotherapy treatment modalities is based.

The demonstration that focal stimulation of the midbrain periaqueductal grey area (PAG) could produce profound analgesia (Reynolds 1969) initiated investigation of stimulation, stress and drug induced analgesia and the methods by which it occurs (Cannon et al 1982, Lewis & Gebhart 1977, Lutfy et al 1993, Nichols & Thorn 1990, Terman et al 1984). Electrical and chemical stimulation of the PAG produces potent analgesia without producing deficits in other sensory systems (Mayer 1979, Terman et al 1984). It can inhibit the nociception produced by a diversity of stimuli in laboratory animals such as paw pinch, electric shock and heat (Lewis & Gebhart 1977), and Hosobuchi et al (1977) also demonstrated its effectiveness in human pain relief. The functional significance of the PAG in analgesia is now well established (Lovick 1991). PAG is involved in both ascending and descending transmission of impulses (Behbehani 1995) and receives afferent input from spinal cord nociceptors and relays projections to and from the cortex, thalamus, amygdala and rostral ventromedial medulla (RVM) as well as the dorsolateral pons (Fields & Basbaum 1994). There are few direct PAG projections to the spinal cord as information is relayed from the PAG to the RVM to the spinal cord via the dorsolateral funiculus. As the RVM receives input from both serotonin (e.g. dorsal raphe nucleus) and noradrenaline-containing neurons (e.g. A5 and A7 cells in the pontine nuclei), this network utilizes both neurotransmitters (Cui et al 1999). Opioid peptides are also located within the PAG. Enkephalin and dynorphin containing cells originate within the PAG. However, endorphinergic cells project to PAG from the hypothalamus (Fields & Basbaum 1994).

The PAG is not a homogeneous structure and according to Morgan (1991), the characteristics of analgesia produced following electrical stimulation of PAG in the rat are dependent on the area stimulated. The terms lateral PAG (lPAG) and ventrolateral PAG (vlPAG) describe functionally distinct columns and these have been the most extensively researched columns. However, it is recognized that there may be overlap in structure and function between these columns and the other parts of the dorsal and ventral regions of the PAG (Bandler et al 1991, Jansen et al 1998).

In addition to the analgesic effects, Lovick (1991) describes a set of complex responses following stimulation of the PAG subdivisions. She noted that stimulation of vlPAG in rodents produces a tripartite effect including inhibition of the sympathetic nervous system, freezing of movement and analgesia which is opioid in nature. Stimulation of lPAG appears to result in a non-opioid form of analgesia accompanied by sympathoexcitation and movement facilitation. Hence she suggested that lPAG coordinates a 'flight or fight' response to threatening or nociceptive stimuli, whereas vlPAG activates more recuperative behaviour involving the opioid system. The 'flight' response usually occurs first and its activity inhibits the vlPAG neurons (Behbehani 1995). A study by Jansen et al (1998) has also confirmed the presence of local connections between the columns of the PAG. As such, it appears that PAG is responsible for coordinating responses which ensure survival rather than solely modulating pain perception (Fanselow 1991).

In addition, connections from higher centres also modulate the activity of the PAG so that learning and memory can influence the responsiveness of the PAG to sensory stimulation (Bandler & Keay 1996). This descending system plays a role in the control of pain in acute inflammatory states (Sluka & Rees 1997) and dysfunction of this system is thought to contribute to widespread pain conditions such as fibromyalgia (Graven-Nielsen et al 1999).

The IASP definition refers to the pain experience as a sensory and emotional one. Although this section of the chapter has predominantly reviewed the neurophysiological mechanisms involved with pain perception, the role of psychological dimensions on pain cannot be underestimated. Attitudes and beliefs about pain can influence the way that pain is perceived and managed by the patient (Unruh et al 1999). Anxiety and distress can be associated with pain and disease and consequent loss of mobility and function (Farrell et al 1996).

Musculoskeletal pain – mechanisms involved in osteoarthritis pain

As mentioned earlier, there are high rates of musculoskeletal pain cited in the literature for aged care residents (Bassols et al 1999). The mechanisms described in the preceding sections underpin the development of chronic or persistent musculoskeletal pain syndromes. For example, in osteoarthritis, breakdown of cartilage and bone can cause the release of inflammatory mediators, in turn causing sensitization of peripheral afferent fibres, spinal and supraspinal centres involved in nociceptive processing. Activation of silent nociceptors and pressure increases within the joint activating high threshold mechanoreceptors summate to increase nociceptive input to the nervous system (Schaible & Grubb 1993). Sensitization of the C-fibre afferents, due to the process of neurogenic inflammation, can cause plasma extravasation and increased joint oedema (Zimmerman 1989).

Central sensitization and convergence of cutaneous, muscle joint input are also mechanisms involved with the perception of joint pain (Schaible & Grubb 1993). Therefore, second order neurons within the dorsal horn would respond to input from these cutaneous and muscular structures to explain superficial tenderness and pain perceived within the muscles surrounding the joint (hyperalgesia). Decreased threshold and increased response to stimulation and larger receptive fields are now evident and as such, previously innocuous movement and touch in areas around and outside the involved joint now promote the perception of pain (Farrell et al 2000).

There is evidence that supraspinal activity counteracts to some extent the increase in spinal and peripheral excitability (Sluka & Rees 1997) as tonic descending inhibitory influences are increased during acute inflammation. In addition to this centrally mediated effect, Stein et al (1999) suggest that there is an increase in peripheral receptors for opioids, which mediate pain relief in response to inflammation. These authors have demonstrated that opioids are released from inflamed tissue and activate opioid receptors located in synovia to decrease the level of pain. Thus both central and peripheral mechanisms are present to decrease the amount of pain experienced in the inflamed arthritic joint.

In addition to the pain involved in osteoarthritis, there is evidence of dysfunction of the muscle and sensorimotor systems. Due to pain, the patient may adopt pain-relieving postures and refrain from painful activity. This may be in part a conscious effort by the patient but may also indicate the effect of pain on motor reflexes as described above. Ferrell et al (1988) have demonstrated that intra-articular inflammation can produce an increase of the flexor withdrawal response possibly responsible for the characteristic flexion deformity of the arthritic knee. Inhibition of the quadriceps muscles might reflect the reduced capacity of the muscle to contract in the presence of pain and joint swelling (Lund et al 1991). Garsden & Bullock-Saxton (1999) demonstrated bilateral deficits in proprioception in unilateral osteoarthritic knees, suggesting the involvement of central control mechanisms of joint proprioception (Sharma et al 1997). There is a potential for deficits in motor control to further compound the situation, adding to the loss of joint control that occurs as a result of pain and injury (Hodges & Richardson 1996).

A surge in research into mechanisms of pain has provided us with important information about the neuroplasticity of the nociceptive system in the presence of injury and disease. Peripheral sensitization can cause an increase in the afferent barrage to the spinal cord as the sensitivity and number of afferent fibres activated is increased in the presence of inflammatory mediators. This increase in input from the periphery drives changes in the spinal cord and higher centres within the central nervous system. Central sensitization may be responsible for the development of referred pain and changes within the motor and autonomic nervous systems that accompany pain. Development of chronic pain is dependent on the relationship between the afferent system, changes in the cellular mechanisms at the level of the spinal cord and the modulation of nociceptive stimuli by the descending inhibitory system. Changes in the motor and sympathetic nervous systems can also contribute to development of chronic pain states, particularly in the case of musculoskeletal pain. Knowledge of how the system changes with injury and the mechanisms involved in pain modulation underpin the strategies for treatment of patients in pain using physiotherapeutic modalities.

In the next sections, assessment and management of pain are covered. Appropriate assessment and the use of relevant outcome measures are essential in the development of a sound management plan for patients in pain.

Assessment of pain in the elderly

Pain, especially chronic pain, can profoundly impact on an older person's quality of life. Some of the consequences of pain in the elderly population include:

- decrease in function and quality of life (Chibnall & Tait 2001, Ferrell 1995, Simmonds & Scudds 2001, Weiner et al 1999)
- increase in agitation (Chibnall & Tait 2001)
- decrease in mobility and independence (Cowan et al 2003, Herr & Mobily 1991)
- increase in emotional distress, depression and anxiety (Chibnall & Tait 2001, Cowan et al 2003)
- increased risk of mortality (Chibnall & Tait 2001)
- disturbed sleeping patterns (Bassols et al 1999, Cowan et al 2003)
- impaired posture and appetite (Cowan et al 2003).

Activity restriction due to pain in the elderly has been found to be as great as that reported by middle-aged people (Brattberg et al 1989). Yet Bowsher (1991) found 55% of people surveyed stated they were unable to lead a normal life because of pain, with the majority of these being over 45 years. This is in contrast to Roy & Thomas (1986) who found that activity levels and use of health care services among elderly people with and without chronic pain do not differ.

Accurate assessment of pain is critical for the identification of appropriate interventions and evaluation of the effectiveness of such interventions (Fig. 15.1) (Herr & Garand 2001). This would require more than a simple question or description of pain intensity (Herr 2002a). The following key points/steps for the assessment of pain in the elderly patient are based on the work of Herr (2000a) and Herr & Mobily (1991):

- a thorough physical evaluation and history, in particular history of pain medication
- detailed assessment of pain – location, quality, intensity, onset, duration, pattern of radiation or variation, manner of expressing pain, relationship to movement or position, time of occurrence, related motor or sensory complaints
- assessment or screening for cognitive impairment, sensorimotor impairment, language, cultural or educational needs
- assessment of any changes in behaviour – vocalizations, body movement or activities of daily living – which will provide clues to the presence of pain
- assessment of functional status, nutrition, sleep patterns, social activity and self-care.

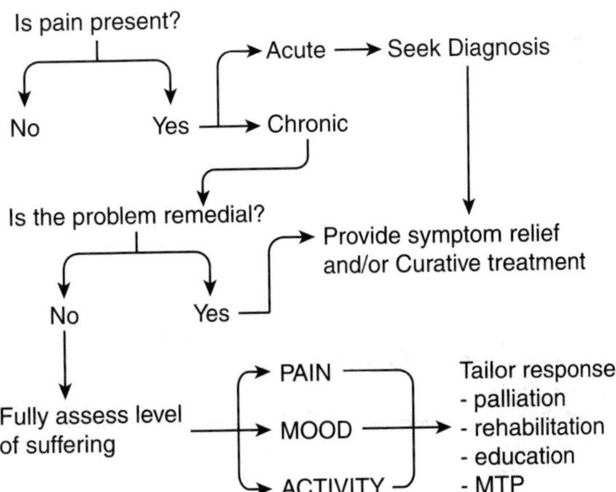

Figure 15.1
Flow diagram of pain assessment and treatment process. MTP, multidisciplinary treatment programme. Adapted from Helme & Gibson (1998) with permission.

Most commonly used tools for assessing pain in the elderly

Prior to selecting a pain scale, the following considerations are needed.

- Demographics of the individual, their educational level, ethnicity and language. Many pain scales are in English and require a level of reading and writing skills.
- If cognitive status or memory is impaired, then the assessment needs to be simple with clear explanations, examples used and demonstrations given. This will ensure the person is attentive and understands what is being asked. It may be necessary to collect all the necessary data over several short sessions rather than one long one.
- Sensory function such as vision and psychomotor skills need to be considered as even mild hearing loss can cause problems with concentration and understanding. If visual impairments are present, it may be necessary to alter the pain scales by enlarging the print, print the questions on one side only to prevent any omissions, insert adequate spacing between questions, and use non-glare paper, simple rather than decorative drawings so as not to confuse, page tabs for those with fine motor coordination problems (Herr & Mobily 1991).
- Consider the person's preference, as some may prefer a pain diagram rather than a pain descriptor scale, and ensure the pain scale has been validated for use with older adults.

Tools

Visual Analogue Scale (VAS)/Verbal Descriptor Scale (VDS)
These consist of a set of numbers with words representing different levels of pain. Patients select the word or number that best represents their intensity of pain. The VAS can be presented horizontally or vertically. The Pain Thermometer is a variation of the vertical VAS. A study of the VAS, VDS, Pain Thermometer and Numerical Rating Scale (NRS) amongst people over 65 years found the failure rate was comparable with the general population. However, the subjects in this study were cognitively alert patients with pain and preferred the VDS of all the scales offered (Herr & Mobily 1993). Gagliese et al (1999) reported that as many as 30% of cognitively intact elderly may be unable to complete the VAS, perhaps due to deficits in abstract reasoning. Kremer et al (1981) also found that increasing age was associated with a higher frequency of incomplete or unscoreable responses on the VAS. In summary, although the VAS is a simple, easy and quick tool to administer, it has not been validated in older adults and may be too abstract for them to use reliably.

McGill Pain Questionnaire (MPQ) and the Short Form-MPQ

These are the most widely used multidimensional pain inventories and measures of pain intensity as well as quality (Herr 2002a, Weiner et al 1998). They are appropriate for use with older adults and those with cognitive impairment. Ferrell et al (1995) assessed pain in 325 nursing home residents with a high prevalence of cognitive impairment. They used five different pain scales – the McGill Present Pain Intensity (PPI), VAS, Verbal 0–10 scale, Memorial Pain Card and the Rand COOP Chart. They found that 83% of the residents could complete at least one of the scales with the highest being the PPI subscale of the MPQ (65%). The MPQ contains a body chart on which the person can indicate the location and type of pain experienced. This is useful for those who have difficulty verbally expressing pain.

Faces Pain Scales

This is an 8-point facial expression scale depicting varying levels of discomfort and has been shown to correlate well with the VAS and the NRS in patients with osteoarthritis of the lower limb joints (Frank et al 1982). It was suggested it could be useful for the elderly with language or mental capacity difficulties. Herr et al (1998) studied the use of a modified version of the Face Pain Scale developed for children. They used 168 cognitively intact adults aged over 65 years. They established preliminary support for its validity and test–retest reliability. This scale was trialled with cognitively impaired adults by Kamel et al (2001). They compared two methods of pain assessment in nursing home residents. In one group, pain was assessed by asking the question 'Do you have pain?' In the second group, pain was assessed with a combination of the VAS, Faces Scale and a Pain Descriptor Scale. The study showed that utilization of the combined scales resulted in an increased frequency of pain reporting. Also, the frequency of diagnosing pain correlated with the level of cognitive functioning. In other words, the less impaired the resident the more likely the pain report. The simple question did not yield the same result as the combination scales as it was considered that older adults may use different terminology to describe pain with terms of 'discomfort' or 'aching' rather than 'pain'. This was clearly demonstrated by Weiner et al (1999) in their pilot study of 158 nursing home residents who responded 'no' when asked if they had pain but would respond to follow-up questions with 'aching or soreness'.

Structured Pain Interview (SPI)

This tool was developed by Weiner et al (1999) who found that cognitive performance had no influence on the stability of self-reported pain. Hence, their study does not support the notion that pain is more difficult to assess in cognitively impaired persons. Chibnall & Tait (2001) likewise found that the amount of pain experienced by older patients did not vary significantly as a function of cognitive impairment. The SPI has been advocated for use with older people (Herr & Garand 2001) with the 0–10 scale (zero means 'no pain' and 10 is 'maximum pain') of limited value in a cognitively impaired population due to its abstract nature.

The SPI basically consists of the questions 'Do you have some pain or discomfort every day or almost every day?' and 'What about aching or soreness?' A positive response to either question is regarded as a positive response to the SPI. Subjects are then asked, 'What part of your body hurts the most today?' and a pain map is shown. The study by Weiner et al (1999) demonstrated considerable miscommunication about pain between residents and staff of the nursing homes investigated. Thus the SPI is a feasible tool for examining pain in the nursing home setting.

Observational and behavioural measures

It has been shown that persons with mild to moderate cognitive impairment can respond to pain scales and provide adequate information about their pain. When the person is unable to use standard self-report measures, information gathered by observing the person's behaviour is useful (Herr 2002b, Herr & Garand 2001). There is much debate in the literature as to whether behavioural observations are sensitive and specific for pain assessment among older persons with dementia. One tool, the Checklist for Nonverbal Pain Indicators, shows preliminary validity and modest reliability with cognitively impaired persons in the acute care setting. This tool requires the clinician to observe the patient both at rest and during movement and to evaluate six pain-related behaviours. Information from family and carers about changes in physical or social behaviours and the impact of pain on activities of daily living is very useful. There have been documented inaccuracies between the assessment of pain by carers and patients, so surrogate reports should not be used until it is determined that the patient's account is unreliable (Cowan et al 2003, Herr 2002b).

The behaviours that may be observed to indicate the presence of pain include vocalizations, facial expressions, restlessness or agitation, groaning and moaning, sleep disturbance, changes in posture as limping or guarding, changes in mobility or uptime or self-care or eating habits. It has been said that clinical observations of facial expressions and vocalizations are accurate means of assessing for the presence of pain but not its intensity (Manfredi et al 2003).

Once the presence of pain has been established in the cognitively impaired person, the next challenge is to identify the source of the pain. Patients may express discomfort from constipation, emotional distress, cold, hunger and fatigue in the same ways - agitation, grimacing and restlessness (Cohen-Mansfield & Lipson 2002). The choice of intervention is thus limited by the inability of the person to cooperate or indicate the effectiveness of the intervention.

Physiotherapy in the management of pain

Changes to nociceptive processing associated with injury or disease can contribute to pain states and as such, it is important for therapists to understand and acknowledge these mechanisms when considering the management of the patient in pain. Treatment of the patient in pain must be tailored to the findings of the physical examination, an understanding of the underlying pathology and knowledge of pain mechanisms. It is important to understand that it is rarely considered appropriate to exacerbate a patient's pain during therapy as this can increase the barrage to the nociceptive system and maintain upregulation and thereby contribute to the painful condition. Addressing sensorimotor and motor deficits is also important to the long-term management of pain and injury. While there has been long-standing anecdotal evidence for a number of physiotherapy modalities for the management of pain conditions, evidence of the effectiveness of spinal manual therapy (SMT), exercise therapy and electrotherapy is now emerging. It is always important to consider possible contraindications to therapy, particularly in the elderly, due to the presence of secondary conditions such as impaired circulation or presence of a cardiac pacemaker.

Physiotherapists commonly use spinal manual therapy techniques to treat conditions of musculoskeletal pain and dysfunction. A number of trials have been conducted that highlight the efficacy of SMT for spinal pain (Aker et al 1996, Koes et al 1992). However, there is only a developing understanding of the mechanisms by which these treatments can exert their effects. The outcomes of SMT have most commonly been described in terms of the biomechanical response to application of the treatment technique. That is, numerous studies have been performed that investigate parameters such as load, deformation, transient vibration assessment and movement of spinal segments following mobilization and manipulation (Allison et al 1998, Herzog 2000, Keller et al 2000, Latimer et al 1998, Lee et al 1993, 1995, Lee & Liversidge 1994, Vicenzino et al 1999). Studies such as these are important to gain a perspective of the nature of the stimulus applied during SMT interventions.

It is implicit in the practice of SMT that the manual contact and movement of the underlying structures produced during the application of techniques provides activation of cutaneous, articular and muscular afferents. Whilst it is tempting to attempt to explain the effects of SMT in terms of the biomechanics of the technique, to underestimate the powerful input to the central nervous system via these afferents would be to fail to appreciate the potential neurophysiological influence of SMT. A multifactorial model to describe the potential neurophysiological effects of SMT was proposed by Wright (Wright 1995, Wright & Vicenzino 1995). In this model, activation of the descending pain inhibitory systems (DPIS) and local segmental pain inhibitory mechanisms as well as psychological effects were suggested as some of the possible mechanisms for the production of SMT-related effects. A number of studies have been performed to evaluate this hypothesis and other possible mechanisms for the effects produced by SMT (Souvlis et al 1999, Sterling et al 2000, Vernon 2000, Vicenzino et al 1996, 1998a, 1998b). Recent studies have also started to determine the mechanisms involved in the hypoalgesia that follows manual therapy to peripheral joints (Paungmali et al 2003a, 2003b).

Transcutaneous electrical nerve stimulation (TENS) has been shown to be effective in producing pain relief. Studies by Sluka et al (1998, 1999, 2000) demonstrate that analgesia following TENS application is related to the release of endogenous opioids. Low-frequency TENS produces pain relief through mu opioid receptors and high-frequency TENS produces antihyperalgesia through delta opioid receptors in the spinal cord (Sluka et al 1999). Furthermore, using an animal model with joint inflammation, the authors were able to show that high frequency TENS (100 Hz) was able to decrease pain in morphine-tolerant rats whereas low frequency

TENS (4 Hz) was not (Sluka 2000). This illustrates that in patients taking opioids for pain relief high frequency TENS may be of more use. In a clinical study by Cheing et al (2002) comparing TENS (100 Hz), isometric exercise and a combination of both to a placebo condition, the authors demonstrated a cumulative reduction in knee pain in chronic knee osteoarthritis patients following 4 weeks of TENS compared to the placebo condition. This pain relief was also demonstrated in a group given TENS and exercise. In a follow-up study, the authors showed that the optimal stimulation period was 40 minutes (Cheing et al 2003).

Osiri et al (2003) in a review for the Cochrane Library concluded that analgesia from high frequency TENS and acupuncture-like TENS treatment was significantly better than placebo treatment. Knee stiffness also improved significantly in the active treatment group compared to placebo. As in the study by Cheing et al (2002), the reviewers concluded that repeated simulation produced a stronger effect (Osiri et al 2003). Electrical stimulation for shoulder pain following stroke was also found to be of value by Cochrane Library evaluation (Price & Pandyan 2003). The authors reviewed four randomized controlled trials (RCTs) including use of TENS and functional electrical stimulation (FES) and concluded that there was no significant change in pain incidence. However, there was a significant treatment effect for FES for improvement in pain-free range of passive humeral lateral rotation. In a review of TENS for rheumatoid arthritis pain in the hand, a review of three RCTs revealed that administration of 15 minutes of acupuncture-like TENS (low frequency, high intensity) per week, for 3 weeks resulted in a significant decrease in rest pain (Brosseau et al 2003).

It is evident that TENS has a therapeutic effect for pain relief in chronic musculoskeletal conditions such as osteoarthritis and rheumatoid arthritis. The use of high or low frequency is dependent on factors such as medication taken by the patient and type of condition.

Application of radiant heat sources such as hot packs and wax baths gives superficial heat to provide relief from pain, muscle spasm and joint stiffness. This type of application is considered to be an effective form of pain relief. However care needs to be taken in the application of heat in patients with impaired sensation or who are cognitively impaired (Ferrell 1996). Appendix 4 provides an overview of the contraindications and precautions in the use of electrophysical agents for pain relief.

Cryotherapy or use of cold can be beneficial for pain relief. It provides effective analgesia by decreasing activity in afferent nerves. However, although effective, it is probably not as well accepted or tolerated in the older patient as heat therapy.

Massage therapy is used frequently to relieve musculoskeletal pain, reduce swelling and for relaxation. In a study by Ferrell et al (1989), the authors were able to demonstrate reduced anxiety and pain perception in cancer patients following massage. Specific trigger point massage may be useful in the presence of myofascial pain syndrome. It has the benefit that it is easily administered by family or caregivers.

Exercise is considered to be an essential tool for use by physiotherapists in the prevention and management of musculoskeletal pain. In the earlier section on neurophysiology of pain, it was highlighted that changes occur in the motor system as a result of both acute and chronic pain. Pain that is not of musculoskeletal origin can produce referred hyperalgesia and change in reactivity in muscles distant from the pain site (Giamberardino et al 1999). Therefore it is essential to assess and treat the motor system to maintain active support and stabilization of joints in pain (Richardson & Hides 2002). Decreasing stress on joint structures may decrease the incidence of pain and improve function. Recent research has demonstrated that there is a decrease in recurrence of pain following the use of specific therapeutic exercise (Hides & Richardson 1996, O'Sullivan et al 1997, 1998). In addition to the supporting or biomechanical effect, there is some evidence that activation of the motor system can provide inhibition of dorsal horn via descending projections from the corticospinal tracts (Galea & Darian-Smith 1995, Galea 2002). In general, exercise is thought to produce many other benefits as well as pain relief such as increasing cardiovascular fitness. Aquatic therapy provides an excellent combination of warmth and exercise and the further therapeutic value and other benefits of aquatic therapy are covered elsewhere in this text. Ahmad & Goucke (2002) advocate the use of 'non-drug treatment options' in the management of patients with neuropathic pain disorders. They consider that adoption of an exercise programme, lifestyle changes and environmental modification together with maintenance of mobility and independence where possible are important adjuncts to drug therapy for pain management.

Summary

- The perception of pain is a complex sensory and emotional experience involving multiple levels of the nervous system.
- In the presence of injury and inflammation, there is upregulation of the nociceptive system so that an increased sensitivity to previously noxious stimuli (hyperalgesia) and decrease in threshold to non-noxious stimulation (allodynia) develop.
- Peripheral and central sensitization of the nervous system occurs to produce these responses, and these mechanisms are also implicated in the development of referred pain. They also underline the transition from acute to chronic pain states.
- Motor and autonomic nervous system changes may occur following injury and these changes can also contribute to the development of chronic or persistent pain syndromes.
- Inhibitory mechanisms mediated by descending pathways from the midbrain are important in modulating spinal processing of nociceptive information. However, psychological

influences play a significant role in the overall pain processing and perception.

- The management of pain by the physiotherapist should be preceded by a thorough assessment of pain, the patient's overall physical presentation and their environment.
- Use of manual therapy techniques such as spinal manual therapy and both specific and general exercise programmes can be valuable to decrease pain.
- Use of adjunct therapies such as massage, heat and cold should be considered in the absence of any contraindications. Research has revealed that TENS can be particularly useful and that the benefits of its use are cumulative over time.
- Further research into the mechanisms of common pain problems in the elderly patient will provide us with the background necessary to develop the most effective therapeutic programmes to manage and hopefully prevent pain.

References

Afable R F, Ettinger W H 1993 Musculoskeletal disease in the aged: diagnosis and management. Drugs and Aging 3(1):49–59

Ahmad M, Goucke C R 2002 Management strategies for the treatment of neuropathic pain in the elderly. Drugs and Aging 19:929–945

Aker P D, Gross A R, Goldsmith C H, Peloso P 1996 Conservative management of mechanical neck pain: systematic overview and meta-analysis. British Medical Journal 313:1291–1296

Allison G, Edmondston S, Roe C et al 1998 Influence of load orientation on the posteroanterior stiffness of the lumbar spine. Journal of Manipulative and Physiological Therapeutics 21:534–538

Ardery G, Herr K A, Titler M G, Sorofman B A, Schmitt M B 2003 Assessing and managing acute pain in older adults: a research base to guide practice. Medsurgical Nursing 12(1):7–19

Bandler R, Keay K A 1996 Columnar organization in the midbrain periaqueductal gray and the integration of emotional expression. Emotional Motor System 107:285–300

Bandler R, Carrive P, Depaulis A 1991 Emerging principles of organisation in the midbrain periaqueductal gray matter. In: Depaulis A, Bandler R (eds) The midbrain periaqueductal gray matter. Plenum Press, New York, p 1-8

Bassols A, Bosch F, Campillo M, Canellas M, Banos J E 1999 An epidemiological comparison of pain complaints in the general population of Catalonia (Spain). Pain 83(1):9–16

Behbehani M M 1995 Functional characteristics of the midbrain periaqueductal gray. Progress in Neurobiology 46:575–605

Bergman S, Herrstrom P, Hogstrom K et al 2001 Chronic musculoskeletal pain, prevalence rates, and sociodemographic associations in a Swedish population study. Journal of Rheumatology 28(6): 1369–1377

Bessou P, Perl E R 1969 Response of cutaneous sensory units with unmyelinated fibres to noxious stimuli. Journal of Neurophysiology 32:1025–1043

Bowsher D, Rigge M, Sopp L 1991 Prevalence of chronic pain in the British population: a telephone survey of 1037 households. The Pain Clinic 4(4):223–230

Brattberg G, Thorslund M, Wikman A 1989 The prevalence of pain in a general population. The results of a postal survey in a county of Sweden. Pain 37(2):215–222

Brattberg G, Parker M G, Thorslund M A 1997 Longitudinal study of pain: reported pain from middle age to old age. Clinical Journal of Pain 13(2):144–149

Bredkjaer S R 1991 Musculoskeletal disease in Denmark. Acta Orthopaedica Scandinavica 62(Supplement 241):10-12

Brosseau L, Yonge K A, Robinson V et al 2003 Transcutaneous electrical nerve stimulation (TENS) for the treatment of rheumatoid arthritis in the hand (Cochrane Review). The Cochrane Library

Burgess P R, Perl E R 1967 Myelinated afferent fibres responding specifically to noxious stimulation of the skin. Journal of Physiology, London 190: 541-562

Cannon J T, Prieto G J, Lee A, Liebeskind J C 1982 Evidence for opioid and non-opioid forms of stimulation produced analgesia in the rat. Brain Research 243:315-321

Carmona L, Ballina J, Gabriel R, Laffon A 2001 The burden of musculoskeletal diseases in the general population of Spain: results from a national survey. Annals of the Rheumatic Diseases 60(11): 1040-1045

Cheing G L, Hui-Chan C W Y, Chan K M 2002 Does four weeks of TENS and/or isometric exercise produce cumulative reduction in osteoarthritic knee pain. Clinical Rehabilitation 16:749-760

Cheing G L, Tsui A Y, Lo S K, HuiChan C W Y 2003 Optimal stimulation duration of TENS in the management of osteoarthritic knee pain. Journal of Rehabilitation Medicine 35:62-68

Chibnall J T, Tait R C 2001 Pain assessment in cognitively impaired and unimpaired older adults: a comparison of four scales. Pain 92(1-2):173-186

Closs S J 1994 Pain in elderly patients: a neglected phenomenon? Journal of Advanced Nursing 19(6): 1072-1081

Coghill R C, Talbot J D, Evans A C et al 1994 Distributed processing of pain and vibration by the human brain. Journal of Neuroscience 14: 4095-4108

Cohen-Mansfield J, Lipson S 2002 Pain in cognitively impaired nursing home residents: how well are physicians diagnosing it? Journal of the American Geriatric Society 50(6):1039-1044

Cowan D T, Fitzpatrick J M, Roberts J D, While A E, Baldwin J 2003 The assessment and management of pain among older people in care homes: current status and future directions. International Journal of Nursing Studies 40(3):291-298

Crook J, Rideout E, Browne G 1984 The prevalence of pain complaints in a general population. Pain 18(3):299-314

Cui M, Feng Y, McAdoo D J, Willis W D 1999 Periaqueductal gray stimulation-induced inhibition of nociceptive dorsal horn neurons in rats is associated with the release of norepinephrine, serotonin and amino acids. Journal of Pharmacology and Experimental Therapeutics 289:868-876

Department of Families Queensland Government 2003 Profile of Older People in Queensland: Health, from www.families.qld.gov.au/seniors/index

Dray A 1995 Inflammatory mediators of pain. British Journal of Anaesthesia 75:125-131

Dray A 1996 Neurogenic mechanisms and neuropeptides in chronic pain. Progress in Brain Research 110:85-94

Fanselow M S 1991 The midbrain periaqueductal gray as a coordinator of action in response to fear and anxiety. In: Depaulis A, Bandler R (eds) The midbrain periaqueductal gray matter. Plenum Press, New York, p 151-173

Farrell M, Gibson S, Helme R 1996 Chronic nonmalignant pain in older people. In: Ferrell B R, Ferrell B A (eds) Pain in the elderly. IASP Press, Seattle, p 81-89

Farrell M, Gibson S, McMeeken J, Helme R 2000 Pain and hyperalgesia in osteoarthritis of the hands. Journal of Rheumatology 27:441-447

Ferrell B A 1991 Pain management in elderly people. Journal of the American Geriatrics Society 39:64-73

Ferrell B A 1995 Pain evaluation and management in the nursing home. Annals of Internal Medicine 123(9):681-687

Ferrell B A, Ferrell B R, Rivera L 1995 Pain in cognitively impaired nursing home patients. Journal of Pain and Symptom Management 10(8):591-598

Ferrell B R 1996 Patient education and non-drug interventions. In: Ferrell B R, Ferrell B A (eds) Pain in the elderly. IASP Press, Seattle, p 35-44

Ferrell B R, Wisdom C, Wenzl C 1989 Quality of life as an outcome variable in the management of cancer pain. Cancer 63:2321-2327

Ferrell W, Wood L, Baxendale R 1988 The effect of acute joint inflammation on flexion reflex excitability in the decerebrate, low spinal cat. Quarterly Journal of Experimental Physiology 73:95-102

Fields H L, Basbaum A I 1994 Central nervous system mechanisms of pain modulation. In: Wall P D, Melzack R (eds) Textbook of pain. Churchill Livingstone, Edinburgh, p 243-260

Fox P L, Raina P, Jadad A R 1999 Prevalence and treatment of pain in older adults in nursing homes and other long-term care institutions: a systematic review. Canadian Medical Association Journal 160(3):329–333

Frank A J M, Moll J M H, Hort J F 1982 A comparison of three ways of measuring pain. Rheumatology and Rehabilitation 21:211–217

Gagliese L, Katz J, Melzack R 1999 Pain in the elderly. In: Melzack R, Wall P (eds) Textbook of pain, 4th edn. Harcourt, London, p 991–1006.

Galea M P 2002 Neuroanatomy of the nervous system. In: Strong J, Unruh A, Wright A, Baxter G D (eds) Pain: a textbook for therapists. Churchill Livingstone, Edinburgh, p 13–41

Galea M P, Darian-Smith I 1995 Voluntary movement and pain: focussing on action rather than perception. Moving in on Pain, Adelaide

Garsden L R, Bullock-Saxton J E 1999 Joint reposition sense in subjects with unilateral osteoarthritis of the knee. Clinical Rehabilitation 3:148–155

Giamberardino M-A, Affaitati G, Iezzi S, Vecchiet L 1999 Referred muscle pain and hyperalgesia from viscera. Journal of Musculoskeletal Pain 7:61–69

Graven-Nielsen T, Sorenson J, Henriksson K G, Bengtsson M, Arendt-Nielsen L 1999 Central hyperexcitability in fibromyalgia. Journal of Musculoskeletal Pain 7:261–271

Harkins S W, Price D D 1992 Assessment of pain in the elderly. In: Turk D C, Melzack R (eds) Handbook of pain assessment. Guilford Press, New York, p 315–331

Harkins S W, Price D D, Bush F M, Small R E 1994 Geriatric pain. In: Wall P D, Melzack R (eds) Textbook of pain, 3rd edn. Churchill Livingstone, Edinburgh, p 769–784

Helme R D, Gibson S J 1998 Measurement and management of pain in older people. Australasian Journal on Ageing 17(1):5–9

Helme R D, Gibson S J 1999 Pain in older people. In: Crombie I K, Croft P R (eds) Epidemiology of pain. IASP Press, Seattle, p 103–112

Herr K 2002a Chronic pain: challenges and assessment strategies. Journal of Gerontological Nursing 28(1):20–27

Herr K 2002b Pain assessment in cognitively impaired older adults. American Journal of Nursing 102(12):65–67

Herr K A, Garand L 2001 Assessment and measurement of pain in older adults. Clinics in Geriatric Medicine 17(3):457–478

Herr K A, Mobily P R 1991 Complexities of pain assessment in the elderly: clinical considerations. Journal of Gerontological Nursing 17(4):12–19

Herr K A, Mobily P R 1993 Comparison of selected pain assessment tools for use with the elderly. Applied Nursing Research 6(1):39–46

Herr K A, Mobily P R, Kohout F J, Wagenaar D 1998 Evaluation of the Faces Pain Scale for use with the elderly. Clinical Journal of Pain 14(1):29–38

Herzog W 2000 Clinical biomechanics of spinal manipulation. Churchill Livingstone, Edinburgh

Hides J, Richardson C 1996 Multifidus muscle recovery is not automatic after resolution of acute, first episode low back pain. Spine 21:2763–2769

Hides J, Stokes M J, Saide M, Jull G A, Cooper D H 1994 Evidence of lumbar multifidus wasting ipsilateral to symptoms in patients with acute/subacute low back pain. Spine 19:165–172

Hodges P W 2001 Changes in motor planning of feedforward postural responses of trunk muscles in low back pain. Experimental Brain Research 141:261–266

Hodges P, Richardson C 1996 Inefficient muscular stabilisation of the lumbar spine associated with low back pain. A motor control evaluation of transversus abdominis. Spine 21:2640–2650

Hosobuchi Y, Adams J E, Linchitz R 1977 Pain relief by electrical stimulation of the central gray matter in human and its reversal by naloxone. Science 197:183–186

Janig W, McLachlan E 1992 Characteristics of function-specific pathways in the sympathetic nervous system. Trends in Neuroscience 15: 475–481

Janig W, Levine J, Michaelis M 1996 Interactions of sympathetic and primary afferent neurons following nerve injury and tissue trauma. Progress in Brain Research 113:161–184

Jansen A S P, Farkas E, Sams J M, Loewy A D 1998 Local connections between the columns of the periaqueductal gray matter: a case for intrinsic neuromodulation. Brain Research 784:329–336

Johansson H, Sojka P 1991 Pathophysiological mechanisms involved in genesis and spread of muscular tension in occupational muscle pain and in chronic musculoskeletal pain syndromes. Medical Hypotheses 35:196–203

Kamel H K, Phlavan M, Malekgoudarzi B, Gogel P, Morley J E 2001 Utilizing pain assessment scales increases the frequency of diagnosing pain among elderly nursing home residents. Journal of Pain and Symptom Management 21(6):450–455

Keller T S, Colloca C J 2000 In vivo transient vibration assessment of the normal human thoracolumbar spine. Journal of Manipulative and Physiological Therapeutics 23:521–530

Koes B W, Bouter L M, Vanmameren H et al 1992 Randomized clinical trial of manipulative therapy and physiotherapy for persistent back and neck complaints – results of one year follow-up. British Medical Journal 304:601–605

Kremer E, Atkinson H J, Ignelzi R L 1981 Measurement of pain: patient preference does not confound pain measurement. Pain 10:241–248

Latimer J, Lee M, Adams RD 1998 The effects of high and low loading forces on measured values of lumbar stiffness. Journal of Manipulative and Physiological Therapeutics 21:157–163

Lee M, Liversidge K 1994 Posteroanterior stiffness at three locations in the lumbar spine. Journal of Manipulative and Physiological Therapeutics 17:511–516

Lee M, Latimer J, Maher C 1993 Manipulation: investigation of a proposed mechanism. Clinical Biomechanics 8:302–306

Lee M, Maher C, Simmonds M J, Kumar S, Lechelt E 1995 Spinal models: use of a spinal model to quantify the forces and motion that occur during therapists' test of spinal motion. Physical Therapy 75:638–641

Lewis V A, Gebhart G F 1977 Morphine-induced and stimulation produced analgesias at coincident periaqueductal central gray loci: evaluation of analgesic congruence, tolerance, and cross-tolerance. Experimental Neurology 57:934–955

Lovick T A 1991 Interactions between descending pathways from the dorsal and ventrolateral periaqueductal gray matter in rats. In: Depaulis A, Bandler R (eds) The midbrain periaqueductal gray matter. Plenum Press, New York

Lund J P, Donga R, Widmer G, Stohler C 1991 The pain-adaptation model: a discussion of the relationship between chronic musculoskeletal pain and motor activity. Canadian Journal of Physiology and Pharmacology 69:683–694

Lutfy K, Hurlbut D E, Weber E 1993 Blockade of morphine-induced analgesia and tolerance in mice by MK-801. Brain Research 616:83–88

Manfredi P L, Breuer B, Meier D E, Libow L 2003 Pain assessment in elderly patients with severe dementia. Journal of Symptom Management 25(1):48–52

Mao J, Price D D, Mayer D J 1995 Mechanisms of hyperalgesia and morphine tolerance: a current view of their possible interactions. Pain 62: 259–274

Mayer D J 1979 Endogenous analgesia systems: neural and behavioral mechanisms. In: Bonica J J (ed) Advances in pain research and therapy. 3. Raven Press, New York, p 385–410

Mayer D J, Mao J, Holt J, Price D D 1999 Cellular mechanisms of neuropathic pain, morphine tolerance and their interactions. Proceedings of the National Academy of Science – USA 96:7731–7736

Melzack R, Wall P D 1965 Pain mechanisms: a new theory. Science 150:171–179

Melzack R, Wall P D 1996 The challenge of pain. Penguin Books, Harmondsworth, Middlesex

Mense S 1993 Nociception from skeletal-muscle in relation to clinical muscle pain. Pain 54:241–289

Merskey H, Bogduk N 1994 Classification of chronic pain: descriptors of chronic pain syndromes and definitions of pain terms. IASP Press, Seattle

Morgan M M 1991 Differences in antinociception evoked from dorsal and ventral regions of the caudal periaqueductal gray matter. In: Depaulis A, Bandler R (eds) The midbrain periaqueductal gray matter. Plenum Press, New York

Nichols D S, Thorn B E 1990 Stimulation-produced analgesia and its cross tolerance between dorsal and ventral PAG loci. Pain 57:347–352

Osiri M, Welch V, Brosseau L et al 2003 Transcutaneous electrical nerve stimulation for knee osteoarthritis (Cochrane Review). The Cochrane Library, Update Software

O'Sullivan P, Twomey L, Allison G 1997 Evaluation of specific stabilising exercise in the treatment of chronic low back pain with radiologic diagnosis of spondylosis or spondylolisthesis. Spine 22: 2959–2967

O'Sullivan P, Twomey L, Alison G 1998 Altered abdominal muscle recruitment in patients with chronic back pain following a specific exercise intervention. Journal of Orthopaedic and Sports Physical Therapy 27:114–124

Paungmali A, O'Leary S, Souvlis T, Vicenzino B 2003a Hypoalgesia and sympathoexcitatory effects of mobilisation with movement for lateral epicondylalgia. Physical Therapy 83(4):374–383

Paungmali A, O'Leary S, Souvlis T, Vicenzino B 2003b Naloxone fails to antagonise initial hypoalgesic effect of a manual therapy treatment for lateral epicondylalgia. Journal of Manipulative and Physiological Therapeutics (in press)

Popp B, Portenoy R K 1996 Management of pain in the elderly: pharmacology of opioids and other analgesic drugs. In: Ferrell B R, Ferrell B A (eds) Pain in the elderly. IASP Press, Seattle, p 21–34

Price C I M, Pandyan A D 2003 Electrical stimulation for preventing and treating post-stroke shoulder pain (Cochrane Review). The Cochrane Library

Price D D, Mayer D J, Mao J R, Caruso Fire Service 2000 NMDA-receptor antagonists and opioid receptor interactions as related to analgesia and tolerance. Journal of Pain and Symptom Management 19:S7–S11

Rexed B 1954 The cytoarchitectonic atlas of the spinal cord in the cat. Journal of Comparative Neurology 100:279–379

Reynolds D V 1969 Surgery in the rat during electrical analgesia induced by focal brain stimulation. Science 164:444–445

Richardson C, Hides J 2002 Exercise and pain. In: Strong J, Unruh A, Wright A, Baxter G D (eds) Pain: a textbook for therapists. Churchill Livingstone, Edinburgh, p 245–266

Roy R, Thomas M 1986 A survey of chronic pain in an elderly population. Canadian Family Physician 32:513–516

Schaible H-G, Grubb B D 1993 Afferent and spinal mechanisms of spinal joint pain. Pain 55:5–54

Sharma L, Pai Y C, Holtkamp K, Rymer W Z 1997 Is knee joint proprioception worse in the arthritic knee versus the unaffected knee in unilateral knee osteoarthritis? Arthritis and Rheumatism 40: 1518–1525

Simmonds M J, Scudds R J 2001 Pain, disability, and physical therapy in older adults: issues of patients and pain, practitioners and practice. Topics in Geriatric Rehabilitation 16(3):12–23

Sluka K A 2000 Systemic morphine in combination with TENS produces an increased antihyperalgesia in rats with acute inflammation. Journal of Pain 1:204–211

Sluka K A, Rees H 1997 The neuronal response to pain. Physiotherapy Theory and Practice 13:3–22

Sluka K A, Willis W D, Westlund K N 1995 The role of dorsal root reflexes in neurogenic inflammation. Pain Forum 4:141–149

Sluka K, Bailey K, Bogush J, Olsen R, Ricketts A 1998 Treatment with either high or low frequency TENS reduces the secondary hyperalgesia observed after injection of kaolin and carrageenan into the knee joint. Pain 77:97–102

Sluka K A, Deacon M, Stibal A, Strissel S, Terpstra A 1999 Spinal blockade of opioid receptors prevents the analgesia produced by TENS in arthritic rats. Journal of Pharmacology and Experimental Therapeutics 289:840–846

Sluka K A, Judge M A, McColley M M, Reveiz P M, Taylor B M 2000 Low frequency TENS is less effective than high frequency TENS at reducing inflammation-induced hyperalgesia in morphine-tolerant rats. European Journal of Pain - London 4:185–193

Souvlis T, Kermode F, Williams E, Collins D, Wright A 1999 Does the initial analgesic effect of spinal manual therapy exhibit tolerance? 9th World Congress on Pain. Book of Abstracts, Vienna

Stanton-Hicks M, Baron R, Boas R 1998 Complex regional pain syndromes: guidelines for therapy. Clinical Journal of Pain 14:155–166

Stein C, Cabot P, Schafer M 1999 Peripheral opioid analgesia: mechanisms and clinical implications. In: Stein C (ed) Opioids in pain control: basic and clinical aspects. Cambridge University Press, New York

Sterling M, Jull G, Wright A 2000 Cervical mobilisation: Concurrent effects on pain, sympathetic nervous system activity and motor activity. Manual Therapy 6:72–81

Sterling M, Jull G, Wright A 2001 The effect of musculoskeletal pain on motor activity and control. Journal of Pain 2:135–145

Sternbach R A 1986 Survey of pain in the United States: the Nuprin Pain Report. Clinical Journal of Pain 2:49–53

Terman G W, Shavit Y, Lewis J W, Cannon J T, Liebeskind J C 1984 Intrinsic mechanisms of pain inhibition: activation by stress. Science 226: 1270–1277

Unruh A M, Ritchie J A, Merskey H 1999 Does gender affect the appraisal of pain and pain coping strategies? Clinical Journal of Pain 15:31–40

Vernon H T 2000 Qualitative review of studies of manipulation-induced hypoalgesia. Journal of Manipulative and Physiological Therapeutics 23: 134–138

Vicenzino B, Collins D, Wright A 1996 The initial effects of a cervical spine manipulative physiotherapy treatment on the pain and dysfunction of lateral epicondylalgia. Pain 68:69–74

Vicenzino B, Collins D, Cartwright T, Wright A 1998a Cardiovascular and respiratory changes produced by lateral glide mobilisation of the cervical spine. Manual Therapy 3:67–71

Vicenzino B, Collins D, Benson H, Wright A 1998b An investigation of the interrelationship between manipulative therapy-induced hypoalgesia and sympathoexcitation. Journal of Manipulative and Physiological Therapeutics 21:448–453

Vicenzino B, Neal R, Collins D, Wright A 1999 The displacement, velocity and frequency profile of the frontal plane motion produced by the cervical lateral glide treatment technique. Clinical Biomechanics 14:515–521

Wall P D, Woolf C J 1984 Muscle but not cutaneous input produces prolonged increases in the excitability of the flexion reflex in the rat. Journal of Physiology - London 356:443–458

Weiner D, Peterson B, Keefe F 1998 Evaluating persistent pain in long term care residents: what role for pain maps? Pain 76(1–2):249–257

Weiner D, Peterson B, Ladd K, McConnell E, Keefe F 1999 Pain in nursing home residents: an exploration of prevalence, staff perspectives, and practical aspects of measurement. Clinical Journal of Pain 15(2):92–101

Woolf C J, Mannion R J 1999 Neuropathic pain: aetiology, symptoms, mechanisms and management. Lancet 353:1959–1964

Wright A 1995 Hypoalgesia post manipulative therapy. Manual Therapy 1:11–16

Wright A, Vicenzino B 1995 Central mobilisation techniques, sympathetic nervous system effects and their relationship to analgesia. Moving in on Pain, Adelaide

Zimmerman M 1989 Pain mediators and mechanisms in osteoarthritis. Seminars in Arthritis and Rheumatism Supplement 2:22–29

16 Physiotherapy in palliative care

Susan R. Hourigan and Diane L. Josephson

This chapter aims to:

- highlight healthy attitudes towards death, dying and ageing
- illustrate how physiotherapy may play a role in palliation
- extend basic knowledge of palliative care.

Introduction

This chapter will illustrate the principles of palliative care and identify aspects of physiotherapy management and practice that are relevant to the palliative care setting. It is important to note that physiotherapeutic assessment and treatment principles are the same for all residents regardless of health status. The major difference in palliative care is that a therapist must prioritize goals directly in relation to the resident's and family's wishes regardless of usual clinical reasoning. Advocacy is the focus and information should be provided to allow residents to make their own choices. Resident comfort and dignity usually comes first - pain management is often the top priority. Communication is of paramount importance during this time to enable a positive focus and to ensure best practice is achieved.

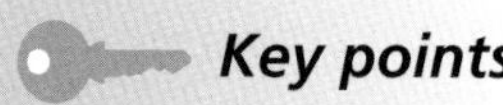

Key points

As birth is a miracle, so is death. We are blessed to be equipped with the skills to help those who are dying.

'Caring for and caring about' – as physiotherapists it is ideal to take an holistic approach – we are not just treating signs and symptoms or an underlying disease but the biopsychosocial needs of an individual and his or her family.

Assessment (as always) should be specific and goal-directed – during palliation it is important to identify patient goals early.

What is palliative care?

Palliative care means a form of care that recognizes that cure or long-term control is not possible; is concerned with the quality rather than the quantity of life; cloaks troublesome and distressing symptoms with treatments whose primary or sole aim is the highest possible measure of patient comfort.

Goals for palliative care have been outlined by the World Health Organization. Palliative care:

- affirms life and regards death as a normal process
- neither hastens nor postpones death
- provides relief from pain and other distressing symptoms
- integrates the psychological and spiritual aspects of pain
- offers a support system to help patients live as actively as possible until death
- offers a support system to help the family cope during the patient's illness and in their bereavement
- uses a team approach to address the needs of patients and their families, including bereavement counselling, if indicated
- will enhance quality of life, and may also positively influence the course of illness
- is applicable early in the course of illness, in conjunction with other therapies that are intended to prolong life, such as chemotherapy or radiation therapy, and includes those investigations needed to better understand and manage distressing clinical complications (WHO 1990, 2002, 2003).

The World Health Organization currently has a large global perspective on palliative care encompassing many different areas such as cancer care, children's care and an African Initiative which is a joint cancer and HIV/AIDS project. WHO's contribution to palliative care, its past, present and future challenges were identified by Sepulveda et al (2002).

Early in the fourth century the original hospices were formed in which matrons opened their homes to the sick and needy. Although a relatively new concept of care within modern medicine, palliative care has foundations in hospices in the UK through the early 1960s and in Australia in the 1980s. Flinders University in South Australia was the first in the world to appoint a Chair in Palliative Care in 1998 (Emeritus Professor Ian Maddocks).

The principles behind palliative care have been suggested by some authors to be those of beneficence, non-maleficence, justice and autonomy:

- beneficence - any act of goodness or kindness
- non-maleficence - not doing harm or not harmful
- justice - fair treatment or conduct; honestly, fairly, accurately
- autonomy - independence or freedom.

Death can be a happy time if a person's needs are met before, during and after their passing. The philosophy of care is such that it encompasses all aspects of a person's make-up. It is the integration of the physical, emotional, intellectual and spiritual components of a person, as illustrated in Figure 16.1.

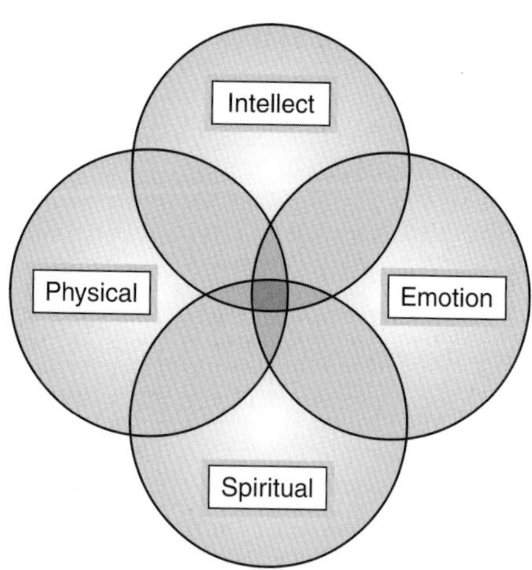

Figure 16.1 *The model of the integration of life aspects.*

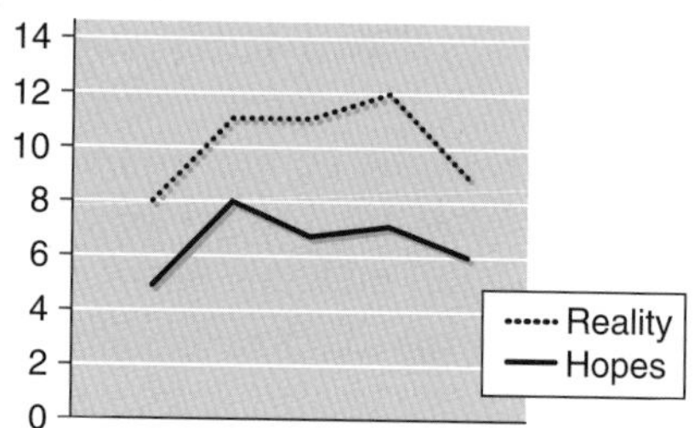

Figure 16.2 *Quality of life as mirrored by hopes and reality.*

Palliative care incorporates principles such as 'wellness' and biopsychosocial models. This clearly relates to a person's quality of life (QOL).

QOL is:

- 'whatever a person says it is'
- subjective satisfaction
- related to the biopsychosocial and spiritual dimensions of a person
- related to the emotional need to feel useful – defines their role
- related to the intellectual ability to remember, concentrate and be able to reframe life events
- related to psychological function (grief, anxiety, depression, peace, acceptance)
- related to social functions such as relationships, intimacy, support and family
- related to spiritual aspects such as finding meaning and transcendence
- related to physical aspects such as mobility and independence
- related to symptoms such as pain, constipation, weakness and shortness of breath.

Quality of life is clearly understood by evaluating the difference between a person's hopes and their reality. If what is experienced matches individuals' hopes, they perceive good quality in their life. Figure 16.2 illustrates this concept. Quality of life may be measured using the McGill Quality of Life questionnaire (Cohen et al 1995).

Patient goals are therefore the ultimate focus. There are many different personality types and each person has had unique and different experiences throughout their life. Palliative care is about providing them with choices and seeing that their decisions are acted upon wherever possible. In aged care many residents will have lost many functions, including intellectual alertness, communication and simple self-care, not to mention the 'social death' which may have surrounded their admission into a facility. Irrespective of this, all the same principles should apply, which encourages participation and decision-making by the resident whenever possible. There are difficulties involved in transparently overlaying the principles of palliative care to aged care due to several factors. Dementia has been a contraindication in the past to hospice admission due to the inability of the person to direct their own care and 'work through their understanding'. Other points which lead to slight modification in the aged care setting involve lack of staff training, hours and expertise and a tendency for symptoms to be dismissed in the aged care setting due to universality and complexity of problems. Regardless of limitations such as these, it is important to achieve best practice in any RACF, and the care provided should be of good quality and embrace the principles of palliative care as outlined.

Physiotherapy and palliative care

Physiotherapy has built up a large research base of techniques and skills that are invaluable to best practices and outcomes in patient care. The choice and use of physiotherapeutic knowledge is of little value without first gaining the trust and cooperation of the patient. Respect for the patient and a deep regard for their feelings and wishes must precede any attempt to offer any form of assistance. In the area of palliative care this is essential. We need the trust and understanding not only of our patient but also of their carer/s and the rest of the team who are involved in each case. Never is there such need for teamwork of the unobtrusive and quiet type. All facets of care must be finely tuned, respected and implemented with minimal fuss and maximum benefit to our patient. We should be like an excellent symphony with all parts coming in and fading out as the music demands.

Communication that reaches across the barriers of race, creed, words and externals must first be gained in order to provide service and support to people at this critical stage in their lives. Palliative care is both sacred and solemn. We need to explore how best to be of service to another in this time when life's journey is drawing to a close.

Good care will depend on good assessment of the physical condition of the person but more importantly we must endeavour to understand the priority of what they perceive to be their needs and desires at this time. We must see this person in the full context of their history and environment. Physical needs may be completely overshadowed and become insignificant for the person compared to the need for love and resolution of their spiritual, emotional or psychological requirements at this time.

This is a time for resolution and finalization of a lifetime's work. It is a period of great power in a person's life when sensitivity and love can facilitate miracles. We are privileged to become part of someone's life at this time because of our knowledge of ageing and physiology, but our skills need to be tempered and refined to the hierarchy of needs of each individual person. If this is not clearly interpreted, our efforts may be destructive rather than constructive at this delicate time.

Our role must be to bring comfort and promote healing of body, mind and spirit, to protect and empower, to teach and re-educate, to alleviate and to assist in whatever way is clinically and humanely possible. We must always be mindful of the acute needs of the patient throughout.

> *It is the centre of our caring being, our humanness which reaches out to others. Caring from the heart uses our reflective knowledge our cognitive thoughts and our action centre to create positive outcomes for the other.*
>
> Roach (1992)

> *As we travel this journey with the resident our lives are changed and enriched and we grow and we learn. All of those experiencing this deeply rewarding and humility provoking pathway of palliative care are able to experience this. To me, the depth of the human soul and spirit is immeasurable and unfathomable.*
>
> In personal interview with S.R. Josephson, August 2002, on 'The positives of working with patients who are dying'

> *Caring gives rise to our meaning and purpose for being in the world.*
>
> Frankl (1959)

> *The caring process can activate a higher power, order or energy in the universe which potentiates healing, health and self-knowledge.*
>
> Keegan & Guzzetta (2000)

The role of physiotherapy

Assessment is essential. As experience is gained intuition takes over from, or enhances, step by step science. The mental process is the same. Closely observe the patient at all times during assessment and history taking. Body language and facial expression may tell you significant things that words do not.

This is the information we need. It can be collected in any order, in any way and in whichever time frame is appropriate.

1. Subjective assessment (may be from family or caregiver)
   - medical history of the patient and course of recent condition
   - family and social history
   - present signs and symptoms
   - previous treatment received and outcome/effects noted

- medications
- goals and desires of the patient
- prescription of aids and comforts.

2. Objective assessment.
3. Physical assessment.

As we collect information we need to clarify our role and our aims with our patient and their family and ensure that we are all working towards the same goals and outcomes. A practical and possible plan of care must evolve for all concerned.

As we evaluate the situation and discuss our findings with other concerned team members, a priority of most urgent needs becomes obvious and leads to a time frame of care and action. It may be that control of pain or emotional distress becomes the first area for attention and very often good drug management can facilitate and greatly enhance future plans and outcomes for good physiotherapy management.

Therapy required may be classified under the model of symptom management and with a view to realizing patient goals and is illustrated in Figure 16.3.

Physiotherapy practice will often encompass:

- rehabilitation, promoting independence, facilitating activities of daily living
- symptomatic treatment (pain/constipation/skin integrity/mobility/independence)
- utilization of treatment modalities such as therapeutic exercise, electrotherapy, joint and soft tissue mobilization, hydrotherapy and equipment prescription

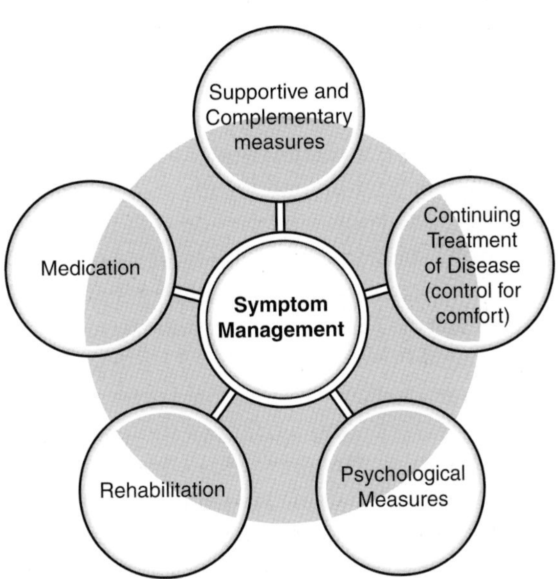

Figure 16.3 *Model of symptom management.*

- education of the resident, carers and families - including disease and health information, health promotion, manual handling, back care, and workplace health and safety and environment auditing
- appropriate exercise plans.

Maintaining or restoring mobility, dexterity and function

Promoting independence and maximizing the full potential of the patient will often be a treatment aim. This may involve some rehabilitation and often a degree of encouragement, reassurance and motivation.

This is the first step in caring and to do this well increases the patient's interest and self-esteem and can take a great deal of the physical burden off the carer or carers.

- Look at the heights of chairs and bed for the patient and see if raising or lowering the height may make life easier for the patient. To get out of bed the person needs to be able to put feet flat on the floor before standing. The correct height chair provides the same easy access and should fully support the thighs. The back support should be straight. If the person is suffering from swollen legs a chair which raises the feet is optimal. Otherwise, if the person is sitting up for a long period of time they will need to elevate their feet. Be careful to ensure the backrest reclines to allow for the length of the hamstring muscles when the feet are elevated. This will reduce the tendency to slide the buttocks forward on the seat and consequently assume a very flexed lumbar spine position that might increase pain in this area. The back of the knees also should be fully supported or the person will experience pain and discomfort in their knee joints.
- Look at the way the person is sitting up from lying in bed. A rope attached to the end of the bed can make life easier and provide independence and exercise for your patient as it assists them to come to a sitting position. A solid pole beside the bed is another good alternative. A hand grasp above the head can make movement around the bed easier but is of little use for sitting up as the angle of pull is incorrect.
- Walking aids can give great support, remove the fear of falling and keep your patient mobile for the maximum length of time. A walking stick gives minimum support and walking frames can provide maximum support. The frame with elbow support promotes good posture and allows more arm strength to be utilized. For someone with lower limb or spinal problems this can be remarkably useful as it decreases the amount of weight-bearing apportioned through the trunk and legs. The walking frame chosen will therefore need to be of a wheeled variety. Pick-up hoppers or 'Zimmer' frames should not be considered for palliative care patients as they greatly load the spine during the 'lift and shift' phase of gait and in so doing are likely to increase bony damage or increase pain.
- Grab rails strategically placed can maximize independence and give confidence. Along the wall, near doorways and on bathroom and shower

walls they can allow greater mobility and independence in confined areas where frames will not fit.

- Handheld retrievers with hooks, magnets, prongs or pincers on the end save the patient bending down and can increase their reach. These can be simply made and can be adapted for your patient's individual needs.
- Cutlery and writing equipment can be easily moulded to be more comfortable and useful by enlarging the area of grip or changing the angle of grip. Home-made bindings can be cleverly modified to suit hand sizes and shapes.
- Clothing can be altered to open down the back to make dressing easier.
- Trays for eating, reading or writing can be made of a piece of light timber that sits across the armrests of a chair.
- Straws are extremely useful to maximize fluid intake and prevent spillage.
- Remote controls and headphones can promote comfort and independence.

The environment needs to be set up to allow the patient easy access to all their aids and comforts. Everything they need should be comfortably within reach.

Providing comfort and protecting skin integrity

In the course of a normal day we all move and readjust our posture many more times than we are aware of. We gesticulate and wriggle and sit and stand incessantly. When someone is unwell these spontaneous movements are seriously minimized. The period of time spent motionless and sedentary can increase to the extent that the areas that take the weight of the body are at risk of breaking down. This is the result not only of direct pressure but it is compounded by the decrease in circulatory efficiency and poorer nutritional intake that often accompany ill health.

The best protection against skin damage is provided by:

1. frequent change of position
2. promoting good skin condition
3. encouraging good circulation with movement and exercise
4. encouraging good nutrition and hydration
5. protecting bony prominences.

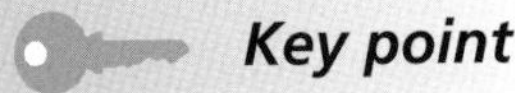

Key point When it comes to pressure areas **prevention** is the answer.

Healing broken skin is difficult and pressure areas are very painful for your patient. The skin integrity will be severely compromised after only one hour of unrelenting pressure. Movement provides the best protection for skin integrity. Varying or reducing the points of pressure by the use of sheepskins or gel pads may assist. Soft cushions or foam should be used to prevent pressure between knees when the patient is lying on their side. Ideally a pressure-varying mattress is also used but these are not always available so we use massage and protection of the vulnerable areas to improve the circulation. Keeping the skin soft and supple by the use of good oils or moisturizers is also invaluable. Aromatherapy oils can be used to promote relaxation and wellbeing as well as for moisturizing.

The main 'risk' areas are the bony prominences and surrounding soft tissues. The most important areas to protect and relieve are:

1. the sacral area and buttocks
2. the elbows
3. the heels
4. the knees
5. the ankles
6. the ears.

Little cradles can be made out of foam to protect the ears. Simply cut the ear shape out of a square piece of foam approximately 8 cm square and 5 cm deep and covered by a pillow case to increase comfort. Socks or soft slippers can be useful for heels and ankles.

Frequent position changes are essential to prevent prolonged pressure on bony prominences. If your patient is physically capable this is not difficult. You can use short walks, vary the time spent in bed resting or up in the chair. You can have comfortable chairs in different rooms or out in the garden. If your patient is dependent this is more challenging and puts a greater onus on the carer.

Education

Manual handling

Walking belts

These belts are made to give carers a 'real' handle on people. Severe damage to joints and skin may be caused by using limbs to move people. Limbs do not give the carer a good grip or indeed any mechanical efficiency but if you put a comfortable belt around the pelvis of your resident a good hold is provided for the carer and greater comfort for the patient. They allow assistance to be directed to the centre of a patient's weight, they facilitate movement patterns and also assist in guiding walking direction.

Slide sheets

These are simply a piece of sail cloth or some other material that is slippery and effectively reduces friction by gliding smoothly on itself. A slide sheet is used in a double layer (either folded or by using two full lengths). The patient's body weight is repositioned by movement of the top layer over the bottom layer. It is important to grasp the top layer or sheet close to your patient's shoulder and hip as these are the key areas for patient movement. Accessing these heavy areas makes movement of the body easy. You can maximize patient comfort by turning their head first in the direction of planned movement (for instance when performing a rolling movement). You can also prepare the patient by bending the top knee to facilitate rolling to the other side and you may prepare by the use of pillows or cushions to support painful or at-risk areas.

The carer must endeavour to follow good back care principles and keep the spine as straight as possible during transfers. This is easy where you have adjustable bed heights but much more difficult to achieve in community care situations.

Mechanical aids

Hoists may be used to reposition fully dependent patients or patients deemed to be unsafe when weight-bearing. These devices dramatically reduce the risk of injury to the carer and indeed to the patient. There are many varieties of hoists on the market and the technique of using each hoist and the appropriate slings must be mastered before any attempt is made to transfer a patient.

Hoists take the full weight of the patient and therefore are of great value in moving patients from bed to chair, bed to bath, chair to chair and maybe from floor back to bed after a fall.

Hoists are expensive items and are not readily available to the wider community. Some community aid programmes will provide hoists for needy cases but these must be prescribed for each individual as the sizes and uses for hoists vary considerably.

In Australia the nurses union has a no-lift policy and this has seen many more hoists available in the workplace than there were previously.

Back care and injury prevention

Anatomically the 'back' is made up of muscles, bones, joints, ligaments, tendons, nerve and discs. All of these structures may be injured. Prevention is the key – we only have one back and backs are notoriously difficult to rehabilitate after injury.

Carers need to know that most back pain comes from frequent, repetitive use of the back in poor positions. The greatest risk factors for back injury are poor posture, sustained postures, poor lifting practices or incorrect manual handling, jerking, twisting and poor personal fitness/wellness. Eighty per cent of disc injury is due to repetitive poor patterns as opposed to one incident. The discs have poor sensation and poor circulation; therefore we often have no indication of injury occurring until the damage is severe. Furthermore intervertebral discs are poorly equipped for healing.

It is important to set up the caring environment so that it is as ergonomically sound as possible. Most caring tasks are repetitive and therefore great care must be taken to ensure safety of the patient and safety of the carer.

Fatigue minimization

Providing palliative care fatigues the carer physically and emotionally. In an RACF carers can share responsibility for residents and thereby reduce the individual burden of care. This luxury is rarely available for a family member caring for another at home. In all instances case discussions involving the patient, carers and all other team members might forestall the possible catastrophic effects from carer fatigue and 'burn-out' by putting into place plans to cope with potentially stressful events that might be predicted for the patient or carer. If not prepared for, the psychological and physical effects from accumulated or one-off events can be far-reaching and make the passing of a resident or loved one more difficult.

Important considerations

- Educate the carer in optimal use of the body and good posture.
- Adjust work heights to facilitate caring and transfers.
- Where possible use mechanical aids and have appropriate training.
- Clear any unnecessary 'clutter' from the area.
- Communicate your intentions, before attempting to move, to both the patient and any assistants.
- Plan the move, and count out loud before beginning.
- Nurse the patient in a well-ventilated and well-lit area. Use cooling or heating as required.
- Carers must look after themselves! Keep fit, strong and well rested. Minimize stress and get help when you need it.

Treatment modalities

Heat/cold therapy

Heat is often a comfort for painful chronic conditions as it improves circulation and promotes relaxation. It is available in many forms from hot water bottles to electric blankets. Very often the frail or neurologically impaired patient has sensory loss and therefore there is a high risk of injury or burns. As with all treatments, the comfort gained must be weighed against the risk of injury and well-informed decisions must be made and monitored. For some arthritic conditions (especially inflammatory subtypes) cold compresses may give relief. Trial and error is often the only way of knowing whether heat or cold may be more effective. If the patient sustains an acute injury or contusion, cold packs applied immediately will result in a better outcome. Limiting circulation to the affected part and decreasing swelling and bleeding into the tissues will reduce the injury response but always be aware of the contraindicating factor to thermal modalities imparted by poor circulation.

Electrotherapy

There are volumes written on the use of electrotherapy and its many positive effects. However, its use may be limited in the area of palliative care. Often if pain is a problem, drug therapy is the chosen treatment. However a multidisciplinary team should not underestimate, and never discount, the possible alternatives such as TENS, magnetic therapy and laser.

Transcutaneous electrical nerve stimulation (TENS)

TENS works on the gate theory of pain control. It may control pain by providing a counter-irritant stimulus through the afferent nerves originating in the skin (it is felt as a mild buzzing or tingling feeling). This ascending sensory information is perceived by the brain rather than the noxious pain information and thereby the pain sensations are blocked before being cognitively perceived. Some research indicated TENS may also stimulate the production of endogenous opioids by the brain and further provide analgesia through this mechanism. The TENS machines are safe and small and have had good effects for some painful conditions. It is easy to apply and teach to the patient or carer.

Laser therapy

This therapy is extremely useful to heal skin lesions. The laser beam used is in the infra-red part of the spectrum and although penetration is not very deep the laser can promote good healing from underneath the lesion. Laser has contraindications and safety rules but in the hands of a trained person it is very useful.

Magnetic therapy

Magnetic therapy may play a role in the treatment of some conditions such as non-uniting fractures, joint pains, healing of ulcers, insomnia and soft tissue injuries. There are many form of magnetic therapy and if it is available can give excellent results. Some forms of underlays for the bed have been trialled successfully and magnetic therapy has the advantage that it can be used with metal in the body and it is very safe. It does have contraindications, e.g. cardiac pacemakers, carcinogenic conditions. The reader is referred to the electrotherapy appendix (Appendix 4).

Ultrasound

This needs to be applied by a trained professional. It is useful for dispersion of bruising, reduction of oedema, promotion of healing and other localized conditions. Precautions must be taken to ascertain sensory feedback – as with most modalities patient feedback is essential to the safety of application. It should be the physiotherapist who applies ultrasound therapy.

Aquatic physiotherapy (hydrotherapy)

The use of warm water immersion to augment and aid treatment through aquatic physiotherapy (hydrotherapy) has been well proven and established in many different cases. This is an excellent modality and the sadness is that it is not more readily available. Hydrotherapy treats the whole person. The body may be wholly or partially immersed in water 32–34°C. The effects of the warmth, buoyancy and hydrostatic pressure make this a treatment of choice for almost all conditions. Most patients and people thoroughly enjoy getting in the warm water, especially those with pain and/or stiffness. The only considerable barrier is those patients who are fearful of water and some cultures which are not used to the concept of water therapy. The contraindications are few, e.g. open wounds, several skin conditions and faecal incontinence. Even the frailest person can benefit from hydrotherapy as floats may be utilized so that the patient need not do anything themselves whilst a therapist is present. Often patients will be independent in their treatment as a programme can be devised to suit the individual and their condition.

The positive effects of water therapy have been known for centuries. There is a great deal of evidence which suggests treatment is very holistic in nature and the benefits are to body and mind promoting relaxation, wellbeing and activity.

The skin is the largest organ in the body and hydrotherapy stimulates and rejuvenates the skin. Joints move freely in water and soft tissues can be lengthened and strengthened. Hydrotherapy stimulates the heart and lungs, assists digestion and aids peripheral circulation and venous return. Muscle spasm and pain are reduced and general wellbeing is enhanced.

Exercise prescription

The numerous benefits of exercise apply to both palliative and non-palliative situations. It is important that an exercise plan is individualized and prioritized and centred around the goals of the client. Some may come into our care after a long period of inactivity and they may be seriously physically deconditioned – there may be a huge physical potential. Others may be physically able with good function and mobility.

Once again the goals and desires of the patient will be the guide to an exercise programme. As with all programmes, goals must be attainable and realistic.

Deep breathing and stretching exercises are always beneficial and the simple exercise of raising both arms above the head while breathing in and then lowering arms while breathing out has long been a favourite. It not only aids the expansion of the lungs but takes the shoulders through a good range of movement. This is also a wonderful form of relaxation incorporating yoga principles and Eastern medicine ideas.

Walking is a great exercise. It benefits the whole body and is good for bladder and bowel maintenance. The goal can be set to suit your patient and progress can be easily seen. It may be that just walking to and from the toilet is all that you and your patient want or you may be able to aim to walk out to the garden.

Gentle passive exercises may be all that is required if your patient is frail and unable to help themselves. Use your hands as scoops and slide one hand under the wrist and one under the elbow and move the arm out to the side and above the head. Always move slowly and never push past resistance. To move the leg slide one hand under the knee and one under the heel and again gently move the leg up and down and out to the side. These simple movements are sufficient to prevent contracture if there is no severe neurological condition.

Exercise may:

- increase circulation
- improve cardiorespiratory status
- improve sleep
- improve mental alertness
- aid in wellness
- control body weight

- control blood sugar levels
- improve skin
- increase quality of life
- provide a sense of wellbeing
- increase muscle strength, joint range of motion, flexibility
- assist in tone management
- decrease or help in the treatment of depression.

Our hands and our heart are our greatest tools of trade and these are our best ways to communicate with and comfort our patient. Hands used sensitively cannot be replaced by an artificial aid.

Massage is very comforting and should always be slow and firm. Gentle stroking back towards the heart in long strokes is very beneficial. Circular movements with the thumbs are excellent if there is swelling around the ankles. This movement is also useful for hand massage. Massage can be done whilst you are talking or it is a nice time to play soft music. Intuition takes over when you are massaging and instinctively you will know what to do. Aromatherapy oils are lovely to use for massage if they are available and again if your patient likes them.

Reflections

Offering a dictaphone has proved helpful to some people who have always wanted to write their life story. The telling of lifetime events can be very healing and allow resolution of old anxieties and hurts. It gives patients goals which may be achievable, realistic and useful. Painting, reading, playing games or the piano or walking certain distances each day can encourage physical activity and satisfaction in the most enjoyable way possible. All of these stimuli provide diversional therapy and improve mental status/ stimulation also.

Constantly remind yourself it is not what you believe to be best but what your patient wants that makes any form of intervention right. It is so important for us not to have an agenda. We will give the best service if we are flexible and sensitive. We are only a part of the big picture and greatly privileged to walk with our patient through these critical days. Be facilitators and be alert to priorities as your patient sees them.

Above all else remember to 'care for and to care about'.

- There is no escaping holistic management if you want to do the best possible job.
- Dealing with grief and loss is inevitable in this field and the ability to communicate is of paramount importance.
- Empathy builds trust, trust gives confidence and helps to restore wellbeing.

Legal and ethical issues

Euthanasia literally means 'good death'. Passive euthanasia is when death is brought about by omission or withdrawal of treatment. Active or voluntary euthanasia is deliberate. It is not within the scope of this text to examine these principles, only to say that we are certainly aiming to achieve a good death for residents by promoting quality not quantity of life through palliative care.

Advance care directives are legal documents which ensure the right to choose or reject cardiopulmonary resuscitation, ventilation, tube or intravenous feeding, antibiotics and operative interventions. Different countries have different laws regarding end-of-life decisions. We have provided a glimpse of the situation in Australia.

Summary

- Death and dying can be a positive and happy experience for all of those involved. This includes the resident, their family, carers and health professionals.
- Palliative care is a total approach to care focusing on quality of life issues and total patient management aimed at physical, emotional and spiritual factors.
- Physiotherapists have a large body of research supportive of their practices in all areas of practice including palliative care.
- Communication may be the key to good management. It is important to get the right information and to re-evaluate it often. Establishing common goals will assist the team to help the resident as much as possible.
- Physiotherapists can assist in many areas of symptom management including pain, mobility, bladder and bowel function and the prevention of pressure areas and skin injury.
- Maintaining or restoring mobility and dexterity may be of priority to the resident. Physiotherapists are the professional of choice to assist in this regard.
- Physiotherapists can play an important role in education regarding back care, manual handling, injury prevention and stress management.
- The principles of good exercise prescription to aid resident management are as important within palliative care as elsewhere. Exercise may help to relieve symptoms and improve quality of life.

References

Cohen S R, Mount B M, Strobel M G, Bui F 1995 The McGill Quality of Life questionnaire: a measure of quality of life appropriate for people with advanced disease. Palliative Medicine 9(3):207–219

Frankl V 1959 Man's search for meaning. Pocket Books, New York

Keegan L, Guzzetta C E 2000 Holistic nursing: a handbook for practice, 3rd edn. Aspen

Roach S 1992 Human act of caring: a blueprint for the health care professional, revised edn. Canadian Health Association Press, Ottawa; Mosby, St Louis

Sepulveda C, Marlin A, Yoshida T, Ullrich A 2002 Palliative care. The World Health Organization's global perspective. Journal of Pain and Symptom Management 24(2):91–96

World Health Organization (WHO) 1990 Cancer pain relief and palliative care. Report of a WHO Expert Committee (WHO Technical Report Series, No. 804). World Health Organization, Geneva

World Health Organization 2002 National cancer control programmes: policies and managerial guidelines, 2nd edn. World Health Organization, Geneva

World Health Organization 2003 URL: www.who.int/cancer/palliative/en/

Further reading

Scheutz B 1995 Spirituality and palliative care. Australian Family Physician 24(5):775–777

Van der Weyden M B 1997 Death, dying and the euthanasia debate in Australia. Medical Journal of Australia 166:173–174

Woodruff R 1996 Palliative medicine. Asperula, Melbourne

Appendix 1 Case studies

Resident 1 (low care example)

Mrs P Age 86

Primary medical diagnosis	Osteoarthritis, osteoporosis, depression
Past medical history	Chronic lumbar spine degeneration, back pain, L2 crush fracture
Past surgical history	Hysterectomy
Social history	Adopted daughter lives nearby
Reason for admission	Social, unable to live safely independently due to pain
Resident's main goal	Stay mobile and independent
Medication list	Celebrex (celecoxib), Fosamax (alendronate sodium), Cipramil (citalopram hydrobromide), paracetamol
Communication ability	Good
Vision and hearing	Wears reading glasses, moderate hearing loss (no aids)
Cognitive state	Good MMSE 26/30
Functional level	Mobilizes with wheelie walker for long distances and outings, uses one stick inside
Mobility and dexterity assessment	Mobile with walker/stick, better in morning, 700 m approx, slow on stairs and uneven surfaces, pain may be a limiting factor at times
Gait assessment	Normal aged
Falls risk assessment	Mild falls risk
Posture/structural deformities	Reasonably erect posture, mild osteoarthritis deformity of knees and fingers
Skin integrity/circulation	Good skin integrity, tends to dryness, circulation good
Pain presentation	Moderate to severe back pain, worse in afternoon/evening, responds well to heat, physiotherapy and TENS
Continence	Mild urinary incontinence, wears a protective pad during the day
Respiratory status	Good
Tone	Normal
Strength	Normal aged
Range of movement	Decreased spinal range in all directions, limbs good
Balance	Slight decrease standing balance, functional reach 15 cm, stops walking whilst talking, stands at rail holding with one hand on one leg approximately 15 seconds
Endurance	One rest stop on an 800 m walk
All aids used	Wheelie walker, stick

Resident 2 (high care – mobile example)

Mrs J Age 92

Primary medical diagnosis	Recurrent falls, dementia
Past medical history	Atrial fibrillation, transient ischaemic attacks (?Cerebrovascular accident), pulmonary oedema, macular degeneration, leg ulcers
Past surgical history	Bowel resection
Social history	Very supportive husband who lives nearby in an independent unit
Reason for admission	Post hospital admission after fall down a flight of stairs (?CVA/TIA), no fractures, moderate visual field loss and (R) neglect (improving)
Resident's main goal	To gain safety in mobility and return home with husband if possible, aid visual return, manage incontinence
Medication list	Apirin, Endep (amitriptyline hydrochloride), Felodur (felodipine)
Communication ability	Good. May mumble occasionally and drift off topic
Vision and hearing	Hears well, able to read small print although confuses some words, poor visuospatial awareness, poor depth perception
Cognitive state	Reasonable, poor short-term memory, ↓attention span and sharing attention between tasks
Functional level	Requires the assistance of two staff to mobilize with wheelie walker, one staff member required for all hygiene needs, dressing, washing, toileting. Able to assist herself with meals once set-up arranged (sits in wheelchair or chair with armrests)
Mobility and dexterity assessment	Rollator, requires two to assist with walk belt, up to 300 m with rest, more able in morning, poor writing (↓coordination, visuospatial and fine control), drinks from normal cup
Gait assessment	Leans backwards and right (able to correct momentarily), lurches at times to the right (choreiform type movement), ballism, lets walker travel off in front of her, impulsive
Falls risk assessment	HIGH (associated with age, mobility, assistance required, incontinence, mental state, visual degeneration and visuospatial losses and medications)
Posture/structural deformities	Thoracic kyphosis
Skin integrity/circulation	Good peripheral pulses, skin integrity good currently, skin fragile
Pain presentation	Nil
Continence	Urinary, wears daytime pad, urge, some nocturnal wetness also becoming more frequent
Respiratory status	Normal for age
Tone	Normal
Strength	Mild–moderate weakness globally associated with disuse
Range of movement	Good

Mrs J continued

Balance	Sitting – tends to drift to right when tired, decreased attention/concentration span Standing – poor, requires assistance of two staff, rail, walker, ballistic movements to right, query related to visuospatial information and depth perception
Endurance	Becomes short of breath, tends to rush in spurts and then rest, walks with assistance and rest up to approximately 300 m
All aids used	Hand rail, manual wheelchair, wheelie walker, rollator, commode, walking belt

Resident 3 (high care – immobile example)

Mrs S Age 91

Primary medical diagnosis	Dementia, severe osteoarthritis, cancer (unknown primary), chronic obstructive airways disease, hypertension, ischaemic heart disease, osteoporosis
Past medical history	Pathological (L) hip fracture, nocturnal confusion
Past surgical history	(L) Total hip replacement
Social history	Very supportive family, two sons married, live nearby and visit regularly
Reason for admission	Post hip fracture, admitted from hospital, non-weight-bearing 6/12
Resident's main goal	Comfort, would love to stand/mobilize if possible
Medication list	Zantac (ranitidine hydrochloride), paracetamol, Coloxyl with senna (docusate sodium; Sennosides A and B), Serenace (haloperidol), Temaze (temazepam), Zyloprim (allopurinol), Lasix (furosemide)
Communication ability	Reasonably good, answers simple questions with ease, requests help for toileting and comfort
Vision and hearing	Moderate hearing loss, mild visual loss
Cognitive state	Orientated to time, place, person. Periods of confusion and poor short-term memory, often very dependent on call buzzer and seeks staff attention persistently. Very anxious during all hygiene and transfer cares (pain with movement)
Functional level	Immobile, chair/bedbound, full hoist or slideboard transfers, slide sheets used for bed mobility, full assistance required for all hygiene needs, full assistance with medications, dressings and transfers. Able to feed herself vitamized meals but requires full assistance with positioning, sitting and set-up of meals and uses spoon only

Mrs S continued

Mobility and dexterity assessment	Immobile, able to assist roll to (R) holding on to bedrail
Gait assessment	n/a
Falls risk assessment	n/a chair or bed bound
Posture/structural deformities	Gross hand and finger deformity (osteoarthritis), swollen OA knees, joint deformity noted in most areas
Skin integrity/ circulation	Peripheral pulses present, no ulcers at present
Pain presentation	Generalized aches 'hurts all over', 5/10 on Visual Analogue Scale, discomfort with transferring, especially when any flexion movement of hips and trunk initiated
Continence	Requests bedpan, wears pad
Respiratory status	Poor, decreased air entry
Tone	No abnormality detected, difficult to assess given joint contractures and soft tissue shortening, resistance to movement is apparent
Strength	Generally very weak, disuse atrophy
Range of movement	Very poor
Balance	n/a
Endurance	Very poor, unable to assess
All aids used	Regency recliner chair (full support/full care), full hoist, slings, slide sheets, slide board, bed cradle, pressure mattress (air alternating), call buzzer, bedpan

Appendix 2

Outcome measures

Measurement required	Measurement tool	Reference
Functional status	Physical Mobility Scale	Nitz J, Brown A, Hourigan S 2004 Using the Physical Mobility Scale to show dependency in frail elderly people: A reliability and validity study (in preparation)
	Elderly Mobility Scale	Prosser L, Canby A 1997 Further validation of the Elderly Mobility Scale for measurement of mobility of hospitalized elderly people. Clinical Rehabilitation 11:338–343
	Clinical Outcomes Variable Scale	Seaby L, Torrance G 1989 Reliability of a physiotherapy functional assessment used in a rehabilitation setting. Physiotherapy Canada 41:264–271
	Functional Independence Measure	Rankin A 1993 The functional independence measure. Physiotherapy 79(12):184
	Motor Assessment Scale	Carr J, Shepherd R, Nordholm L, Lynne D 1985 A Motor Assessment Scale for stroke. Physical Therapy 65:175–180
	Katz Index of Independence in ADL	Katz S, Down T D, Cash H R et al 1970 Progress in the development of the index of ADL. Gerontologist 10:20–30
	Barthel Index	Mahoney F I, Barthel D 1965 Functional evaluation: the Barthel Index. Maryland State Medical Journal 14:56–61. http://www.strokecenter.org/trials/scales/barthel.html Wade D T 1992 Measurement in neurological rehabilitation. New York, Oxford University Press
Balance	Functional reach	Duncan P W, Weiner D K, Chandler J, Studenski S 1990 Functional reach: a new clinical measure of balance. Journal of Gerontology 45:M192–M197
	Lateral reach	Brauer S G, Burns Y R, Galley P 1999 Lateral reach. A new clinical measure of medio-lateral balance. Physiotherapy Research International 4:81–88
	Timed 'Up and Go'	Podsiadlo D, Richardson S 1991 The timed 'up and go': a test of basic functional mobility for frail elderly persons. Journal of the American Geriatrics Society 39:142–148

table continues

Measurement required	Measurement tool	Reference
	Timed 'Up and Go' (manual)	Lundin-Olsson L, Nyberg L, Gustafson Y 1998 Attention, frailty, and falls: the effects of a manual task on basic mobility. Journal of the American Geriatrics Society 46:758–761
	Timed 'Up and Go' (cognitive)	Shumway-Cook A, Brauer S, Woollacott M 2000 Predicting the probability of falls in community-dwelling older adults using the timed up and go. Physical Therapy 80:896–903
	'Stops Walking to Talk'	Nitz J C, Thompson K 2003 'Stops walking to talk': A simple measure of predicting falls in the frail elderly. Australasian Journal on Ageing 22(2):97–99
	Functional Step Test	Hill K, Bernhardt J, McGann A, Maltese D, Berkovits D 1996 A new test of dynamic standing balance for stroke patients: reliability and comparison with healthy elderly. Physiotherapy Canada 48:257–262
	Clinical test for sensory integration of balance	Shumway-Cook A, Horak F B 1986 Assessing the influence of sensory interaction on balance. Physical Therapy 66(10):1548–1550
	Balance and mobility assessment	Tinetti M 1986 Performance-oriented assessment of mobility problems in elderly patients. Journal of the American Geriatrics Society 34:119–126
Gait	Definitions/descriptions	Eliopoulos C 1987 Gerontological nursing, 2nd edn. J B Lippincott, Philadelphia Bates B 1991 A guide to physical examination and history taking, 5th edn. J B Lippincott, Philadelphia
Gait speed	10 metre walk (timed)	Wade D T 1992 Measurement in neurological rehabilitation. Oxford University Press, New York
Falls risk	'Stops walking when talking'	Lundin-Olsson L, Nyberg L, Gustafson Y 1997 'Stops walking when talking' as a predictor of falls in the elderly. Lancet 349:617
	Timed 'Up and Go'	Shumway-Cook A, Brauer S, Woollacott M 2000 Predicting the probability of falls in community-dwelling older adults using the timed up and go. Physical Therapy 80:896–903
	Falls Efficacy Scale	Tinetti M, Richman D, Powell L 1990 Falls efficacy as a measure of fear of falling. Journal of Gerontology 45:P239–P243
	Berg Balance Scale	Berg K, Wood-Dauphinee S, Williams I J, Maki B 1992 Measuring balance in the elderly: validation of an instrument. Canadian Journal of Public Health 83(suppl):57–61

Measurement required	Measurement tool	Reference
Pressure risk and skin integrity	Norton Scale	Norton D, McLaren R, Exton-Smith A N 1975 An investigation of geriatric nursing problems in hospitals. Churchill-Livingstone, Edinburgh
	Braden Scale	Bergstrom N, Braden B, Boynton P, Bruch S 1995 Using a research based assessment scale in clinical practice. Nursing Clinics of North American 30:539–551
	Waterlow	Waterlow J 1991 Waterlow pressure sore prevention/treatment policy. Professional Nurse 6(5):258–264 (see www.woundcarehelpline.com)
Circulation	Peripheral pulses Skin colour and integrity	See surface anatomy text for revision on where to palpate arteries in superficial areas (radial artery, carotid artery, dorsalis pedis artery, posterior tibial artery, femoral artery, brachial artery) Objectively/draw diagrams
Posture/deformities	Kyphosis measure (tragus to wall)	Grimmer K 1997 An investigation of poor cervical resting posture. Australian Journal of Physiotherapy 43:7–16
Range of motion and strength	Joint range measurement Manual muscle strength	Clarkson H M, Gilewich G B 1989 Musculo-skeletal assessment. Williams & Wilkins, Baltimore
Flexibility	Neural tension tests	Butler D 1991 Mobilisation of the nervous system. Churchill Livingstone, Edinburgh
Tone	Ashworth Scale	Bohannon R W, Smith M B 1987 Inter-rater reliability of a modified Ashworth scale of muscle spasticity. Physical Therapy 67:206–207
Endurance	3, 6 or 10 minute walk Heart rate	Wade D T 1992 Measurement in neurological rehabilitation. Oxford University Press, New York
	Respiratory rate Recovery heart rate	Skinner J S (ed) 1993 Exercise testing and exercise prescription for special cases: theoretical basis and clinical application. Lea and Febiger, Philadelphia
	RPE – perceived exertion rate	Borg G A 1982 Psychophysical bases of perceived exertion. Medicine and Science in Sports and Exercise 14:377–387
Respiratory function	Respiratory function test Expiratory peak flow	Webber B A 1988 The Brompton Hospital guide to chest physiotherapy, 5th edn. Blackwell Scientific Publications, Oxford

table continues

Measurement required	Measurement tool	Reference
Dexterity	Nine hole peg test	Wade D T 1992 Measurement in neurological rehabilitation. Oxford University Press, New York
Pain	McGill Pain Questionnaire Visual Analogue Scale	Melzack R, Wall P 1982 The challenge of pain. Basic Books, New York
Life satisfaction	SF 36	Ware J E, Sherbourne C D 1992 The MOS 36-item short-form health survey (SF-36): 1. Conceptual framework and item selection. Medical Care 30:473–483
Cognitive	MMSE Mini Mental State Examination	Folstein M F, Folstein S E, McHugh P R 1975 Mini mental state. A practical method for grading the cognitive state of patients for the clinician. Journal of Psychiatric Research 12:189–198

These are references for some outcome measures that might be useful for recording change in residents' status. The list is by no means complete and many other measures might be used to show particular aspects regarding a resident. These measures have been chosen because they are relatively simple and appropriate to the scope of problems encountered in residents of aged care facilities.

Appendix 3 Suggestions for successful case conferences

The purpose of case conferences is to review and develop the plan of care necessary for, and provided to, a given resident. The involved parties often include the resident, their family or representative, the care and support staff, the resident's general practitioner, the physiotherapist and other health professionals as deemed necessary. Appropriate notification and organization well in advance will ensure that as many of these individuals as possible are present at the meeting. It may be considered inappropriate or unnecessary for the resident to be in attendance at this meeting but largely the resident or their family or representative should decide this themselves, with advice from the health professionals involved. Best practice would suggest the resident should be present for the meeting, which should be totally focused on their particular needs.

Case conferences are an effective and efficient way to gather all of the important and necessary people involved in resident care so that they can strive for excellence in achieving total resident needs, in consultation with the individual. It is considered that after the resident assessment, review of findings and conference is conducted, interventions will be made to change, improve or maintain the care given in order to deliver an holistic individualized approach which targets the given resident's particular needs. Communication channels should be open between all interested parties at all times and a case conference is an excellent way to orientate all caregivers to a particular resident's need. Further, case conferences allow health professionals and caregivers greater insight into all aspects of patient management and knowledge of how their individual responsibilities tie into the 'whole' picture. Multidisciplinary care should have *a team approach* by way of a clear common goal and an understanding of different individuals' responsibilities and how their role influences and relates to other team members' work.

The timetabling of case conferences ensures adequate development of care plans and appropriate assessment, planning, implementation and evaluation on an initial and ongoing basis. The meetings enable a thoroughly resident-centred approach to be developed and give an excellent opportunity for the care recipient to speak freely about any of their concerns or wishes.

It is important that all aspects of care be examined at the case conference and that the physiotherapist is in attendance for this. Other health professionals who may be involved include registered nurses, doctors, occupational therapists, speech pathologists, pharmacists, audiologists, dietitians and podiatrists. Often nursing assistants, enrolled nurses and diversional therapists (or activities officers) contribute an important part in the conference also. Physiotherapists may have input into many of the key areas raised, which often include but are not limited to the following:

- communication
- mobility
- meals and drinks
- personal hygiene
- toileting
- bladder and bowel management
- understanding activities of daily living
- wandering and intrusive behaviours
- physical aggression
- emotional dependence
- danger to self or others
- other behaviours
- social and human needs of the resident and family or friends
- medications
- technical nursing procedures
- therapy (physiotherapy, occupational therapy, social work, speech therapy, diversional therapy)
- sleep
- pain management
- other services (music, aromatherapy, dietitians, podiatrists).

At the time of the case conference it is important to thoroughly review any aspects of care also related to injury prevention, health promotion and life satisfaction. Falls prevention may be illustrated as a key topic within a case conference and information related to medication review, behaviour management, bladder management and/or the need for review of walking aids and/or exercise programmes will therefore be very important.

Best practice around the time of a case conference would be reflected by the physiotherapist undergoing a total review of the resident's assessment and treatment before the meeting. The physiotherapist at the very least should outline, during the case conference, all aspects of resident management in relation to assistance required for mobility, dexterity and therapy or exercise needs. It may be useful to outline strengths and weaknesses (or problem areas) discovered by your physical assessment so others involved can gain an insight into physiotherapy care of the resident. It is useful to everyone involved to outline the desired aim of any therapy programme that is being undertaken.

A case conference is an excellent forum in which to discuss ideas for trialling new equipment, such as a new chair, with families and caregivers. Goal setting in this setting is enormously worthwhile when all stakeholders and motivators are present. Certainly a case conference is an excellent forum in which to stress the benefits of appropriate exercise and the difference it can make to health and life satisfaction. The promotion of physiotherapy input into residential aged care can be a well-intended goal of our participation in case conferencing.

Appendix 4

Electrotherapy considerations in aged care practice (EPAs – electrophysical agents)

Equipment	Contraindications/ Precautions	Uses (examples)	Application
Heat – deep (SWD, MW, US)	*Contraindications* Unreliable patients Inbuilt stimulator (e.g. pacemaker, SWD not to be used within 3 m) Poor circulation (DVT, PVD, haemorrhage, varicose veins) Any rapidly dividing tissue where there is risk of spread (e.g. acute infection, cancer, tumours, TB, osteomyelitis) Inability to communicate Sensory loss Risk of exacerbating existing conditions (e.g. fever, inflammatory or infective conditions, skin problems, recent radiotherapy, cardiac failure) Application to eyes or testes Pregnancy	Pain management Promote healing Promote circulation Increase comfort Facilitate joint nutrition and movement Very useful for OA	Skin test (hot/cold) Warning given Check for erythema during and after application Read manufacturer's instructions regarding application Ensure safety of resident and others Ensure good equipment maintenance as per instructions Record all contraindication checks, machine checks, warnings given, treatment parameters utilized, immediate reactions, treatment effects, plans, etc. MW/SWD – contraindicated if metal within field (implants, jewellery) or within 3 m of electrical stimulation or biofeedback. Take precautions to ensure there is little moisture within the field and that movement is minimal
Heat – superficial (wax baths, infra-red, hot packs)	*Contraindications* Circulatory insufficiency (PVD, atherosclerosis, arterial/venous	Pain Muscle spasm To provide warmth or warm-up before treatment	Skin test every site of application (hot/cold) Warning given Check erythema at 3, 6, 9 minutes of a 15-minute

table continues

Equipment	Contraindications/ Precautions	Uses (examples)	Application
	insufficiency) Risk of spread of infection or rapidly dividing tissue (i.e. acute infection, tumours, TB, osteomyelitis) Risk of exacerbating pre-existing ailments (e.g. unstable cardiac condition, acute swelling, open wounds, skin conditions) Application to testes or eyes Wax contraindicated if skin is broken *Precautions* Sensory loss Inability to communicate Heat intolerance Careful of photo-sensitivity with IRR	OA/RA Promote healing Promote circulation Increase comfort Skin moisturizing (wax) Colles fracture (wax often useful in rehabilitation stage)	application and afterwards where possible Follow manufacturer's instructions regarding application and maintenance of equipment Hydrocollators to be kept at 76–80°C Refer to textbooks listed for dosage parameters
Cryotherapy (cold)	*Contraindications* Circulatory problems (PVD, vasopastic disease, e.g. Raynaud's) Fear of cold Risk of exacerbating pre-existing condition Sensory loss – peripheral nerve injury Hypersensitivity (allodynia) *Precautions* Inability to communicate Sensory loss	Acute injuries Swelling Chronic musculoskeletal pain Muscle spasm Spasticity Chronic inflammatory oedema Cellulitis Muscle strengthening	Skin test – ice sensitivity, hot/cold Warning given Inspect after 2–5 minutes. Generally 20-minute application
TENS	*Contraindications* Pacemaker or other inbuilt stimulator	Acute pain Chronic pain Post surgical	Sharp/blunt test Warning given

Equipment	Contraindications/ Precautions	Uses (examples)	Application
	Pregnancy (contraindicated over or near the uterus) *Precautions* Circulatory insufficiency Risk of spread Risk of exacerbating pre-existing conditions (e.g. cardiac failure, skin conditions) Sensory loss		See manufacturer's instructions and given texts for dosage parameters Example: Chronic pain (a) Conventional type 80–120 Hz high frequency 0–30 mA low intensity Pulse width 0.05 ms, 30 min (b) Acupuncture type 2–10 Hz low frequency High intensity (as tolerable 30 mA++) Pulse width 0.2 ms, 30 min++ Endogenous opioid release (c) 'Burst' 2–5 Hz/70–100 Hz moderate intensity (0–30 mA) 30 min
Ultrasound (no or low heat)	*Contraindications* Inbuilt stimulator (e.g. pacemaker or other) Application near or over a pregnant uterus or to eyes or testes *Precautions* Circulatory problems Risk of spread or dissemination Risk of exacerbating pre-existing conditions Inability to communicate Sensory loss	Treatment of swelling Treatment of pain Shortened soft tissue Promotion of healing	Skin test sharp/blunt Warning given Check manufacturer's instructions Check texts referred to for dosage parameters Examples: Acute swelling (low intensity, pulsed) e.g. 1:4, 30 s/ERA, 0.5 W/cm^2 (Avoid treatment in initial bleeding phase of an injury) Chronic swelling (medium intensity, continuous) e.g. 2 min/ERA, 0.8–1.0 W/cm^2 Acute pain (low intensity, pulsed) e.g. 30 s/ERA, 0.5 W/cm^2

table continues

Equipment	Contraindications/ Precautions	Uses (examples)	Application
			Healing (low intensity, pulsed) e.g. 0.5 W/cm^2 Lengthening (medium–high intensity, continuous) e.g. 1:1, 5–15 min, 0.8–1.5 W/cm^2
Magnetic therapy	See manufacturer's guidelines Pacemakers Be aware of metal implants Rapidly dividing cells Metastates/sepsis	Chronic pain Acute swelling Chronic swelling Promote circulation and healing	See equipment directions and manufacturer's guidelines Check output with magnet supplied e.g. Acute 2–4 Hz Chronic 10–25 Hz Pain syndromes 50 Hz
Laser (LLLT)	*Contraindications* Irradiation of the eye area Pregnancy (no application over or near pregnant uterus)	Wound healing Pain Acupuncture type Immunosuppressive effect Increase nerve sprouting and regeneration (?)	Check manufacturer's guidelines and instructions (machines vary widely) (in J/cm^2) <0.5 Acupuncture 0.5–1.0 Acute conditions 1.0–2.5 Subacute conditions 2.0–4.0 Chronic conditions
	Precautions Rapidly dividing cells, e.g. metastases, TB where there is risk of spread or dissemination Risk of exacerbation of pre-existing conditions (e.g. skin problems, infection, photosensitized patients) (antimalarial, antibiotics, gold) Over glands (endocrine/thyroid) Inability to communicate	*Precautions* ***Always ensure exposure is less than 8–9 J/cm^2 in any one session*** Do not use near SWD Well-lit enclosed room Class 3B lasers – safety glasses *required* for therapist and resident Safety glasses are recommended for all applications and types Use a warning sign	Acute – daily Rx for 3 days, then 3 times per week. Low doses. After 3–6 treatments, and after increasing the dose, if there is no change – then cease treatment Chronic – daily for 3 days, then 2 times per week. Higher doses, less often to avoid inhibition Chronic pain 0.9–1.8 J/radiant area Pulsed lasers Stimulations <1000 Hz (wound treatment) Inhibition >100 Hz (pain, OA, RA, post-surgical treatment)

Equipment	Contraindications/ Precautions	Uses (examples)	Application
			Treatment time = energy density (mJ/cm^2) × treatment area (cm^2)/laser average power (mW) Laser average power (mW) = pulse frequency × pulse width × peak power
Electrical stimulation (TENS, FES, NMES, FNS, IF, HV, etc.)	*Contraindications* Contraindicated over inbuilt stimulators (e.g. pacemaker) Transthoracic applications Long duration direct current Use within 3 m of SWD Contraindicated over or near a pregnant uterus *Precautions* Circulatory problems Risk of spread (e.g. neoplasm, infection) Risk of exacerbating pre-existing conditions (e.g. heart problems, hypertension, skin problems) Inability to communicate Sensory loss (may use low intensity treatments with care) Unreliable residents Broken skin (careful – decreased impedance leads to concentration in current flow)	Acute swelling Promote circulation and healing Pain management Motor or sensory stimulation Stiffness Wound treatment	See manufacturer's guidelines and instructions Machines vary widely Skin test – sharp/blunt Check skin impedance, outputs, stimulation, suction devices, dosage parameters Ensure records kept including checks, treatment details, immediate results of treatment, etc. Take care with machine maintenance; repeated uses of electrodes, sponges and covers can change their conductivity and therefore resultant treatment parameters
UV	*Contraindications* Application to eyes Eye protection required for therapist and resident	Increase immune response Kill bacteria Increase vitamin D synthesis Acne Ulcer management	Erythemal skin test (E1) Treatment frequency will vary between daily to once every 3 days depending on degree of erythema achieved (related to dosage required). Light to

table continues

Equipment	Contraindications/ Precautions	Uses (examples)	Application
	Precautions Confirm photo-sensitivity status unaltered (i.e. check for photosensitizing agents, medical conditions, photoallergies) Acute skin condition or infection Skin grafts Skin damage Infra-red radiation treatment		stimulative doses are useful for healing of open wounds. A stronger reactive dosage may be useful for germicidal purposes Ensure coverage of area not being treated Warm up lamp
Pressure pumps	*Contraindications* Circulatory insufficiency (arterial) Risk of exacerbating pre-existing conditions (e.g. acute muscle haematoma, DVT, skin condition, acute infective process, cardiac failure) Unreliable patient *Precautions* Inability to communicate Sensory loss	Swelling/oedema Increase interstitial pressure Stimulate venous and lymphatic flow Partial venous stasis and ulceration (with care)	Check skin/pain, sensitivity to pressure Follow manufacturer's guidelines and read given protocols Ensure equipment maintenance Example: Acute 30–35 mmHg Chronic 45–50 mmHg Vascular 30–40 mmHg Lymphoedema (arm) 40–60 mmHg, (leg) 60–80 mmHg Adjust rest periods depending on age, tissue being compressed (5–30 s); e.g. young/muscle injury 5–7 s rest, poor vascular function 20–30 s rest

SWD, short wave diathermy; MW, microwave; IRR, infra-red radiation; ERA, effective radiation area; FES, functional electrical stimulation; NMES, neuromuscular electrical stimulation; FNS, functional nerve stimulation; IF, interferential; HV, high voltage; DVT, deep vein thrombosis; PVD, peripheral vascular disease; OA, osteoarthritis; RA, rheumatoid arthritis; TB, tuberculosis.

The physiotherapist must ensure that their duty of care responsibilities are maintained. Ensure familiarity with the specific equipment selected, the manufacturer's guidelines and that the equipment satisfies relevant national standards. Choose the appropriate modality based on good clinical reasoning and known effects of the equipment. At all times be aware of infection control considerations and utilize high standards of practice in this regard.

A full explanation should be given to the resident about the modality, how it works, its perceived benefits for them and what to expect during and after treatment.

Position the resident comfortably and prepare them, the treatment area and the equipment. Ensure contraindications are checked as detailed above and also that sensitivity tests are completed.

Appropriate warnings must be given and understood (and recorded as such), usually as (WGAU). Full outlines of these are available in the given references - refer to Robertson et al (2001).

Standard practice in application:

1. Check contraindications.
2. Prepare - give the resident a full explanation and instructions, check treatment area and equipment.
3. Give appropriate warning.
4. Apply the treatment - remain within call.
5. Complete treatment and checks.
6. Document treatment.
7. Re-evaluate effects and effectiveness before next treatment and modify accordingly.

References and further reading

Cameron M H (ed) 1999 Physical agents in rehabilitation. WB Saunders, Philadelphia

Forster A, Palastanga N (eds) 1981 Clayton's electrotherapy: theory and practice, 8th revised edn. Baillière Tindall, London.

Lehmann J F (ed) 1982 Therapeutic heat and cold. Williams & Wilkins, Baltimore

Low J, Reed A 2000 Electrotherapy explained: principles and practice, 3rd edn. Butterworth Heinemann, Oxford

Nelson R, Hayes K, Currier D (eds) 1999 Clinical electrotherapy. Appleton and Lange, Stamford

Robertson V J, Chipchase L S, Laakso E L et al 2001 Guidelines for the clinical use of electrophysical agents. Australian Physiotherapy Association, St Kilda, Victoria. Email: national.office@physiotherapy.asn.au

Wells P E, Frampton V, Bowsher D (eds) 1998 Pain: management and control in physiotherapy. Heinemann Physiotherapy, London

Wadsworth H, Chanmugan A P P 1983 Electrophysical agents in physiotherapy, 2nd edn. Science Press, NSW

Appendix 5

Mobility aids

Aids to be reviewed:

- walking sticks or canes (single, tripod, four-point)
- hopper, Zimmer frame or 'pick up' frame (standard, with wheels)
- wheelie walkers (three-wheeled, four-wheeled, seated, easy walker (low and high))
- rollator (easy-walker type, standard)
- mechanical devices such as the standing hoist (with walking adaptation).

For each aid we need to examine the following factors:

- maintenance and other safety issues
- individual fitting
- suitability and recommendations for use
- patient education with the aid
- cost
- availability.

The prescription of suitable aids to maximize function, safety and mobility is one of the biggest tasks a physiotherapist must do. A broad spectrum of devices is available from the walking stick through to a rollator (Fig. A5.1) and furthermore through the use of mechanical equipment such as the standing/walking hoist for rehabilitation. It is extremely important to educate patients in the correct use of the chosen aid. No doubt everyone has seen the wandering patient carrying a hopper frame above the ground and wondered how long it would be before an injury would occur if no suggestions for change were made and implemented. It is surprising how often walking sticks contribute to a poor gait pattern largely when used on the incorrect side. Stairs are a particular hazard and if encounters are planned then the physiotherapist will spend time practising with a resident to ensure safety and confidence.

Walking sticks

Maintenance and other safety issues

It is imperative to check the rubber stopper/s on a regular basis to see that there has not been too much wear and therefore loss of gripping ability. Ensure the stick is inherently stable and that the grip is in good order and suitable for the resident.

Individual fitting

A stick should be fitted to ensure correct height. This is usually with the hand level equivalent with that of the greater trochanter (with the elbow

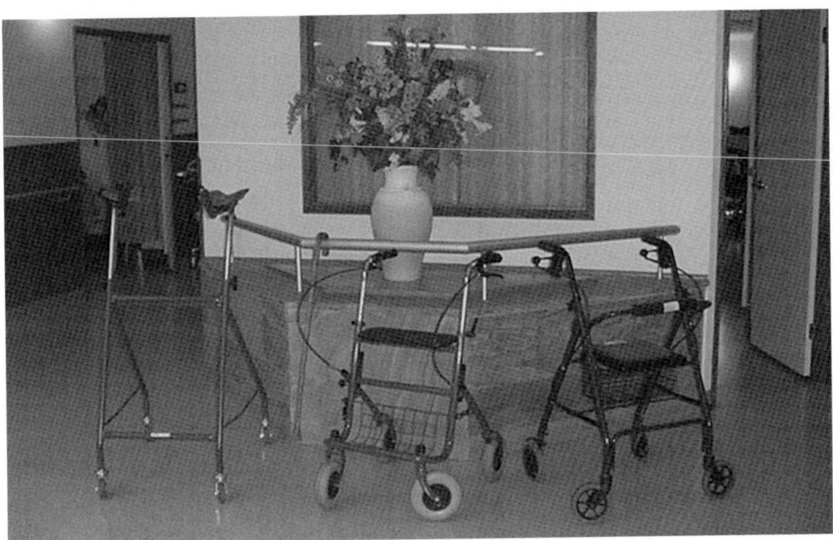

Figure A5.1
Various walking aids (from left to right): rollator, walking stick, wheeled walker with tray and pneumatic tyres, and four-wheeled walker with seat and lockable hand brakes.

comfortably bent) and the stick placed on the ground approximately 10 cm lateral to the fifth toe. A physiotherapist should check and recommend the height initially as bad habits and heights are often difficult to correct at a later date when the person has become accustomed to them. Moulded and foam handles are available for residents with arthritic and other such complaints who have deformity or weakness in the hand.

Suitability and recommendations for use

The walking stick provides the least assistance available and generally provides little assistance aside from being a confidence booster. It may give slight assistance for balance and have some effect on weight-bearing also as long as it is used correctly. Two sticks can be prescribed for residents requiring extra assistance. Two sticks may be useful for residents with ataxia or some lower extremity amputees wearing prostheses. Some patients will benefit from three- or four-pronged sticks that are intrinsically more stable on the ground and do not require as much stability to be provided from the individual, but only if used correctly so that all prongs are in contact with the ground at the same time. All too often only the prongs adjacent to the resident are in contact, thus causing the walking stick to be unstable and unsafe.

Patient education with the aid

A stick should be utilized on the *opposite side* to any weakness or disability present. Firstly the resident may use a three-point pattern (e.g. stick, weak leg, strong leg or conversely right stick, left leg, right leg) but they should work towards a two-point pattern (stick and opposite leg together, then strong leg), which is closer to a normal gait pattern. Two sticks may also be prescribed and either a two- or four-point pattern is then utilized. The physiotherapist should be careful to teach these patterns correctly. A four-point pattern with two sticks (e.g. right stick, left leg, left stick, right leg) is slower and proffers more assistance and stability although it is a little more disjointed. The two-point pattern (e.g. left stick and right leg together, then right stick and left leg together) is a more flowing and 'normal' pattern.

Cost and availability

Walking sticks are relatively cheap devices and are widely available. They are made from many different products including wood, metal and plastics. Some can be folded up in segments for easier carriage and storage.

Hopper frames (Zimmer frames or 'pick up' frames)

Maintenance and other safety issues

The biggest drawback of a standard hopper frame is the requirement of the person operating it to be able to step, stop, lift the frame, place the frame down further ahead, and step again. This is a very staccato and disjointed movement pattern, which does not reflect the smooth and transient phases succinctly followed through in a normal gait pattern. Using the hopper frame requires the ability to stand (even though momentarily) unassisted whilst balancing and carrying the frame forwards. All these requirements place increased demand on the systems, lead to an abnormal gait pattern and do not allow for momentum and the learned repetitious pattern of walking which is so innate as a primary reflex since birth. Furthermore, this requires a pattern that is inherently more dangerous with increased periods of unsupported stance and therefore greater risk of falls and injury.

Other safety issues that need to be addressed are again related to maintenance of rubber stoppers and handgrips.

Individual fitting

A hopper frame should be fitted such that the resident's hands are at the level of the greater trochanters with the elbows comfortably bent.

Suitability and recommendations for use

Hoppers may provide a reasonable amount of stability when on the ground and may be suitable for residents who are unable to control the forward momentum of a wheeled aid. As alluded to above, it is very important to assess the safety of the resident utilizing the hopper as they do need to be able to stand unsupported momentarily in order to place the hopper frame forwards. During this movement the resident is potentially unstable in the posterior and lateral directions and the risk of a fall is high, with consequent fractured neck of femur or pelvis the outcome.

Hopper frames are widely available and relatively cheap.

Wheeled hopper frames

Maintenance and other safety issues

All rubber stoppers, slides and wheels should be checked on a regular basis. Rubber stoppers and slides can become worn or loose. Wheels can become worn, loose or blocked in movement by dust and hair picked up off the floor and environment.

These frames are useful for those who need to go a little slower and need more stability than that provided by a wheelie walker. The wheeled hopper frame plus or minus rear slides is useful for some residents, especially those who would not be able to control the increased forward momentum of a wheelie walker.

Wheelie walkers

These are often the aid of choice for many reasons. For low care residents especially who are ambulant and active within the community they are an excellent device. Wheelie walkers provide moderate assistance to balance, can be relied upon often as a seat when fatigue sets in, come with the option of brakes (push-down, or hand brakes which lock), fold up easily into a car, and tend to operate smoothly around corners and over small bumps. Obviously they are a big drawback if residents need to negotiate stairs and in these cases most people would require the assistance of a carer. The model with the seat, brakes and carry basket is always popular.

It is important to note that pieces of equipment such as these should be chosen with the resident, who often takes great care over which colour and model is chosen. It is important to involve the resident as much as possible in these decisions – after all a mobility aid becomes a close friend after many years of good use and reliance. Patient acceptance is at the heart of effective use and a therapist must gather in support from the resident, carers and family members for the good use of walking aids to occur.

Maintenance and other safety issues

It is important to check tyres, wheels, brakes, handgrips, seats and structure regularly. Brakes are often in need of attention on wheelie walkers as worn tyres, broken or maladjusted cables can often lead to brakes not working.

Individual fitting

Wheelie walkers should be fitted to enable comfortable reach to the handles by the resident at approximately the height of the greater trochanters. Occasionally handles may be adjusted at a higher level to counteract poor walking posture and a flexed thoracic position, thereby facilitating more erect standing. It is important to consider how a resident will use the brakes (and indeed if they can) and to make a decision regarding what type of brakes, if any, would be more suitable for them. Several options exist in relation to brakes including a 'push-down' variety that applies rubber stoppers to the floor, regular bicycle type brakes, and brakes that can be locked into position either by a small push-in button or by a lever lock-down mechanism. Residents require varying abilities in order to use these mentioned devices and their appropriateness must be assessed.

Patient education with the aid

It is important to teach residents how to use the brakes and to encourage them to be involved in maintenance and checking of the aid at regular intervals. Residents should be encouraged to walk as upright as possible and not to let the aid 'get away from them'. A poor flexed posture that is largely unsafe should be avoided.

Cost

Wheelie walkers are more expensive than sticks or hoppers but generally offer increased options and incorporate extra design features.

Availability

Wheelie walkers are widely available from both pharmacies and equipment suppliers.

Easy walkers

Easy walkers are very sturdy; some consider even 'heavy' aids. For this reason they seem particularly useful for very tall and/or very heavy (often male) residents. Because of their weight they do have increased stability but for frailer, weaker residents this seems to hinder rather than assist. The shorter easy walkers support mobile residents to the same degree as the wheelie walkers discussed above, yet do not have the benefits of easy packing into a car and providing a seat. Taller easy walkers (with forearm support) are another option for those requiring more support and stability.

Tri-wheeled walkers

Another variation on the wheelie walker theme, three-wheeled walkers are useful as they can be made narrower to fit through doorways or around furniture. The drawback is that this decreases the stability provided and may indeed create an accident as the person attempts to manipulate the walker whilst balancing and walking, and talking, and meeting all other criteria for standing and getting around. Additionally they do not provide as much mediolateral support in front and therefore are less reliable stability-wise. The therapist would do better in most instances to prescribe a four-wheeled walker and adjust the environment where necessary, and where possible.

Rollators

Rollators provide increased stability and safety when mobilizing for those with acute mobility difficulties and those requiring maximal assistance. As forearm support is proffered they rely on the ability of the person to grasp with two hands or at least to weight-bear through both upper limbs. Unlike wheelie walkers, rollators generally facilitate better posture as support is offered closer to the person's centre of gravity rather than leaning forward to gain support and control at waist height.

Maintenance and other safety issues

It is important to check the wheels, handgrips, forearm supports (or gutters) and structure of rollators regularly as poor maintenance can lead to injury and poor use.

Individual fitting

Rollators should be adjusted in order to correctly fit residents' heights and arm lengths. The forearm support should be at the level of the elbow in a flexed position with the resident standing tall. The length and angle of the forearm support can also be adjusted for individual fit.

Rollators are widely available and although more expensive than other aids are often utilized by more than one resident, especially in a high care facility.

Mechanical devices

Technology is always progressing, or at least offering new options. Recently a standing hoist which brings a person into standing through a more physiologically appropriate trajectory (of increased trunk flexion) was introduced. Older hoists would bring a person into weight-bearing in a position leaning backwards rather than through trunk flexion. Recent anecdotal evidence has pointed towards residents gaining strength in the lower limbs and benefiting functionally from being transferred in this new machine. Additionally under-leg supports and suspender straps can be used after removing the footplate of the machine to mobilize a resident. Even more appropriately, designers are now working on attaching forearm supports so the person walks as if in a rollator frame whilst having the safety of the harness attached.

Maintenance and other safety issues

As with all mechanical devices and mobility aids, routine maintenance is important for safety. Individual residents should be assessed for suitability and appropriate sling size recommended. Residents requiring assistance such as this are much more dependent and require a great deal of support; two staff members must be in attendance for this type of mobilization. These hoists are very expensive comparably and usually only available for a large number of residents in reasonably well-equipped facilities; they may be prescribed for their dual use as a walker and a standing hoist.

Index

Note: Page numbers in *italics* refer to illustrations or tables.